RCSI HANDBOOK OF CLINICAL SURGERY FOR FINALS

RCSI HANDBOOK OF CLINICAL SURGERY FOR FINALS

Fifth Edition

Gozie Offiah and Arnold Hill

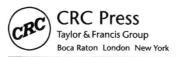

CRC Press
Taylor & Francis Group
Boca Raton London New York

CRC Press is an imprint of the
Taylor & Francis Group, an **informa** business

Fifth edition published 2022
by CRC Press
6000 Broken Sound Parkway NW, Suite 300, Boca Raton, FL 33487-2742

and by CRC Press
2 Park Square, Milton Park, Abingdon, Oxon, OX14 4RN

ISBN: 9781032074955 (hbk)
ISBN: 9781032074948 (pbk)
ISBN: 9781003207184 (ebk)

DOI: 10.1201/9781003207184

Typeset in Minion
by KnowledgeWorks Global Ltd.

Access the companion website: www.routledge.com/cw/Offiah

CONTENTS

Preface	xxxiii
Acknowledgements	xxxv
Disclaimer	xxxvii
List of Contributors	xxxix
Eponymous Microvignette	xli

Chapter 1 PRINCIPLES OF SURGERY 1

History Taking–Common Surgical Symptoms 3

Introduction 3
Presenting complaint 3
History of presenting complaint–pain 3
Past medical history 4
Drug history 4
Allergies 4
Family history 4
Social history 4
Systems review 5
Summary 5

Upper GI Symptoms 5

Dyspepsia 5
Dysphagia 5
Gastro-oesophageal reflux disease (GORD)/heartburn 5
Haematemesis 5

Lower GI Symptoms 6

Altered bowel habit 6
Rectal bleeding 6
Tenesmus 6

Hepatobiliary Symptoms 6

Jaundice 6

Peripheral Arterial Disease Symptoms 6

Claudication 6
Rest pain 6

Urology Symptoms 7

Dysuria 7
Haematuria 7

Differential Diagnosis of the Acute Abdomen **7**

Key points   7
Differential diagnosis of epigastric pain   7
Differential diagnosis of right upper quadrant (RUQ) pain   11
Differential diagnosis of LUQ pain   11
Differential diagnosis of umbilical pain   12
Differential diagnosis of right/left flank pain   12
Differential diagnosis of diffuse abdominal pain   12
Differential diagnosis of right iliac fossa (RIF) pain   12
Differential diagnosis of left iliac fossa (LIF) pain   14
Differential diagnosis of suprapubic pain   14

Surgical Incisions/Scars **16**

Drains **17**

Key points   17
Complications   17
Types of drains   18

Nutrition in Surgical Patients **18**

Key points   18
Poor nutrition leads to the following   18
Body mass index (BMI)   18
Types of nutritional support   19

Medications in Surgery **21**

Pre-operative drug alterations   21
Patients on warfarin   21
Reversing warfarin   22

Fluids in Surgical Patients **23**

Common indications   23
Assessing fluid balance   23
Fluid requirements   24
Fluid compartments   24
Fluid types   24
Fluid challenge   26
Special circumstances   26
Special surgical circumstances   26
Administration of blood products   27

Sepsis **27**

Diagnosis of sepsis   27
Adjunctive investigations   28
Severe sepsis management   28
Septic shock   28
Management of septic shock   29

Chapter 2   HERNIAS   31

General Principles   33
Definition   33
Incidence (relative)   33
Uncommon hernia types   33
General pathology   34

Inguinal Hernia   34
Epidemiology   34
Types of inguinal hernia   35
Surgical anatomy   36
Clinical presentation   37
Differential diagnosis   37
Investigations   37
Management   37
Complications of inguinal hernia repair   38

Femoral Hernia   38
Epidemiology   38
Surgical anatomy   39
Clinical features   39
Differential diagnosis   39
Management   39

Umbilical Hernia   40
Aetiology   40
Types of umbilical hernia   40
Management   40

Incisional Hernia   40
Aetiology   40
Clinical presentation   41
Management   41

Spigelian Hernia   41
Key points   41

Obturator Hernia   42
Key points   42

Chapter 3   UPPER GASTROINTESTINAL SURGERY   43

Benign Oesophageal Disorders   45
Gastro-Oesophageal Reflux Disease (GORD)   45
Definition   45
Key facts   45
Epidemiology   45
Risk factors   45

Pathophysiology 45
Clinical features 45
Investigations 45
Management 46
Complications 46

Barrett's Oesophagus **46**
Definition 46
Aetiology 47
Management 47

Hiatus Hernia **47**
Definition 47
Key facts 48
Investigations 48
Management 49
Complications of hiatus hernia 49

Peptic Ulcer Disease **50**
Definition 50
Key facts 50
Aetiology 50
Clinical features 50
Investigations 51
Management 51
Complications 51
Managing complications of peptic ulcer disease 52

Upper Gastrointestinal Bleeding **53**
Definition 53
Key facts 53
Clinical presentation 53
Physical exam 53
Investigations 54
Management of unstable upper GI bleed 54
Rockall score 55

Dysphagia and Odynophagia **55**
Definition 55
Causes of dysphagia 55
Causes of odynophagia 56

Oesophageal Motility Disorders **57**
Primary 57
Secondary 57

Achalasia **57**
Definition 57
Key facts 58

Epidemiology 58
Pathogenesis and aetiology 58
Investigations 58
Complications 59
Management 59

Diffuse Oesophageal Spasm 59
Presentation 59
Investigations 59
Management 59

Chagas Disease 59
Definition 59
Key facts 59

Scleroderma and Oesophageal Dysmotility 60
Key points 60

Oesophageal Cancer 60
Key facts 60
Adenocarcinoma 60
SCC 60
Clinical features 61
Investigations 61
Management 62

Gastric Cancer 63
Key facts 63
Classification and aetiology 63
Pathophysiology 63
Risk factors for adenocarcinoma 64
Investigations 64
Management 64
Partial/total gastrectomy complications 65
Prognosis 66

Consent for Oesophago-Gastro-Duodenoscopy 66
Explain to patient what the procedure involves 66
Intravenous sedation used 67
Preparation for the OGD 67
Risks associated with OGD 67

Chapter 4   HEPATOBILIARY SURGERY 69
Jaundice 71
Definition 71
Aetiology 71
Pathophysiology 71
Differential diagnosis 73

Investigations 73
Management 75
Prognosis 76

Gallstone Disease **76**
Key facts 76
Aetiology 76
Pathophysiology of gallstones 76

Asymptomatic Gallstones **78**
Key points 78

Biliary Colic **78**
Pathogenesis 78
Clinical features 78
Investigations 79
Management 79

Acute Cholecystitis **79**
Definition 79
Pathophysiology 80
Clinical presentation 80
Investigations 80
Management 80

Gallbladder Empyema **81**
Definition 81
Presentation 81
Investigations 81
Management 82

Gangrene of the Gallbladder **82**
Presentation 82
Diagnosis 82
Management 82

Perforated Gallbladder **82**
Clinical presentation 82
Investigations 83
Management 83

Chronic Cholecystitis **83**
Presentation 83
Investigations 83
Management 83
Complications 83

Mucocoele **83**
Aetiology 83

Presentation 84
Management 84

Gallstone Ileus **84**
Aetiology 84
Clinical presentation 84
Diagnosis 84
Treatment 84

Obstructive Jaundice **84**
Pathophysiology 84
Clinical presentation 85
Diagnosis 85
Management 85

Ascending Cholangitis **85**
Definition 85
Aetiology 85
Pathophysiology 85
Clinical presentation 86
Investigations 86
Treatment 86
Prognosis 87

Acute Pancreatitis **87**
Definition 87
Key facts 87
Aetiology 87
Pathophysiology 88
Clinical presentation 88
Differential diagnosis 88
Investigations 89
Risk scoring 89
Complications 90
Management 91
Prognosis 92

Chronic Pancreatitis **92**
Definition 92
Key facts 92
Aetiology 92
Pathophysiology 93
Differential diagnosis 93
Investigations 93
Management 94
Prognosis 95

Pancreatic Cancer **95**
Key points 95

Aetiology   95
Pathophysiology   95
Differential diagnosis   96
Investigations   96
Management   96
Prognosis   97

Chapter 5   COLORECTAL SURGERY   99

Acute Appendicitis   101
Key facts   101
Pathophysiology   101
Clinical features   101
Special tests   102
Differential diagnosis   102
Investigations   102
Appendicitis scoring system–Alvarado score   103
Management   103
Complications of acute appendicitis   104
Carcinoid tumour of the appendix   104

Diverticular Disease   104
Definition   104
Key facts   104
Epidemiology   104
Aetiology   105
Clinical presentation   105
Complications   105
Pericolic/paracolic abscess   105
Peritonitis   105
Diverticular fistula   106
Stricture formation   106
Investigations for acute diverticulitis   106
Classification of diverticular disease   107
Management   107

Colorectal Cancer   108
Key facts   108
Risk factors   108
Pathophysiology   108
Morphology   108
Clinical presentation   109
Emergency presentations   109
Investigations   109

Staging 109
Pathological staging 110
Management 110
 Potentially curative treatment 110
 Surgical options based on tumour location 110
 Chemotherapy 110
 Palliative treatment 111
 Follow-up 111

Bowel Obstruction **111**
Definition 111
Classification 111
Obstruction can be complicated or uncomplicated 111
Clinical presentation 112
Aetiology 112
Other causes of bowel obstruction 113
Investigations 113
Management 114
Specific management 114

Perianal Disorders **114**
Key anatomical facts 114

Haemorrhoids **115**
Definition 115
Aetiology 115
Four degrees of haemorrhoids 115
Complications 115
Investigations 116
Management 116

Anal Fissure **117**
Definition 117
Aetiology 117
Types of anal fissure 117
Clinical features 117
Examination 117
 Acute anal fissure 117
 Chronic fissure 118
Management 118

Anorectal Abscess **118**
Definition 118
Classification 118
Clinical features 118
Investigations 119
Management 119

Anal Fistula   **119**

  Definition   119

  Key facts   119

  Aetiology   119

  Clinical features   119

  Investigations: examination   119

  Clinical assessment   119

    Types of anal fistula (Parks' classification)   120

  Management   121

  Surgical management options   121

Pilonidal Sinus and Abscess   **121**

  Definition   121

  Aetiology   121

  Pathogenesis   121

  Clinical features   122

  Examination   122

  Investigations   122

  Management   122

    Acute   122

    Definitive   122

Anal Cancer   **123**

  Risk factors   123

  Anal intraepithelial neoplasia (AIN)   123

  Anatomy of the anal canal defining the types of tumours   123

  Lymphatic drainage   123

  Types of anal canal tumours   123

  Clinical features   123

  Investigations   124

  Management   124

  Treatment   124

Stomas   **124**

  Definition   124

Loop Ileostomy   **124**

  Clinical features   124

  Clinical relevance   125

  Associated Colorectal Surgery   125

End Ileostomy   **126**

  Clinical features   126

  Associated colorectal surgery   126

End Colostomy   **127**

  Clinical features   127

  Associated colorectal surgeries   127

Loop Colostomy   **128**
Key points   128
Defunctioning Stoma   **128**
Stoma Complications   **128**
Stoma Stenosis   **129**
Definition   129
Aetiology   129
Clinical presentation   129
Management   129

Stoma Retraction   **129**
Definition   129
Aetiology   129
Clinical features   129
Management   130

Necrosis   **130**
Aetiology   130
Clinical features   130
Management   130

Parastomal Hernia   **130**
Definition   130
Aetiology   130

High-Output Stoma   **131**
Definition   131
Aetiology   131
Complications   131
Management   132

Skin Complications   **132**
Key facts   132
Aetiology   132
Management   132

Chapter 6   INFLAMMATORY BOWEL DISEASE   **133**
Definition   **135**
Key Points   **135**
Epidemiology   **135**
Pathophysiology   **136**
Ulcerative Colitis Clinical Features   **137**
Crohn's Disease Clinical Features   **138**
Extraintestinal Manifestations   **139**

Extraintestinal manifestations of CD and UC 140
Investigations 140
Management 141
Surgical Management of UC **142**
Types of surgery for UC 143
Surgical Management of CD **143**
Pre-operative preparation 144

Chapter 7   PERIPHERAL VASCULAR DISEASE   145

Peripheral Arterial Disease (PAD) **147**
Definition 147
Aetiology 147
Signs and symptoms 147
Differential diagnoses for PAD 148
Investigations 148
Management 149
Acute Lower Limb Ischaemia **150**
Definition 150
Aetiology 150
Complications 150
Types of amputation 150
Management 151
Complications of reperfusion 151
Abdominal Aortic Aneurysms **151**
Definition 151
Key facts 152
Risk factors 152
Surveillance 152
Clinical features 152
Differential diagnosis 153
Investigations: imaging 153
Management: elective repair 153
Complications of AAA repair 154
Endoleak 155
Other types of aneurysm 155
Ruptured AAA **156**
Clinical features 156
Management 156
Varicose Veins **157**
Definition 157
Aetiology 158
Clinical features 158

Complications 158
Diagnosis and investigations 158
Trendelenburg test 159
Management 159
Complications of surgery 159

Deep Vein Thrombosis (DVT) 160
Definition 160
Aetiology 160
Risk factors 160
Clinical features 160
Investigations 161
Prophylaxis 161
Management 161
Thrombolysis 161

Carotid Artery Disease 162
Definitions 162
Clinical features of symptomatic carotid artery disease 162
Investigations 162
Management 162
Carotid endarterectomy 163

Leg Ulcers 163
Definition 163
Causes 165

The Diabetic Foot 165
Features of the diabetic foot 165
Aetiology 166
Risk factors 166
Clinical features 166
Investigations 166
Management 166
Neuropathic ulcers 167

Chapter 8   BREAST DISORDERS 169
Breast Cancer 171
Key facts 171
Aetiology 171
Pathological features 171
Invasive ductal carcinoma 172
Invasive lobular carcinoma 172
Ductal carcinoma in situ 172
Clinical features 172
Investigations 173

Triple assessment 173
Surgical management 175
Medical management 177

Breast Cancer Screening **178**
BreastCheck 178

Benign Breast Disease **179**
Fibroadenoma 179
Breast cysts 179
Fibrocystic disease 179
Breast infections 179
Fat necrosis 180
Gynaecomastia 180

Chapter 9   ENDOCRINE DISORDERS **181**
Anatomical Review **183**
Thyroid gland 183
Parathyroid glands 183
Important nearby structures 183
Central control 184

Types of Thyroid Disease **185**
Differential Diagnosis of Neck Swelling **186**
Investigation of Thyroid Disorders **187**
Bloods 187
Imaging 188
Surveillance of a single nodule 189
Biopsy 189

Thyroidectomy **189**
Thyrotoxicosis **189**
Definition 189
Investigation of thyrotoxicosis 190
General management of thyrotoxicosis 191
Definitive management of thyrotoxicosis 191

Graves' Disease **192**
Definition 192
Investigations of Graves' disease 193
Management of Graves' disease 193
Medical 193
Radioactive iodine 193
Surgery 193
Thyroid Cancer **194**

Papillary Thyroid Cancer   **194**

   Pathological features   194

   Metastatic activity   194

   Prognostic factors   194

Follicular Thyroid Cancer   **195**

   Pathological features   195

   Metastatic activity   195

Medullary Thyroid Cancer   **195**

   Definition   195

Anaplastic Thyroid Cancer   **196**

   Definition   196

   Aetiology   196

   Treatment   196

   Investigations   196

   Treatment   196

Primary Hyperparathyroidism   **197**

   Aetiology   197

   Diagnosis   197

   Treatment   198

   Presentation   198

Secondary and Tertiary Hyperparathyroidism   **199**

Phaeochromocytoma   **199**

   Definition   199

   Aetiology   199

   Presentation   200

   Investigations   200

   Treatment   200

Cortisol Excess and Cushing's Disease   **200**

   Causes   201

   Investigations   201

   Treatment   201

   Post-operative management   201

Conn's Syndrome (Primary Hyperaldosteronism)   **202**

   Definition   202

   Investigations   202

   Treatment   203

Chapter 10   UROLOGY   **205**

Common Urological Devices   **207**

   Urinary catheters   207

   Suprapubic catheter   208

   Nephrostomy   209

JJ ureteric stent   209
Urostomy or ileal conduit   210

Acute Urinary Retention (AUR)   **211**
Epidemiology   211
Aetiology   211
Clinical presentation   211
Investigations   212
Treatment   212

Benign Prostatic Hyperplasia   **213**
Definition   213
Key facts   213
Clinical presentation   213
Investigations   214
Treatment   214
Complications of surgery   215

Urinary Tract Stones   **215**
Aetiology   215
Clinical presentation   216
Investigations   217
Complications of urolithiasis   217
Management of acute episode   217
Surgical   218
Emergency   218

Renal Cell Carcinoma   **219**
Epidemiology   219
Aetiology   219
Clinical presentation   219
Symptoms   219
Signs   219
Paraneoplastic syndromes associated with RCC   219
Investigations   220
Treatment   221

Bladder Cancer   **221**
Epidemiology   221
Aetiology   221
Clinical presentation   222
Investigations   222
Treatment   223
Prognosis   223

Prostate Cancer   **223**
Epidemiology   223
Aetiology   223
Clinical presentation   224

Investigations 224
Histology grading 224
Treatment 224
Testicular Tumours 225
Epidemiology 225
Aetiology 225
Clinical presentation 226
Investigations 226
Treatment 226
Prognosis 227
Acute Testicular Pain 227
Differential diagnosis 227
Testicular Torsion 227
Epidemiology 227
Clinical presentation 227
Management 227
Torsion of the Appendix Testis/Hydatid of Morgagni 228
Aetiology 228
Clinical presentation 228
Management 228
Acute Epididymo-Orchitis 228
Definition 228
Aetiology 228
Clinical presentation 229
Investigations 229
Management 229
Renal Transplant 229
Key facts 229
Aetiology 229
Contraindications to renal transplant 229
Pre-transplant workup 230
During heterotopic transplant 230
Maintenance immunosuppressive therapy 230
Complications of renal transplant 231
Signs of acute rejection 231

Chapter 11   CARDIOTHORACIC SURGERY 233
Pre-Operative Investigations for Cardiothoracic Surgery 235
Coronary Artery Bypass Grafting (CABG) 235
Indications for surgery 235
Procedure 235
Selection of conduits 236

Complications 236
Prognosis 236

Valvular Heart Disease 237
Choice of valve type 237

Aortic Stenosis (AS) 238
Aetiology 238
Clinical presentation 238
Investigations 238
Indications for surgery 238
Surgical approach 238
Prognosis 239

Mitral Regurgitation (MR) 239
Aetiology 239
Clinical presentation 239
Investigations 239
Indications for surgery 239
Surgical approach 239
Prognosis 239

Mitral Stenosis (MS) 240
Key facts 240
Clinical presentation 240
Investigations 240
Surgical approach 240
Prognosis 240

Aortic Regurgitation (AR) 240
Key facts 240
Aetiology 240
Clinical presentation 240
Investigations 241
Indications for surgery 241
Prognosis 241

Pneumothorax 241
Definition 241
Classification 241

Primary Spontaneous Pneumothorax 241
Key facts 241
Clinical features 242
Investigations 242
Complications 242
Management 243
Surgery 243

Secondary Spontaneous Pneumothorax   **243**
Aetiology   243
Notes on thoracic surgery   243
Chest Tube Insertion   **243**
Definition   243
Key facts   244
Chest tube insertion technique   244
Confirmation of tube placement   244

Chapter 12   MAJOR TRAUMA   247

Major Trauma   **249**
Definition   249
Common aetiology   249
Global burden of fatal injury   249
Global injury mortality by cause   249
Advanced Trauma Life Support (ATLS®) System (Tenth Edition)   **250**
General information   250
Key points   250
The trauma triad of death   253
Adjuncts to primary survey   254
Secondary survey   254
Thoracic Trauma   **254**
Key features   254
Management–ATLS protocol   254
Underwater seal drain   256
Management–secondary survey   257
Abdominal Trauma   **258**
Key features   258
Categories of abdominal trauma   258
Initial examination   259
Indications for resuscitative laparotomy   261
Indications for urgent laparotomy   261

Chapter 13   PLASTIC SURGERY   263

Malignant Melanoma   **265**
Definition   265
Incidence   265
Risk factors: environmental and genetic   265
Clinical presentation   265
Differential diagnosis   266
Pathological subtypes   266
Staging   266
Management   267

Basal Cell Carcinoma versus Squamous Cell Carcinoma   **268**

Burns   **270**
Aetiology   270
Emergency burn care   270
Severity of burn injury depends on multiple factors   270
Assessing depth of the burn   270
Burn resuscitation   271
Management   272
Complications   273

Wound Healing   **273**
Classification   273
Disordered wound healing   275
Wound management   276

Dupuytren's Disease   **278**
Definition   278
Epidemiology   278
Aetiology   278
Presentation   278
Dupuytren's diathesis (DD)   279
Surgical indications   279
Complications (surgery)   280

Hand Trauma   **280**
Tendon injuries   280
Fractures   281
Amputations   281

Upper Limb Compression Neuropathy   **281**
Median nerve   281
Ulnar nerve   282
Radial nerve   283

Compartment Syndrome   **283**
Description   283
Presentation   284
Causes   284
Diagnosis   284
Management   285
Complications   285

Infectious Flexor Tenosynovitis   **285**
Definition   285
Key points   285

Complications 285
Kanavel's cardinal signs 285
Management 285
Trigger Finger (Stenosing Flexor Tenosynovitis) 286
Key points 286
Management 286
Complications from surgery 286

Chapter 14   ORTHOPAEDIC SURGERY 287
Principles of Orthopaedics 289
Definitions 289
General fracture management 290
Principles in fracture treatment 290
Why do we reduce fractures? 290
Fracture reduction 290
The principles of fracture fixation 291
Stages in fracture healing 291
Upper Limb Injuries 292
Distal Radial Fracture 292
Key facts 292
Risk factors 292
Presentation 292
Eponyms 292
Treatment 294
Complications 295
Humeral Fracture 295
Key facts 295
Mechanisms of injury 295
Presentation 296
Neer classification 296
Treatment 296
Complications 296
Clavicle Fracture 297
Key facts 297
Treatment 298
Complications 298
Anterior Shoulder Dislocation 298
Key facts 298
Treatment 298
Posterior Shoulder Dislocation 299
Key facts 299
Management 299

Scaphoid Fracture   **300**
   Key facts   300

Lower Limb Injuries   **301**

Hip Fracture   **301**
   Key facts   301
   Presentation   301
   Complications   302

Slipped Upper Femoral Epiphysis (SUFE)   **303**
   Key facts   303
   Clinical presentation   303
   X-ray features   303
   Management   304

Ankle Fractures   **304**
   Key facts   304
   Clinical presentation   304
   Classifications   304
   Maisonneuve fracture   306
   Complications of ankle fractures   306

Tibial Fracture   **307**
   Key facts   307
   Treatment   307

Open Fractures   **307**
   Definition   307
   Key points   308
   Management   308

Compartment Syndrome in Orthopeadics   **308**
   Key facts   308
   Clinical features   309
     Symptoms   309
     Signs   309
   Treatment   309

Pelvic Fractures   **309**
   Key facts   309
   Types   310
   Initial management   310
     Complications   310

Septic Arthritis   **311**
   Key facts   311
   Investigations   311
   Treatment   311

Back Pain   **312**
   Key facts   312

Cauda Equina Syndrome   **312**
Definition   312
Clinical presentation   312
Diagnosis   312
Treatment   312
Sciatica   **313**
Defintion   313
Clinical presentation   313
Investigations   313
Management   313
Osteoarthritis   **313**
Key facts   313
Clinical presentation   314
Investigations   314
Characteristics of osteoarthritis on radiographs   314
Management   314
Total hip arthroplasty (THA)   314
Total knee arthroplasty (TKA)   315

Chapter 15   NEUROSURGERY   **317**
Cranial Trauma   **319**
Key points   319
Scalp layers   319
Concussion   320
Skull fractures: classification   320
Aetiology of head injuries   320
Cerebral blood flow   320
Munro-Kellie doctrine   321
Application in head injury   321
Cerebral herniation   321
Assessment of head injury   322
Investigations   324
Management   324
Extradural Haemorrhage   **325**
Mechanism of injury   325
Clinical presentation   325
Management   325
Subdural Haemorrhage   **326**
Key facts   326
Mechanism of injury   326
Clinical presentation   326
Risk factors   326
Treatment   327

Subarachnoid Haemorrhage (SAH)   **328**
Definition   328
Investigations (non-traumatic)   328
Management of aneurysmal SAH   329

Spinal Injury   **329**
General principles   329
General anatomy pointers   330
Assessment of injuries to vertebral column   330
Clinical examination   330

Spinal Cord Injury   **332**
Spinal cord syndromes   332
Initial management of spinal injuries   334

Brain Tumours   **334**
Key facts   334
Clinical presentation   335
    Clinical presentation of supratentorial tumours   335
    Clinical presentation of infratentorial tumours (posterior fossa tumours)   335
Pathogenesis   337
Investigations   337
Pathophysiology   337
Management   338

Chapter 16   OTORHINOLARYNGOLOGY (ENT)   **341**

General ENT   **344**
Foreign body in the ear   344
Foreign body in the nose   344
Foreign body in the upper oesophagus   345

Acute Tonsillitis   **345**
Definition   345
Key facts   345
Pathogens   346
Clinical presentation   346
Investigations   346
Complications of acute tonsillitis   347
Management   347

Head and Neck Masses   **347**
Peritonsillar abscess (quinsy)   347
Parapharyngeal abscess   348
Retropharyngeal abscess   348

Otology   **348**

Pinna (Auricular) Haematoma   **348**

Key facts   348
Clinical presentation   349
Management   349

Prominent Ears   **349**

Definition   349
Key facts   349
Clinical presentation   349
Management   349

Otitis Externa   **349**

Definition   349
Key facts   349
Risk factors   350
Pathogens   350
Clinical presentation   350
   Symptoms   350
   Signs   350
Management   350

Acute Otitis Media (AOM)   **350**

Definition   350
Key facts   350
Pathogens   351
Clinical presentation   351
   Symptoms   351
   Signs   351
   Management   351
Complications of AOM   351

Otitis Media with Effusion (OME)   **351**

Definition   351
Key fact   352
Risk factors   352
Clinical presentation   352
   Symptoms   352
   Signs   352
Investigations   352
Management   352
Complications of OME   352

Chronic Suppurative Otitis Media   **352**

Definition   352
Key facts   353
Management   353

Cholesteatoma   **353**
   Definition   353
   Key facts   353
   Classification   353
   Aetiology   353
   Clinical presentation   353
      Symptoms   353
      Signs   353
   Investigations   354
   Management   354

Acoustic Neuroma   **355**
   Definition   355
   Key facts   355
   Clinical presentation   355
   Investigations   355
   Management   356

Rhinology   **356**

Epistaxis   **356**
   Local causes   356
   Systemic causes   356
   Clinical presentation   356
      Symptoms   356
      Signs   356
   Blood vessels involved   356
   Investigations   357
   Management   357

Allergic Rhinitis   **357**
   Definition   357
   Key facts   357
   Typical allergens   357
   Clinical presentation   358
      Symptoms   358
      Signs   358
   Investigations   358
   Management   358

Nasal Polyps   **358**
   Key facts   358
   Clinical presentation   358
      Symptoms   358
      Signs   358
   Investigations   359
   Management   359

Sinusitis — 359
Key facts — 359
Local causes — 359

Acute Rhinosinusitis — 359
Definition — 359
Key facts — 359
Clinical presentation — 360
  Symptoms — 360
  Signs — 360
Investigations — 360
Management — 360

Chronic Rhinosinusitis — 360
Definition — 360
Key facts — 360
Clinical presentation — 360
  Symptoms — 360
  Signs — 360
Investigations — 361
Management — 361
Complications of sinusitis — 361

Head and Neck Anatomy — 361
Oral cavity subsites — 361
Larynx (voice box) — 362
Pharynx — 362
Risk factors — 362
Aetiological factors — 363

Human Papilloma Virus — 363
Key facts — 363
Investigations — 364
Nutritional status — 364
Airway concerns — 364
Speech rehabilitation — 364
Staging — 364
Management — 365

Laryngeal Cancer — 365
Function of the larynx — 365
Histological subtypes — 365
Management — 366
Surgical options — 366

Oral Cancer — 366
Histological subtypes — 366
Treatment — 367

Oropharyngeal Cancer   **367**
  Key facts   367
  Management   367
Nasopharyngeal Carcinoma (NPC)   **368**
  Definition   368
  Key facts   368
  Clinical presentation   368
  Staging   368
  Investigation   368
  Management   368
Surgical Procedures   **368**
Tonsillectomy   **368**
  Indications   368
  Complications   369
  Management of tonsillectomy bleed   369
Ventilation (Tympanostomy) Tubes   **369**
  Definition   369
  Indications   369
  Types   369
  Complications   370
Mastoidectomy   **370**
  Definition   370
  Indications   370
  Types   370
  Complications   371
Parotidectomy   **371**
  Indications for superficial parotidectomy   371
  Indications for total parotidectomy   371
  Complications   371
Neck Dissection   **372**
  Definition   372
  Key facts   372
  Types   372
  Complications   373

Surgical Scores and Classification Systems   **375**

Further Reading   **385**

Index   **395**

PREFACE

The *Handbook of Clinical Surgery* is designed for RCSI medical students in their final year attending the three RCSI medical schools in Dublin, Bahrain and Malaysia to address the knowledge and skills that a student needs to pass surgery final medical year exams. These core knowledge and skills are the same needed to be a competent doctor in clinical practice. There has been excellent feedback from the book's four editions from students in RCSI, other Irish medical schools and internationally.

Several experts reviewed this new edition of the RCSI Handbook of Clinical Surgery for Finals. We have also added relevant surgical anatomy, videos and multiple-choice questions for self-assessment to the chapters that will be useful and add context to your reading. This *RCSI Handbook of Clinical Surgery for Finals* should be used as an adjunct to all clinical placements and formally taught programme material. It has been designed as a handbook, rather than a textbook, to be helpful at the patient bedside and in the library. We are proud to be part of the *RCSI Handbook of Clinical Surgery for Finals* and wish you the best of luck with your final exams.

Gozie Offiah and Arnold Hill

ACKNOWLEDGEMENTS

The editors are grateful for the contribution of colleagues to the fifth edition of the book. We would like to thank all the patients who consented to use their images in this handbook. We would also like to extend our gratitude to the RCSI graduate-entry students who provided feedback via a survey and focus group sessions. This has formed a vital part of our endeavour to provide a comprehensive and up-to-date text.

DISCLAIMER

The information in this book is the opinion of many different authors and contributors and is derived from multiple references at each contributing author and reviewer's discretion. Clinical surgery and medicine are ever-changing fields. The editors, authors and contributors to the *RCSI Handbook of Clinical Surgery for Finals* have made every effort to provide accurate and complete information as of the date of publication. However, given the rapid changes occurring in medical science and the possibility of human error, there may be some technical inaccuracies, typographical or other errors. The information contained herein is provided "as is" and without warranty of any kind. The contributors to this book, including the RCSI, disclaim responsibility for any errors or omissions or results obtained from the use of the information contained herein.

SENIOR EDITORS

Dr Gozie Offiah–Clinical Senior Lecturer, Royal College of Surgeons in Ireland, Dublin

Prof Arnold Hill–Professor and Chair of Surgery, Royal College of Surgeons in Ireland, Dublin

ASSISTANT EDITORS

Dr Juliette Duff, Royal College of Surgeons in Ireland, Dublin

Dr Jaclyn Croyle, Royal College of Surgeons in Ireland, Dublin

Dr Aqeel Alameer, Royal College of Surgeons in Ireland, Dublin

EDITORIAL ADVISORS

Prof Tom Walsh, Royal College of Surgeons in Ireland, Bahrain

Prof Frank Cunningham, Royal College of Surgeons in Ireland, Dublin

COMPANION WEBSITE: www.routledge.com/cw/Offiah

CONTRIBUTORS

Dr Tahir Abbasi

Dr Niamh Adams

Dr Mohammed Al Azzawi

Mr Firas Ayoub

Dr Azlena Ali Beegan

Mr Mohammed Ben Husien

Prof Ciaran Bolger

Mr Waqas Butt

Dr Kira Casey

Dr Matthew Common

Dr Liz Concannon

Dr Arielle Coomara

Prof Martin Corbally

Mr Andrew Coveney

Dr Daniel Creegan

Dr Melanie Cunningham

Mr Niall Davis

Dr Sheila Duggan

Dr Evan Fahy

Dr Celia Fernandez

Dr Eilish Galvin

Dr Ann Marie Gavin

Dr Syama Sundar Gollapalli

Mr Enda Hannan

Dr Bronagh Harrington

Dr Grace Hennessy

Dr Claire Hevican

Mr Anthony Hoban

Mr Ahmed Hussain

Mr Edrin Iskander

Mr Ghazi Ismael

Dr Daniel Kane

Dr Amr Kazim

Dr Gerard Kelly

Dr Areeg Khair

Mr Moataz Khogali

Dr Ramy Khojaly

Dr Fiona Kiernan

Dr Nauar Knightly

Dr Donata Lankaite

Dr Lie Shien Laski

Dr Joan Lennon

Mr Muhammad Hamid Majeed

Dr Sherif Mamdouh

Mr Nawar Masarani

Mr Seamus McHugh

Dr Mena Megally

Dr Raluca Mitru

Dr Amira Mohammed

Mr Wail Mohammed

Dr Jill Mulrain

Prof Frank Murray

Mr Peter Naughton

Dr Kulsoom Nizami

Mr Amr HA Nour

Prof John O'Byrne

Mr Peter O'Leary

Prof James Paul O'Neill

Mr Barry O'Sullivan

Dr Aoibhlinn O'Toole

Dr Cyrille Payne

Dr Carolyn Power

Prof Colm Power

Dr Kevin Quinlan

Dr Michael Quirke

Dr Ryan Roopnarinesingh

Dr Emily Rutherford

Mr Monim Salih

Dr Anneela Shah

Dr Lindi Snyman

Dr Hamzah Soleiman

Mr Igor Soric

Dr Ciaran Stanley

Mr Thavakumar Subramaniam

Dr Emma Tong

Dr Roisin Tully

Dr Mark Twyford

Prof Raghu Varadarajan

Mr Prasanna K Venkatesh

Dr Criona Walshe

Dr Christopher White

Dr Rachel Wu

Dr Hind Zaidan

EPONYMOUS MICROVIGNETTE

Vignette	Sign	Who were they?
A 42-year-old man gets struck in the chest with a baseball bat during an assault. He presents to the Emergency Department, and it is noted that he has decreased heart sounds on auscultation, hypotensive and distension of the JVP is noted in the neck.	Beck's Triad of Cardiac Tamponade	**Claude Schaeffer Beck** was a pioneer American cardiac surgeon, famous for innovating various cardiac surgery techniques and performing the first defibrillation in 1947.
A 35-year-old woman presents to the Emergency Department with RUQ pain. She is of increased adiposity, is noted to have scleral icterus and has been complaining of some recent fevers and intermittent chills at home.	Charcot's Cholangitis Triad	A French neurologist and professor of anatomical pathology. Charcot has been referred to as 'the father of French neurology and one of the world's pioneers of neurology.' His name has been associated with at least 15 medical eponyms.
A 50-year-old man presenting with RUQ pain for the last 24 hours. Upon examining his abdomen, the doctor firmly placed a hand at the costal margin in the right upper abdominal quadrant and asked him to take a deep breath in. However, this caused the patient to catch his breath due to pain.	Murphy's sign of cholecystitis	An American physician and abdominal surgeon noted for advocating early surgical intervention in appendicitis appendectomy. In addition to general surgical operations, such as appendectomy, cholecystostomy, bowel resection for intestinal obstruction and mastectomy, he performed and described innovative procedures in neurosurgery, orthopaedics, gynaecology, urology, plastic surgery, thoracic surgery and vascular surgery.
A 20-year-old man presented with generalised abdominal pain, nausea and vomiting over 12 hours localised to the right iliac fossa. Upon examination, the physician pressed on a point 1/3 the way on a line from the ASIS to the umbilicus, which elicited a pain response.	McBurney's point	**Charles Heber McBurney, MD,** was an American surgeon who described the point of most significant tenderness in appendicitis, which is now known as McBurney's point.

Vignette	Sign	Who were they?
An 82-year-old elderly woman presented after falling on an outstretched hand, having tripped getting out of her pew in church. On examination, she had a 'Dinner fork deformity' of her left wrist. An X-ray confirmed an extracapsular fracture of the distal radius with dorsal angulation (apex volar).	Colles' fracture	**Abraham Colles** (23 July 1773–16 November 1843) was professor of anatomy, surgery and physiology at the Royal College of Surgeons in Ireland. His teaching career was highly successful and drew crowds of students to RCSI. He enhanced the surgical profession's reputation so that it was no longer considered inferior to medicine. This was the era of surgery before anaesthesia, antisepsis and antibiotics, so treatments were relatively crude with high mortality from bleeding and infections.
A 37-year-old woman presented to the clinic with symptoms of fatigue, constipation and weight gain. She had also noticed a central neck lump which has been getting more prominent over the last few months and has become quite large. On examination, the surgeon asked her to raise her hands over her head and hold them there. After about 1 minute, the woman's neck veins began to protrude, her face became flushed, and she became short of breath.	Pemberton's sign	**Dr Hugh Pemberton,** an English physician who was a pioneer for diabetes, thyrotoxicosis and peripheral vascular disease in England in the 1920s.
A 62-year-old man presented to the orthopaedic clinic with pain, swelling and stiffness behind his right knee. There was a visible and palpable mass in the popliteal fossa and some joint line tenderness on examination. Ultrasound confirmed a popliteal cyst.	Baker's cyst	**William Morrant Baker** was an English physician and surgeon. Baker became Sir James Paget's assistant for many years, perfecting his trade. He resigned from his post as a surgeon in 1892 due to his locomotor ataxia condition.

Vignette	Sign	Who were they?
A 64-year-old woman smoker was referred to the Breast Clinic with recent eczematous changes to her left nipple and areolar area. She underwent Triple Assessment, and results came back, showing a DCIS of her left breast.	Paget's disease of the nipple	Sir James Paget was an English surgeon and pathologist and is considered, together with Rudolf Virchow, as one of the founders of scientific medical pathology. There are several medical conditions named after him, including: • Paget's disease of bone. • Paget's disease of the nipple (a form of intraductal breast cancer spreading into the skin around the nipple). • Paget's abscess, an abscess that recurs at the site of a former abscess which had resolved.
A 72-year-old man slipped on ice while out walking on New Years' Eve. He landed on the dorsum of his hand and wrist, and in the Emergency Department, someone said it was a 'Garden Spade' deformity. X-ray showed a distal radial fracture with volar angulation (apex dorsal).	Smith's fracture	Smith was an Irish surgeon and pathologist in the 1800s. He received his Licentiate of the Royal College of Surgeons in Ireland in 1832 and became a Fellow of the Royal College of Surgeons in Ireland in 1844. He is known to be the person who corrected Colles' description of the Colles' fracture. He co-founded the Dublin Pathological Society in 1838 with Abraham Colles, Sir Dominic Corrigan and William Stokes.
An 80-year-old man presented to the general surgery OPD with painless jaundice. History and exam were performed by the medical student attached to the team. On examination, the student palpated a mass in the RUQ. They reported their findings to the Consultant, who stated, 'in the presence of a palpably enlarged gallbladder which is non-tender and accompanied with mild, painless jaundice, the cause is unlikely to be gallstones.'	Courvoisier's law	Ludwig Georg Courvoisier was a surgeon from Basel, Switzerland. He was one of the first doctors to remove gallstones from the common bile duct.

Chapter 1

PRINCIPLES OF SURGERY

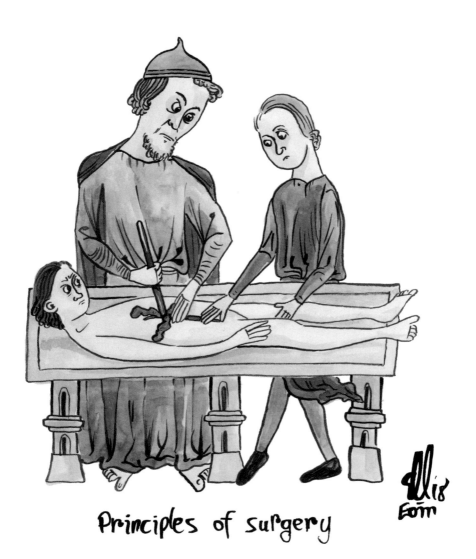

Principles of surgery

DOI: 10.1201/9781003207184-1

CONTENTS

History Taking–Common Surgical Symptoms	3
Upper GI Symptoms	5
Lower GI Symptoms	6
Hepatobiliary Symptoms	6
Peripheral Arterial Disease Symptoms	6
Urology Symptoms	7
Differential Diagnosis of the Acute Abdomen	7
Surgical Incisions/Scars	16
Drains	17
Nutrition in Surgical Patients	18
Medications in Surgery	21
Fluids in Surgical Patients	23
Sepsis	27

HISTORY TAKING–COMMON SURGICAL SYMPTOMS

INTRODUCTION

- Introduce yourself: State your name and your job title.
- Identity: Make sure you are speaking to the correct patient (name and date of birth), ask the patient where they are from, job occupation/retired.
- Permission: Confirm the reason for seeing the patient ("I'm going to ask you some questions about your abdominal pain/what brought you to the emergency department today, would that be OK?").
- Positioning: Make sure the patient is comfortable, try to sit at the same level as them.

 Always wash your hands/disinfect before greeting the patient.

PRESENTING COMPLAINT

- Ask the patient to describe their problem using open questions (e.g. "What's brought you into hospital today?").
- The presenting complaint should be expressed in the patient's own words (e.g. "I have pain in my lower abdomen.").
- Use ICE to explore the patient's ideas, concerns and expectations (ICE).

HISTORY OF PRESENTING COMPLAINT–PAIN

- **SR.COPD.SARAH** mnemonic works for all causes of pain and can be used for other symptoms, too–Use it while you work out your differential diagnoses.
  - Alternatively, you can use the mnemonic SOCRATES (Site, Onset, Character, Radiation, Associations, Time, Exacerbating/relieving factors, Severity).
- **Site**
  - "Where is the pain?" "Can you point to where the pain is?"
- **Radiation**
  - "Does the pain move or spread out anywhere?"
    - Gallbladder disease: Around to right side of your back or shoulder-tip.
    - Pancreatic disease: Straight through to the back.
    - Ureteric disease: Loin to the groin.
- **Character:** If necessary, give examples but avoid leading questions.
  - "How would you best describe this pain?"
    - Sharp like a needle/burning or stinging/dull or throbbing.
    - Restless/prefer to lie still (colicky pain).
- **Onset**
  - When did it start?
  - Suddenly/gradually?

- **Periodicity**
  - Time of day: Night (PUD vs gallstone)
  - Worse after eating fatty food
  - "Does the pain build up and get worse over minutes/hours?" (crescendo pain)
    - Always at the same? Improving/getting worse?
- **Duration**
  - "How long have you experienced the pain?"
- **Severity** (out of 10)
  - Maximum pain and baseline pain
- **Associated symptoms**
  - Vomit: Quantity/quality.
  - PR bleed/melaena: Black, tarry and sticky stool.
  - Hematemesis: Vomit any bright red blood? Small black bits like tea leaves or coffee grounds in your vomit?
  - Dysuria: Stinging when you urinate.
    - Tenesmus: Feeling of not fully emptying bowels after a bowel motion.
- **Relieving factors**
  - Pancreatitis: Relieved when sitting forward
    - Analgesia/Food
- **Aggravating factors**
  - Worse after a deep breath? Worsened by walking or moving?
- **History of this symptom**
  - "Have you experienced this type of pain before?"
  - Don't forget to ask about weight loss

PAST MEDICAL HISTORY

- Explore childhood, medical, surgery, obstetrics/gynaecological, psychiatric conditions/disease.
- Ask about specific risk factors relevant to their presenting complaint.

DRUG HISTORY

- Dose, frequency, route
- Intravenous drug use
- Over-the-counter (OTC) medications
- Recreational drugs

ALLERGIES

- Specify what type of reaction the patient had to the drug: Rash/nausea/anaphylaxis.

FAMILY HISTORY

- Ask the patient about any family diseases or conditions relevant to the presenting complaint and the age of onset of the disease (e.g. were they deceased before age 65).

SOCIAL HISTORY

- Alcohol intake (units/week).
- Smoking history: What do they smoke? Current or ex-smoker? (establish the pack-year)
- Home environment: Is the patient managing at home?

- Travels: Any recent travels abroad, long haul flights, infectious diseases risk
- Occupation: This can be asked at the beginning of the history when identifying the patient. Working at present or retired?

SYSTEMS REVIEW

- Run through a full list of symptoms from major systems: **Cardiovascular, Respiratory, Gastrointestinal, Genitourinary, Neurological, Psychiatric, General Review** (if not already explored earlier in the history, ask about weight loss, rashes, joint pain, lumps, appetite changes).

SUMMARY

- Name and age of the patient, presenting complaint, relevant medical history.
- Give a differential diagnosis.
- Explain a brief investigation and management plan.
- **"I would like to introduce/present Mr Joe Bloggs, a 73-year-old retired accountant from Clontarf, who presented with a 1-day history of intermittent right upper quadrant pain …."**

UPPER GI SYMPTOMS

DYSPEPSIA

- Persistent or recurrent abdominal pain or abdominal discomfort centred in the upper abdomen.
- "Discomfort" refers to a subjective, negative feeling that does not reach the level of pain according to the patient.

DYSPHAGIA

- Subjective sensation of difficulty or abnormality of swallowing.
  - New or long-standing?
  - Worsening or staying the same?
  - Able to swallow fluids/solids only?
  - Able to swallow saliva?

GASTRO-OESOPHAGEAL REFLUX DISEASE (GORD)/HEARTBURN

- Bitter-tasting/sour fluid in throat or mouth.
  - Ask how frequently it occurs.
  - Is it associated with food?
  - Relieving factors (lying flat, food avoidance).

HAEMATEMESIS

- Coffee grounds represent old or low-volume gastric bleeding.
- Dark red blood is either variceal or arterial.
- Blood appearing only after repeated vomiting ("blood-streaked vomitus") usually represents traumatic oesophageal cause or gastritis.

LOWER GI SYMPTOMS

ALTERED BOWEL HABIT

- May indicate underlying bowel cancer or inflammatory bowel disease.
- May be change in frequency, constipation or change in stool consistency.

RECTAL BLEEDING

- Haemorrhoids or anal bleeding: Bright red in colour and only on wiping.
- Rectal bleeding: On the surface of the stool.
- Colonic bleeding: Dark red in colour, mixed up with the stool, or with clot.
- Proximal colonic bleeding: Is stool maroon red in colour and loose?
- Dyschezia: "Is it painful?" Painful bleeding would suggest an anal fissure.
- Haemorrhoids are not typically painful unless thrombosed.

TENESMUS

- Feeling of not fully emptying bowels after a bowel motion.
  - Suggests low rectal tumour.

HEPATOBILIARY SYMPTOMS

JAUNDICE

- Yellow discolouration of the sclera and skin due to hyperbilirubinaemia.
  - Ask for itch, dark urine and pale stool in every case.
  - Itch suggests **post-hepatic** obstruction.
- Ask when the patient last felt well.

PERIPHERAL ARTERIAL DISEASE SYMPTOMS

CLAUDICATION

- Pain in calf, thigh or buttock precipitated by exercise and relieved by rest due to inadequate blood flow.
  - Claudication distance: "How far can you walk before needing a rest?"
  - "How long do you typically rest for before recommencing walking?"
  - "When did the pain on walking first begin?"
  - "Did your leg suddenly go cold and then recover with the onset of calf pain on walking?"

REST PAIN

- Severe, burning pain in limb affected by inadequate arterial flow, present at rest. Pain is neuropathic in nature due to neuronal ischaemia.
  - "Worse at night-time?"

- "Do you have to hang your leg over the side of the bed?"
- "Do you have to walk around your room at night to relieve the pain?"

UROLOGY SYMPTOMS

DYSURIA

- Pain on micturition.
  - Burning when you pass water?
  - Pain in lower abdomen?
  - Nocturia, frequency.

HAEMATURIA

- Blood in the urine
- "Does the blood occur at the start of urination?" (suggests bladder origin)
- "Does the blood appear at the end of urination, or during urination?" (suggests prostatic or penile origin)

DIFFERENTIAL DIAGNOSIS OF THE ACUTE ABDOMEN
FIGURE 1.2 AND TABLE 1.1

KEY POINTS

- Formulate a differential diagnosis as the history progresses. Figure 1.1
- Ask targeted questions which help to rule in or rule out your differential diagnoses as you proceed through your history.
- You should ask 2–3 questions about each differential diagnosis to show the examiner that you are considering the likely causes for the patient's presentation.
  - These are all "leading questions" for typical symptoms of each disease. With practice you will be able to frame them with "open questions" and use your own style of history taking.

DIFFERENTIAL DIAGNOSIS OF EPIGASTRIC PAIN

- **Peptic ulcer disease/gastritis**
  - Constant pain, aggravated by movement (inflammation).
  - Heartburn.
  - Melaena.
  - Haematemesis/Coffee-ground vomit.
  - Duodenal ulcer: Usually woken up with pain. Eating/Milk relieves pain.
- **Pancreatitis**
  - Epigastric pain radiating through to the back.
  - Constant pain, aggravated by movement (inflammation).
  - Relieved when sitting forward.
  - History of this pain before? After alcohol? History of gallstones?

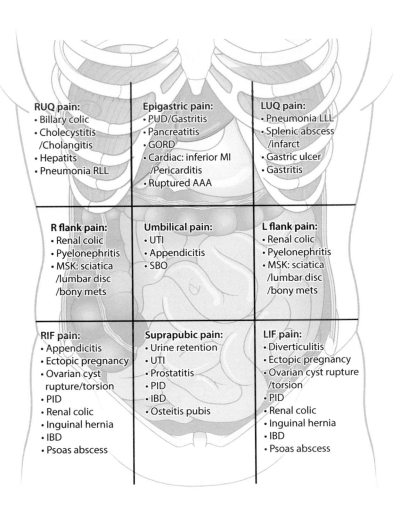

RUQ pain:
- Billary colic
- Cholecystitis /Cholangitis
- Hepatits
- Pneumonia RLL

Epigastric pain:
- PUD/Gastritis
- Pancreatitis
- GORD
- Cardiac: inferior MI /Pericarditis
- Ruptured AAA

LUQ pain:
- Pneumonia LLL
- Splenic abscess /infarct
- Gastric ulcer
- Gastritis

R flank pain:
- Renal colic
- Pyelonephritis
- MSK: sciatica /lumbar disc /bony mets

Umbilical pain:
- UTI
- Appendicitis
- SBO

L flank pain:
- Renal colic
- Pyelonephritis
- MSK: sciatica /lumbar disc /bony mets

RIF pain:
- Appendicitis
- Ectopic pregnancy
- Ovarian cyst rupture/torsion
- PID
- Renal colic
- Inguinal hernia
- IBD
- Psoas abscess

Suprapubic pain:
- Urine retention
- UTI
- Prostatitis
- PID
- IBD
- Osteitis pubis

LIF pain:
- Diverticulitis
- Ectopic pregnancy
- Ovarian cyst rupture /torsion
- PID
- Renal colic
- Inguinal hernia
- IBD
- Psoas abscess

Figure 1.1 Regional differential diagnosis of an acute abdomen.

- **GORD**
  - Heartburn
  - Epigastric pain radiating to the chest.
  - Relieved with Gaviscon or cool drinks.
- **Cardiac (Myocardial Infarction [MI]/Pericarditis)**
  - Chest pain, tightness or discomfort.
  - Radiation to left arm, shoulder or jaw.
  - Short of breath/Sweaty (diaphoretic)/anxious.
  - Any history of heart trouble such as a heart attack or angina?

Table 1.1 Acute Abdomen Investigations

Acute Abdomen Investigations (to Consider If Indicated)	To Rule-in
Bedside	
Vitals	Shock
Urine output	Hypovolaemia, retention
Urine dipstick	UTI, haematuria, bilirubinuria
ECG	MI
Capillary glucose	DKA
Urine	
Urine culture and sensitivity	UTI
β-hCG	Ectopic pregnancy
Amylase	Pancreatitis
Stool/Swab	
Culture and sensitivity	If indicated
Blood	
FBC	**Hb:** Anaemia **WCC:** Infection **Platelets:** Surgery prep
CRP	Infection
Blood culture and sensitivity	Sepsis/SIRS
U&E	Urea and creatinine: AKI, dehydration
Ca²⁺	Ureteric stone, pancreatitis
LFTs	Hepatobiliary causes, pancreatitis (may be deranged, more commonly in obstructive causes of pancreatitis [e.g. gallstone disease]) **Bilirubin:** Liver damage, bile duct obstruction, haeme breakdown **ALT:** Liver, skeletal muscle, kidney (small amounts) **AST:** Liver, kidney, cardiac muscle, brain **ALP:** Liver, bile ducts, bone **GGT:** Bile duct obstruction, alcohol, drugs **Albumin:** Malnutrition, pancreatitis **PTT:** Coagulation screen **LD:** Anaemia, kidney disease, liver disease, cardiac muscle injury, pancreatitis, infections, cancer **Total protein**
Coagulation screen	Surgery prep, liver dysfunction
Type and screen	Surgery prep, blood loss
Amylase, lipase	Pancreatitis (3× upper limit of normal)
Troponin	Myocardial Infarction
Glucose	Diabetic Ketoacidosis (DKA)
ABG	**Lactate:** Ischaemia, sepsis
β-hCG	Pregnancy, ectopic pregnancy

(continued)

Table 1.1 Acute Abdomen Investigations (*continued*)

Acute Abdomen Investigations (to Consider If Indicated)	To Rule-in
Imaging	
Ultrasound (US)	**Abdomen:** Hepatobiliary, AAA, appendicitis, complicated pancreatitis **Pelvis:** Ectopic pregnancy, ovarian cyst
CXR–erect	Perforated viscous
PFA	Obstruction: Small bowel normally: <3 cm Large bowel normally: <6 cm Caecum/sigmoid normally: <9 cm
CT +/– Contrast	Abdomen/pelvis: Obstruction, perforation site Angiography: Mesenteric ischaemia KUB: Renal/Ureteric stone, AAA
MRCP	If no common bile duct (CBD) stone seen on US
Invasive	
Endoscopic US/ERCP	If no CBD stone, but dilated CBD on MRCP
Percutaneous cholangiography	If ERCP fails
OGD/colonoscopy	PUD/IBD
Diagnostic Laparoscopy	If still unknown

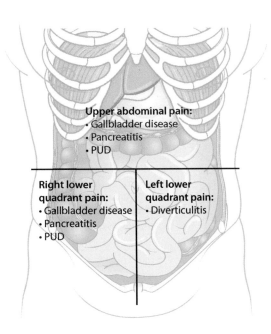

Figure 1.2 Essential components of the regional differential diagnosis of an acute abdomen.

- **Ruptured AAA**
  - Abdominal pain radiating to the back.
  - Dizzy, light-headed, or sweaty.
  - Collapse/loss of consciousness.
  - Any history of poor circulation to your legs or heart disease?
  - Ever diagnosed with an aneurysm?

DIFFERENTIAL DIAGNOSIS OF RIGHT UPPER QUADRANT (RUQ) PAIN

- **Biliary colic**
  - Ingestion of a fatty meal prior to pain.
  - Crescendo: Pain waxes and wanes.
  - Colicky: Restless with rapid escalation pain, bending over or moving to find a position of comfort.
  - Pain usually lasts less than 6 hours.
- **Cholecystitis/cholangitis**
  - Ingestion of a fatty meal prior to pain.
  - Radiation around the right side to the back/right shoulder/shoulder-tip.
  - Pain lasts >24 hours.
  - Constant pain, aggravated by movement (inflammation).
  - Jaundice: Dark urine, pale stools, yellowing of eyes and skin, pruritus.
  - *Cholangitis*
    - Charcot's triad: (1) Pain, (2) fever/chills, (3) jaundice.
    - Reynold's pentad: (4) Shock, hypotension, (5) confusion.
  - Murphy's sign: (+ve in cholecystitis) Tenderness and inspiratory arrest upon deep palpation of the costal margin along the mid-clavicular line as the patient takes a deep breath in.
- **Hepatitis**
  - Constant pain, aggravated by movement (inflammation).
  - Medication history, travel history and social history (alcohol and recreational drug use).
- **Pneumonia**
  - Diaphragmatic irritation from lower lobe pneumonia may cause RUQ or LUQ pain.
  - Short of breath.
  - Productive cough.
  - Chest/RUQ/LUQ pain; pleuritic and sharp/knife-like.

Cholangitis Signs

Charcot's Triad: Pain, fever/chills, jaundice.

Reynold's Pentad: Above + shock/hypotension, confusion.

DIFFERENTIAL DIAGNOSIS OF LUQ PAIN

- Left lower lobe pneumonia
- Splenic abscess/infarction
- Gastritis
- Gastric ulcer
- Herpes zoster

DIFFERENTIAL DIAGNOSIS OF UMBILICAL PAIN

- **Appendicitis** (see right iliac fossa [RIF] pain).
- **Small bowel obstruction (SBO)**–Diffuse abdominal pain.
- **UTI**–Cystitis
  - Lower abdominal/pelvic pressure.
  - Dysuria, pyuria, haematuria, frequency.

DIFFERENTIAL DIAGNOSIS OF RIGHT/LEFT FLANK PAIN

- **Renal colic** (as per ureteric colic–see RIF pain)
- **Pyelonephritis**
  - UTI and systemic features: Fever, rigors, nausea, vomiting.
  - Constant dull pain (inflammatory).
- **Musculoskeletal**
  - Sciatica
  - Lumbar disc
  - Bony metastases

DIFFERENTIAL DIAGNOSIS OF DIFFUSE ABDOMINAL PAIN

- **Gastroenteritis**
  - Diarrhoea +/– blood/mucus.
  - Vomit.
- **Acute mesenteric ischaemia**
  - Risks: elderly, atrial fibrillation, cardiovascular disease, history of chronic mesenteric ischemia.
  - Ask for associated vomiting, diarrhoea, ileus.
  - Typically very severe pain unrelieved by analgesia.
- **Chronic mesenteric ischaemia**
  - Post-prandial pain.
  - Weight loss.
  - Change in bowel habit.
- **Bowel obstruction**
  - Vomit–Green in colour (bilious) or brown (faeculent).
  - Constipation/obstipation (no flatus in complete obstruction).
  - Distension.
  - Perforation (sudden).
    - On exam: decreased resonance on percussion.
  - **SBO (high):** First, bilious vomit; later, constipation.
  - **LBO (low):** First, constipation; later, faeculent vomit. On exam: distension, tympanic abdomen, high-pitched bowel sounds.

DIFFERENTIAL DIAGNOSIS OF RIGHT ILIAC FOSSA (RIF) PAIN

- **Appendicitis**
  - Migratory umbilical pain to RIF pain.
  - Worse on movement or coughing (inflammation).
  - Fever, chills, rigors.
  - Nausea/vomiting.
  - Anorexia i.e. lack of appetite.

- Deep tenderness at McBurney's point: 1/3 distance from ASIS to the umbilicus. Also rebound tenderness (peritonitis).
- Rovsing's sign: LIF palpation increases RIF pain.
- Obturator sign: Lie supine, flex hip and knee 90 degrees Examiner passively internally rotates the hip, causing pain. Retrocaecal appendicitis can inflame the obturator internus, which stretches with this manoeuvre.
- Psoas sign: Lie on side with knees extended. Examiner passively extends thigh, causing abdominal pain. Retrocaecal appendicitis can inflame ileo-psoas. Differential diagnosis: psoas abscess.

- **Ectopic pregnancy**
  - Full menstrual history
    - LMP (first day of last menstrual period).
    - Illicit normal cycle for the patient.
    - Menorrhagia?
    - Period late/irregular bleeding?
    - Pregnant?
    - PV bleeding between periods?
  - Dizzy/faint/hypotensive.
  - Dyschezia: Painful bowel motion due to blood collecting and irritating the Pouch of Douglas.

- **Ruptured ovarian cyst**
  - Full menstrual history
    - LMP (first day of last menstrual period).
    - Period late/irregular bleeding?
    - Pregnant?
    - PV bleeding between periods?
  - Sudden onset (unlike appendicitis).
  - Vomit–vomiting with severe pain suggests ovarian torsion.

- **Pelvic inflammatory disease (PID)**
  - Ask for symptoms associated with ruptured ovarian cyst.
  - Fever.
  - Vaginal discharge.
  - Full sexual history necessary.

- **Inguinal hernia**
  - "Lump in the area before this pain began?"
  - "Lump there all the time or does it come and go?" (incarcerated or not).
  - "Lump swollen and tender now?"
  - "Lump gone in the morning and appears during the day?"
  - Dragging sensation.
  - Strangulation: Constant pain. On exam: Fever, tachycardia, localized tenderness, irreducible hernia.

- **Ureteric stone**
  - Severe pain.
  - Radiates from "loin to groin."
  - Restless with the pain.
  - Haematuria.
  - Dysuria, urgency.
  - Vomiting.

- **Inflammatory bowel disease**
  - Change in bowel motion. What is normal for you?
  - Haematochezia/Bloody diarrhoea.
  - Systemic symptoms
    - Weight loss.
    - Joint pain.
    - Eye trouble.
    - Skin rash.

DIFFERENTIAL DIAGNOSIS OF LEFT ILIAC FOSSA (LIF) PAIN

- **Diverticulitis**
  - Change in bowel motion. What is normal for you?
  - Haematochezia/Bloody diarrhoea.
  - Fever, chills, rigors. Anorexia.
  - Prior colonoscopy? Any abnormalities found?
- **Ectopic pregnancy** (as above)
- **Ruptured ovarian cyst** (as above)
- **Pelvic inflammatory disease** (as above)
- **Inflammatory bowel disease** (as above)
- **Ureteric stone** (as above)

DIFFERENTIAL DIAGNOSIS OF SUPRAPUBIC PAIN

- **Urine retention** (as above)
- **UTI** (as above)
- **Prostatitis** (as above)
- **Pelvic inflammatory disease** (as above)
- **Inflammatory bowel disease** (as above)
- **Osteitis pubis** (as above)

Table 1.2 Evaluation and Management of Acute Abdomen

Acute Abdomen Treatment (to Consider If Indicated)	To Treat
Bedside (Ins/Outs)	
O_2	Hypoxia
Urine output	Hypovolaemia, retention
Urine dipstick	UTI, haematuria, bilirubinuria
ECG	MI
Capillary glucose	DKA
Urine	
Urine culture and sensitivity	Urinary Tract Infection (UTI)
β-hCG	Ectopic pregnancy
Amylase	Pancreatitis
Stool/Swab	
Culture and sensitivity	If indicated

Table 1.2   Evaluation and Management of Acute Abdomen

Acute Abdomen Treatment (to Consider If Indicated)	To Treat
Blood	
FBC	**Hb:** Anaemia **WCC:** Infection **Platelets:** Surgery prep
CRP	Infection
Blood culture and sensitivity	Sepsis/SIRS
U&E	Urea and creatinine: AKI, dehydration
Ca²⁺	Ureteric stone, pancreatitis
LFTs	Hepatobiliary causes, pancreatitis (may be deranged, more commonly in obstructive causes of pancreatitis [e.g. gallstone disease]) **Bilirubin:** Liver damage, bile duct obstruction, haeme breakdown **ALT:** Liver, skeletal muscle, kidney (small amounts) **AST:** Liver, kidney, cardiac muscle, brain **ALP:** Liver, bile ducts, bone **GGT:** Bile duct obstruction, alcohol, drugs **Albumin:** Malnutrition, pancreatitis **PTT:** Coagulation screen **LD:** Anaemia, kidney disease, liver disease, cardiac muscle injury, pancreatitis, infections, cancer **Total protein**
Coagulation screen	Surgery prep, liver dysfunction
Type and screen	Surgery prep, blood loss
Amylase, lipase	Pancreatitis (3× upper limit of normal)
Troponin	MI
Glucose	DKA
Nil per os (NPO)	Preparation for surgery
IV Access	Fluids/medications
Urine catheter	Retention, monitor output
IV Fluids	• Hartmann's (Na⁺ lactate) • 0.9% NaCl and 20 mmol KCl (if vomiting) • 5% Dextrose 2 L As either/both of: 1 Replacement IV fluids 2 Maintenance IV fluids
Nasogastric tube (NGT)	**Wide bore**—to decompress obstruction/relieve vomiting **Fine bore**—to feed
Medical	
Anti-emetic	Vomiting.
Analgesia (as per WHO ladder)	Contraindications: • Opioids in SBO (constipation) • NSAIDs in PUD, AKI, asthma
Antibiotics (empiric then specific)	Infection

(continued)

Principles of Surgery 15

Table 1.2   Evaluation and Management of Acute Abdomen

Acute Abdomen Treatment (to Consider if Indicated)	To Treat
Prophylactic	
PPI	Prevent Peptic Ulcer Disease (PUD) /Gastritis
Anti-coagulation	Venous thrombo-embolism (VTE) • Thrombo-embolic deterrent stockings (TEDs) • Low Molecular Weight Heparin (LMWH) (e.g. enoxaparin 20–40 mg SC OD)
Management Order	
Conservative	
Medical	
Endoscopy	
Interventional Radiology	
Surgery	

SURGICAL INCISIONS/SCARS

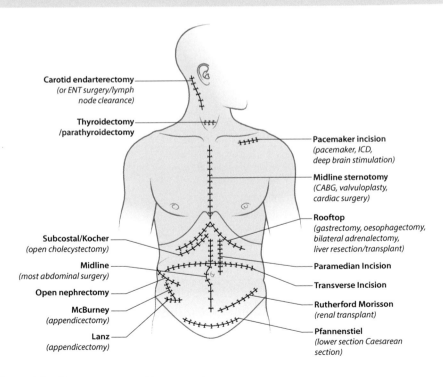

Figure 1.3   Common open and laparoscopic scars.

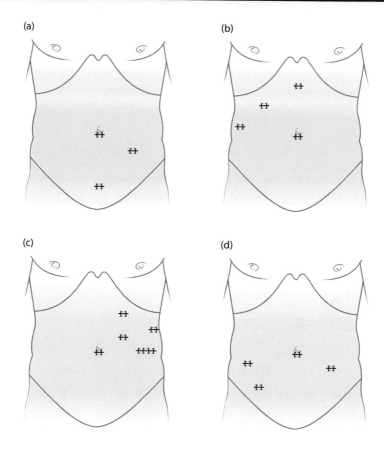

Figure 1.4 Laparoscopic port sites and scar locations.

DRAINS

KEY POINTS

- Drains remove collections of **blood** (drainage of haemothorax), **fluid** (ascitic drain), **pus** (drainage of empyema or subphrenic abscess) or **air** (pneumothorax).
- Drains prevent accumulation of fluid around the operative site (e.g. bile after biliary surgery).
- Generally, drains are removed when nothing further is coming out or when contents of the drain fall below 30–50 ml depending on the site in 24 hours.

COMPLICATIONS

- Damage to underlying structures by migration or misplacement.
- A route for infection.

TYPES OF DRAINS

- **Open passive drains:** Provide a conduit for drainage of secretions.
  - Yates, Penrose.
- **Closed passive drains:** Siphon effect of gravity and capillary action.
  - Robinson, NGT, ventriculoperitoneal shunt, chest tube (tube thoracostomy).
- **Closed active drains:** Generate active suction.
  - "Redivac" drain, "Minivac" drain.
- **T Tube**
  - Rarely used. Post-open exploration of the bile duct after intraoperative cholangiogram.
  - Superseded by Endoscopic retrograde cholangiopancreatography (ERCP).
  - Decompresses the bile duct system and makes sure there are no further stones.
  - It is percutaneous drain.
  - Draining 600 ml per day initially and slowly reduce.
  - After 10 days the tube will form a fibrotic reaction with the skin and it will close.
  - Before removing it, clamp it for 24 hours and look for signs of obstructive jaundice.

NUTRITION IN SURGICAL PATIENTS

KEY POINTS

- Timely nutrition reduces catabolic state and skeletal muscle wasting.
- Pre-existing malnutrition is common in surgical patients.
- Advanced malignancy, sepsis from appendicitis or diverticulitis, prolonged vomiting and bowel obstruction while the patient is NPO, all lead to excessive catabolic states and require early nutritional support.
- Albumin and transferrin levels are poor indicators of nutritional state.
- Prealbumin has been shown to be a useful test of nutritional status and progress, although not routinely done in clinical practice.

POOR NUTRITION LEADS TO THE FOLLOWING

- Impaired albumin production.
- Impaired wound healing and collagen deposition.
- Skeletal muscle weakness (ICU myopathy).
- Reduced neutrophil and lymphocyte function.

BODY MASS INDEX (BMI)

- Most commonly used measure of nutrition.
- Weight in kg/height^2.

- 18–25 kg/m^2 is normal, <15 underweight, >30 obese.
- Grip strength is a useful measure of skeletal muscle strength.

TYPES OF NUTRITIONAL SUPPORT

- **Oral**
  - Always the preferred route.
  - Start oral feeding early and avoid excessively long pre-operative fasting and post-operative fasting.
  - Promotes normal GI flora and mucosal balance.
  - Chewing gum has been found to stimulate and improve GI function.
- **Nasogastric or nasojejunal**
  - Nasojejunal tubes used if NGT is not possible, e.g. severe vomiting, gastric resection, gastric outlet obstruction.
- **Feeding gastrostomy or jejunostomy**
  - **Gastrostomy:** For patients with functioning GIT but cannot swallow/anorexia (PEG = percutaneous endoscopic gastrostomy). Figure 1.5
  - **Jejunostomy:** To bypass stomach, e.g. ulcers.
- **Total parenteral nutrition (TPN)**
  - May be given to patients in whom the oral and NG/NJ route is not possible.
  - E.g. extensive bowel resection, severe catabolic state with fistula and bowel resection such as in Crohn's disease, pancreatitis.
  - Peripheral TPN must be given through a large diameter vein–most commonly given via central vein.
  - Hyperosmolar solution can lead to tissue damage if extravasation occurs.

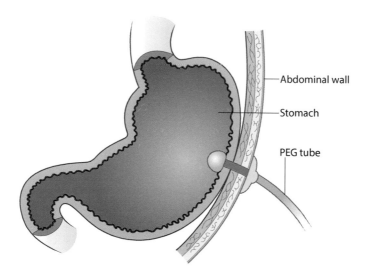

Figure 1.5   Gastrostomy.

- **Central TPN**
  - Hickmann line: Dedicated tunnelled catheter.
  - PICC line (peripherally inserted central venous catheter). Figure 1.6
  - Risks of central venous catheterisation include:
    - Haematoma/haemorrhage.
    - Line superinfection, infection to surrounding soft tissues.
    - Line obstruction/kinking/malplacement.
    - Damage to surrounding structures from malplacement
      - Pneumothorax
      - Air embolism
      - Cardiac dysrhythmias
      - Carotid artery dissection
- **TPN-associated complications**
  - Hyperosmolarity.
  - Lack of glycaemic control.
  - Nutrient deficiencies.
  - Liver dysfunction, cholestasis and pancreatic atrophy.
  - Fluid overload.
- **Patients on TPN require:**
  - Daily U&E and glucose until stabilised on TPN.
  - LFTs twice weekly.
  - Magnesium, copper, manganese, zinc, phosphate weekly.

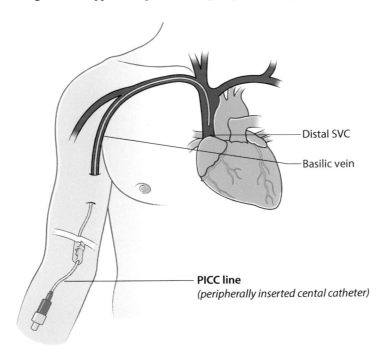

Distal SVC

Basilic vein

PICC line
(peripherally inserted cental catheter)

Figure 1.6   PICC line.

MEDICATIONS IN SURGERY

PRE-OPERATIVE DRUG ALTERATIONS

- Most drugs can be continued during surgery because of the risk of losing disease control if stopped suddenly. Table 1.3
- **Calcium channel blockers and beta blockers must be continued.**
- Patients on long-term steroids are at risk of adrenal atrophy and therefore unable to mount a physiological stress response to surgery. Severe hypotension can occur if steroids are discontinued.
- **"Sick day rules"**: Patient's steroid dose is doubled to counter the increased steroid requirement when patient is ill. In surgery, at induction of anaesthesia, the patient should be given IV steroids.

Table 1.3   Pre-Operative Guidelines for Medications Prior to Surgery

Drug	When to Stop before Surgery
Combined oral contraceptive pill (COCP) and human replacement therapy (HRT)	4 weeks before surgery
K-sparing diuretics and ACE-inhibitors	Day of surgery
Lithium	Day before surgery
Anticoagulants (warfarin/heparin including prophylactic dose), antiplatelets	Variable (occasionally continued during surgery)
Oral hyperglycaemic drugs and insulin	Variable

PATIENTS ON WARFARIN

- Normal target INR 2.5
- In patients with mechanical valve or recurrent thromboembolism while on warfarin, target INR 3.5
- Generally, hold warfarin 5 days prior to surgery
- LMWH e.g. enoxaparin 40 mg SC OD starts 24–36 hours after last dose of warfarin
- Stop LMWH 24 hours prior to procedure
  - Check INR (general should be <1.5)
- Restart warfarin 12–24 hours post-procedure. Table 1.4
- 24 hours post-procedure restart LMWH, continue until INR therapeutic

Table 1.4   Guidelines for Warfarin Administration

If No Major Bleed, the Following Can Be Applied	
INR	Action
<6*	Reduce dose of warfarin
6–8*	Omit warfarin for 2 days then reduce dose
>8*	Omit warfarin and give 1–5 mg of oral vitamin K

* If minor bleeding with INR >5 give 1–3 mg IV instead of PO vitamin K.

REVERSING WARFARIN

- If there is risk of severe bleed, causing bleeding into a confined space or hypotension, warfarin should be stopped and IV vitamin K 5–10 mg given. Prothrombin complex can also be administered.

Table 1.5 Medications Used in Surgical Patients

DVT Prophylaxis	
LMWH	**TEDS/Compression Stockings**
• Enoxaparin 40 mg SC OD	• Contraindicated in peripheral arterial disease
OR	
• Dalteparin 5000 units SC OD	
OR	
• Tinzaparin 3500–4500 units SC OD	
Anti-Emetic Medication	
If Nauseated, Prescribe Regular:	**If No Nausea, Prescribe PRN:**
• Cyclizine 50 mg TDS IM/IV/PO except in patients with fluid retention	• Cyclizine 50 mg TDS IM/IV/PO except in patients with fluid retention
OR	• Metoclopramide 10 mg TDS IM/IV if heart failure
• Metoclopramide 10 mg TDS IM/IV if heart failure	• Ondansetron 4–8 mg TDS PO/IV TDS
OR	
• Ondansetron 4–8 mg TDS PO/IV if vomiting	

Analgesia		
If No Pain, Prescribe PRN:	**If Mild Pain, Prescribe Regular:**	**If Severe Pain, Prescribe Regular:**
• Paracetamol 1 g QDS PO	• Paracetamol 1 g QDS PO • Codeine 30 mg QDS PO (tramadol is a suitable alternative)	• Co-codamol 30/500 mg, 2 tablets QDS PO AND PRN • Morphine sulphate 10 mg QDS PO

Cyclizine is a good first-line nausea treatment for almost all cases except in fluid retention (heart failure), metoclopramide can be used as an alternative.
  Avoid metoclopramide (a dopamine antagonist) for patients with Parkinson's disease due to the risk of exacerbating symptoms.

Patients on long-term NSAIDs should be prescribed a regular PPI (e.g. omeprazole) alongside this to prevent risk of GI bleed.

Table 1.6   Laxatives Used in Surgical Patients

Laxative Type	Name	For Use in	Notes
Stool softener	Docusate sodium Arachis oil (rectal)	Contraindicated in patients with nut allergy	Good for feaecal impaction
Bulking agents	Methylcellulose	Faecal impaction and colonic atony	Can take days to deliver effect
Stimulant laxatives	Senna Bisacodyl	Bisacodyl: acute abdomen	May exacerbate abdominal cramps
Osmotic laxatives	Lactulose Phosphate enema	Phosphate enema (acute abdomen)	May exacerbate bloating

FLUIDS IN SURGICAL PATIENTS

COMMON INDICATIONS

- Daily maintenance (2.5 L)
- **Replace any fluid deficit**
  - Hypovolaemia
    - Shock, dehydration, low urine output, excess fluid loss (e.g. vomiting), third space losses.
    - Reduced fluid intake: NPO status pre-/post-operatively, reduced Glasgow Coma Scale (GCS).
  - Sepsis
- **Replace ongoing losses**
  - Vomiting, diarrhoea
  - Stoma, fistula
  - Burns
  - Fever

ASSESSING FLUID BALANCE

- **Hypovolaemic signs**
  - End of bed charts: Reduced urine output, tachycardia, postural hypotension, low blood pressure (late).
  - Patient's peripheries: Reduced capillary refill time, cool peripheries, reduced skin turgor.
  - Patient's face: Sunken eyes.
  - U&E: Higher urea and creatinine; higher Na^+.
- **Hypervolaemic signs**
  - Increased resp. rate, tachy, hypertension, increased central arterial pressure and pulmonary artery pressure due to increased mean arterial pressure (MAP) and circulatory overload.
  - Patient's neck: Raised jugular venous pulse.
  - Patient's chest: Bibasal crepitations.
  - FBC: Low haematocrit, low Hb.
  - U&E: Lower urea and creatinine; lower Na^+.
  - CXR: Pulmonary oedema.

FLUID REQUIREMENTS
- **Normal daily fluid intake** = 2.5 L
- **Normal daily losses** = 2.5 L
  - Urine = 1.5 L
  - Insensible = 0.8 L (e.g. from skin, lungs)
  - Stool = 0.2 L
- **Electrolytes**
  - Na^+ 120–140 mmol
  - K^+ 70 mmol

FLUID COMPARTMENTS
- H_2O = 2/3 of body mass
  - 70 kg male = 45 kg H_2O
- Rule of thirds (breakdown of fluid compartments):
  - Extra-cellular fluid (ECF) = 1/3
    - Intravascular = 1/3
    - Interstitial = 2/3
  - Intra-cellular fluid (ICF) = 2/3

FLUID TYPES
- **Colloids**
  - Types
    - Natural: Blood, fresh frozen plasma (FFP), albumin.
    - Synthetic: Gelofusine (gelatin-based), Voluven (starch-based).
  - Mechanism of action
    - Higher osmotic pressure
    - Initially remains in intravascular volume and intravascular expansion (larger molecules don't pass easily through vascular endothelium)
  - Uses
    - Replacement fluids due to major haemorrhage/intravascular loss. Table 1.8
  - Disadvantages
    - NOT for usual hydration
    - Expensive
    - Risks: Anaphylaxis and coagulopathy (latter more associated with starch-based colloids)
- **Crystalloids**
  - Mechanism of action
    - Equal distribution across all fluid compartments (smaller molecules dissolve easily and pass freely through vascular endothelium).
  - Types
    - Hartmann's or normal saline is usually used for fluid maintenance and majority of fluid resuscitation. Table 1.7
- Advantages
  - Cheaper
  - Less risks

Table 1.7 Types of Crystalloid Fluids

	Normal Saline (0.9% Na⁺ Cl⁻)	Hartmann's (Na⁺ Lactate, Ringer's Lactate)	5% Dextrose
Contents	Na^+ 154 mmol/L Cl^- 154 mmol/L	Na^+ 131 mmol/L Cl^- 111 mmol/L K^+ 5 mmol/L Ca^+ 2 mmol/L Lactate 29 mmol/L	50 g dextrose
Mechanism of action	ECF: Equilibrates rapidly (1/3 intravascular) ICF: Takes longer to get to ICF	Similar fluid distribution as normal saline. Considered more physiological than normal saline. Lactate metabolised to HCO_3^- and can buffer acidosis (e.g. in: sepsis; post-operatively)	Equilibrates across all fluid compartments. Only 1/9th will remain in intravascular space (85 ml). Hence, NOT suitable for fluid resuscitation.
Uses	Fluid resuscitation Vomiting patients Fluid maintenance	Fluid resuscitation Fluid maintenance	Fluid maintenance only
Risks	Hyperchloraemic metabolic acidosis		Fluid overload Hyponatraemia
Prescription for a 70 kg male	1 L normal saline + 20 mmol K^+Cl^- +/– replace deficit/ ongoing losses		1 L 5% dextrose + 20 mmol K^+Cl^- +/– replace deficit/ ongoing losses

Table 1.8 IV Fluid Prescription Rates and Indications

	Rate	Fluid Type
Resuscitation	If hypotensive or tachycardic 500 ml (Hartmann's or normal saline) bolus (over 10–15 min) or 250 ml in heart failure, reassess patient, especially heart rate, blood pressure and urine output.	• Blood • Normal saline • Hartmann's • Colloid
Hypovolaemic/acutely Ill	1 L/4–6 hours	• Normal saline • Colloid
Maintenance	1 L/9–10 hours (as a general rule, adults require 3 L per 24 hours, elderly 2 L per 24 hours.	• Normal saline • 5% Dextrose
Elderly/mild overload/ overload risk (heart/renal failure)	1L/10–18 hours 250 ml bolus for resuscitation (see above)	• Normal saline • 5% Dextrose

FLUID CHALLENGE

- Indications: Shock, low urine output.
- Prescription: 500 ml of normal saline/30 min (250 ml if frail/overload risk).
- Result: If urine output improves, this suggests that hypovolaemia was the cause of low urine output.

> Bolus 250–500 ml crystalloid over 10–15 min.

SPECIAL CIRCUMSTANCES

- Children
    - Dextrose/saline (calculate according to guidelines).
- GI loss
    - Replace K^+ if patient profusely vomiting or has diarrhoea or high output stoma.
- Heart failure
    - Slow rate
- Renal failure
    - Slow rate
    - Caution with electrolytes, especially K^+
- Liver failure
    - Predisposed to raised Na^+ and low albumin
    - Consider albumin-based solution
    - Avoid normal saline

SPECIAL SURGICAL CIRCUMSTANCES

- Acute blood loss
    - Wide bore cannulae
    - Prescribe colloid/normal saline until blood if available
    - Consider O-negative blood until crossmatched blood is available.
- Low urine output
    - Aim for 0.5–1 ml/kg/hr (equivalent to 30 ml/hr).
    - Ensure catheter inserted correctly and not blocked
    - Fluid challenge indicated
- Pancreatitis
    - Large third space fluid losses
    - Aggressive fluid resuscitation indicated
- Post-operative
    - Check operative notes for documentation of intra-operative losses–replace losses
    - Replace losses from drains etc.
- Shock
    - Replace with colloid or normal saline.
- Burns
    - Parkland formula = 4 ml Hartmann's solution × body weight (kg) × % TBSA (rule of 9's)
    - More information found in Chapter 13

ADMINISTRATION OF BLOOD PRODUCTS

- In the non-haemorrhaging patient, the rate of transfusion will depend on age, clinical scenario and cardiac status.
- From starting the infusion to completion, the total transfusion time should not exceed 4 hours for 1 unit of RBCs; average 2–3 hours.
  - Both plasma and platelets are transfused over 30–60 minutes
- Monitoring for reactions
  - Severe reactions are most likely to occur within the first 15 min/50 ml.
  - The most common problem associated with transfusion is a temperature, which may not be related to the transfusion process
  - In general, if the temperature rises >1.5°C, the transfusion should be stopped and a reaction assessed for/ruled out before completing the transfusion.
- Elderly patients or those with compromised cardio-respiratory function will require closer monitoring.
  - Consider the need for furosemide (20–40 mg) after every 1–2 units of RBCs.
    - Always assess clinically before administration.
- In general, the rule is that 1 unit of RBC increases Hb by 1 g (based on a 70 kg patient).
  - For smaller, elderly, frail patients, it may actually increase by 1.5–2 g.
- Assess post-transfusion Hb levels
  - In the non-bleeding patient, a Hb check can be done 15 min after the transfusion has been completed.

SEPSIS

DIAGNOSIS OF SEPSIS

- **Old method:**
  - Two or more of systemic inflammatory response syndrome (SIRS) criteria:
    - Acutely altered mental status
    - Respiratory rate > 20 breaths/minute
    - Heart rate > 90 beats/minute
    - Temperature < 36°C, or > 38.3°C
    - WCC $< 4 \times 10^6/L$, or $> 12 \times 10^6/L$.
  - AND a suspected infection
- **Newer method:**
  - **Sequential Organ Failure Assessment (SOFA) score**: Looking at respiration, coagulation, liver, cardiovascular, central nervous system and renal parameters (or quicker method **qSOFA score**). A SOFA score ≥ 2 indicates sepsis. Table 1.9

Table 1.9 qSOFA Score for Sepsis

qSOFA
Respiratory rate of 22 breaths/min or greater
Altered mentation
Systolic blood pressure of >100 mmHg

Sepsis 6

Take 3
Urine output hourly
Bloods–FBC, U&E (to guide fluids), CRP (to monitor trend) and lactate
Blood cultures (before antibiotics)

Give 3
Oxygen–maintain SpO$_2$ >94% (88–92% in COPD)
IV fluids (up to 30 ml/kg)
IV antibiotics (according to local guidelines, e.g. for an inpatient: piperacillin-tazobactam 4.5 g TDS +/– stat of gentamicin depending on severity or response)

ADJUNCTIVE INVESTIGATIONS

- Look for cause
  - Dipstick urine and urinalysis
  - Culture of indicated sample–urine/stool/wound/skin/IV lines/CSF/aspirate (joint, pleural, ascitic, abscess)/bone
  - CXR
- Don't ever forget glucose–diabetes predisposes infection and diabetic patients often have abnormal glucose levels during infection

Table 1.10   Diagnosis of Severe Sepsis

Diagnosis of Severe Sepsis If Any of the Following Present	
Clinical Signs	Laboratory Results
Acutely altered mental status	Platelets < 100 × 10^6/L
New oxygen requirement	Lactate > 2 mmol/L after IV fluids
Systolic BP < 90 mmHg OR > 40 mmHg below patient's normal range OR MAP < 65 mmHg	Creatinine > 177µmol/L
	Bilirubin > 34µmol/L
	INR >1.5 OR aPTT > 60 s
Urine output <0.5 ml/kg for 2 hrs	Glucose >7.7 mmol/L (in non-diabetic)

SEVERE SEPSIS MANAGEMENT

- Senior review immediately (registrar/consultant)
- Reassess frequently in first hour
- Consider other investigations/management
- Consider critical care consult

SEPTIC SHOCK

- A subset of sepsis in which particularly profound circulatory, cellular and metabolic abnormalities are associated with a greater risk of mortality than with sepsis alone.
- Look for signs of septic shock after fluid challenge.

- Patients with septic shock can be clinically identified by a vasopressor requirement to maintain a MAP of ≥65mmHg and serum lactate level >2 mmol/L (>18 mg/dL) in the absence of hypovolemia.
- Septic shock is associated with hospital mortality rates greater than 40%.
- Patients with suspected infection have poor outcomes if they have at least two or more signs from the qSOFA score.

MANAGEMENT OF SEPTIC SHOCK

- Consultant referral
- Critical care consult
- Consider transfer to higher level of care.

MCQs FOR SELF-ASSESSMENT

Chapter 2

HERNIAS

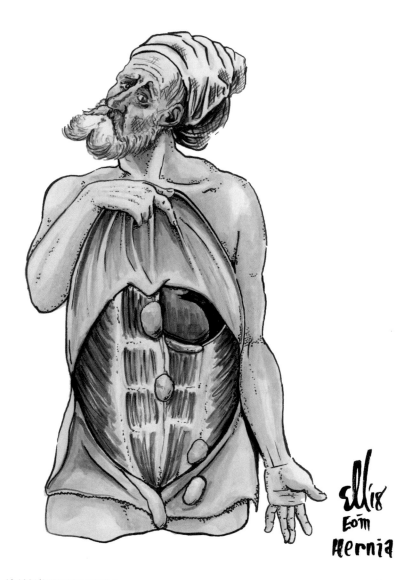

DOI: 10.1201/9781003207184-2

CONTENTS

General Principles	33
Inguinal Hernia	34
Femoral Hernia	38
Umbilical Hernia	40
Incisional Hernia	40
Spigelian Hernia	41
Obturator Hernia	42

GENERAL PRINCIPLES

DEFINITION

- A hernia is an abnormal protrusion of an organ (or part of an organ) through its containing body wall Table 2.1.

Table 2.1 Classification of Hernias

Classification According to Anatomical Location		Classification According to Aetiology	
Ventral	Umbilical/periumbilical, parastomal, epigastric, spigelian	Congenital	Defect is present from birth (+perinatal repair) • Persistent processus vaginalis–risk of indirect inguinal hernia • Gastroschisis–risk of periumbilical hernia • Omphalocoele–risk of umbilical hernia
Groin	Inguinal, femoral, pantaloon	Acquired–primary	Increased abdominal pressure or weakened abdominal wall
Pelvic	Obturator, sciatic, perineal		Risk factors: Ageing, smoking, steroid use, pregnancy, obesity, chronic cough, connective tissue disorders, heavy lifting
Flank	Superior/inferior lumbar triangle hernias	Acquired–incisional (secondary)	Iatrogenic wall damage • Post-surgical–surgical site infection increases risk

INCIDENCE (RELATIVE)

- Groin > ventral > pelvic > flank
- Classical distribution (statistics are always changing)
  - Inguinal (~75% of all hernias repaired)
  - Femoral (~10% of all hernias repaired)
  - Umbilical (~5% of all hernias repaired)
- Ventral: 33% incisional, 67% primary

UNCOMMON HERNIA TYPES

- **Richter's hernia**
  - Partial thickness of bowel trapped within sac Figure 2.1.
  - Leads to partial bowel obstruction with vomiting but the patient continues to pass flatus.
- **Sliding hernia**
  - A peritoneal covered structure such as the colon or urinary bladder *slides* down extra-peritoneally with the peritoneum adjacent to it and forms the wall of the hernial sac.

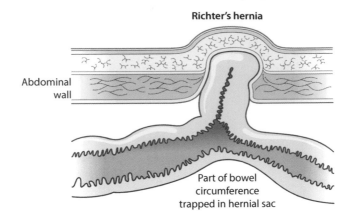

Richter's hernia

Abdominal wall

Part of bowel circumference trapped in hernial sac

Figure 2.1   Richter's hernia.

- **Pantaloon hernia**
  - Both a direct and indirect hernia occurring simultaneously.

GENERAL PATHOLOGY

- **Reducible**
  - Contents re-enter their containing cavity (usually the abdomen) either spontaneously or with manipulation.
- **Irreducible or incarcerated**
  - Hernia persists despite manipulation
  - Leads to obstruction (i.e. bowel)
  - Narrower neck of hernia (i.e. femoral) increases risk
  - At risk of strangulation
- **Strangulated**
  - Ischaemia and necrosis of hernia contents
  - Decreased venous/lymphatic flow → increased bowel oedema → impeded arterial flow → infarction → necrosis

INGUINAL HERNIA

EPIDEMIOLOGY

- Male:female = 8:1
- Median age at presentation
  - Men: 50–70 years old
  - Women: 60–80 years old

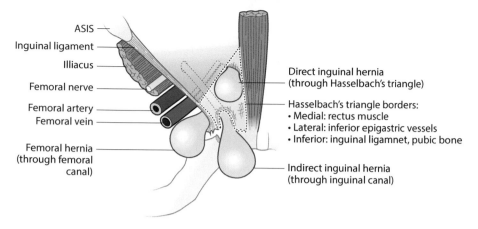

ASIS

Inguinal ligament

Illiacus

Femoral nerve

Femoral artery

Femoral vein

Femoral hernia
(through femoral
canal)

Direct inguinal hernia
(through Hasselbach's triangle)

Hasselbach's triangle borders:
• Medial: rectus muscle
• Lateral: inferior epigastric vessels
• Inferior: inguinal ligamnet, pubic bone

Indirect inguinal hernia
(through inguinal canal)

Figure 2.2   Hernia types.

TYPES OF INGUINAL HERNIA

- Can be direct or indirect according to their anatomical relationship to the inferior epigastric artery, inguinal canal, and Hesselbach's triangle Figure 2.2.
- *IN*direct hernias pass *IN* the inguinal canal
  - Leave the abdomen via the deep inguinal ring to follow an oblique course through the inguinal canal
  - Emerges through the superficial ring, may descend into scrotum
  - May extend to the tunica vaginalis surrounding the testis
  - The peritoneal sac may derive from a patent or re-opened processus vaginalis
- **Direct hernias** protrude directly through (anteriorly) the transversalis fascia in Hesselbach's triangle
- **Pantaloon hernia** describes a combination of both

KEY POINT

Inguinal hernia can be indirect–passes in the inguinal canal (through deep inguinal ring and emerges through the superficial ring), or direct–protrudes through the transversalis fascia

---

KEY POINT

A direct inguinal hernia occurs medially to the inferior epigastric vessel, while an indirect inguinal hernia occurs laterally to the inferior epigastric vessels

---

SURGICAL ANATOMY

- **Inguinal ligament:** Runs from ASIS to pubic tubercle.
- **Hesselbach's triangle**
  - Inferior–inguinal ligament.
  - Lateral–inferior epigastric artery.
  - Medial–rectus sheath.
- **Deep inguinal ring**
  - Made from an fv fascia.
  - Lies 1–2 cm superior to the *midpoint* of the inguinal ligament.
- **Superficial inguinal ring**
  - V-shaped defect in external oblique aponeurosis.
  - Lies superomedial to the pubic tubercle.
  - **Inguinal canal:** Runs from the deep to superficial ring.
  - **Anterior wall**
    - Entire canal–external oblique aponeurosis.
    - Lateral third–internal oblique.
  - **Posterior wall**
    - Entire canal–transversalis fascia.
    - Medially–conjoint tendon.
  - **Superior wall**
    - Internal oblique, external oblique, and transversus abdominis (conjoint tendon).
  - **Inferior wall**
    - Inguinal ligament (rolled external oblique aponeurosis).

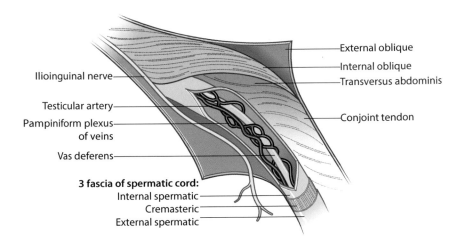

Figure 2.3 Inguinal canal.

Table 2.2   Contents of the Inguinal Canal

Three Vessels	Four Nerves
• Testicular artery and vein (pampiniform venous plexus) • Artery and vein to the vas deferens • Cremasteric artery and vein	• Nerve to the cremaster • Sympathetic nerves • Ilioinguinal nerve • Genital branch (genitofemoral nerve)
Three Fasciae	Three Others
• External spermatic fascia • Cremasteric muscle and fascia • Internal spermatic fascia	• Spermatic cord • Vas deferens • Lymphatics

CLINICAL PRESENTATION

- Can often be incidental/asymptomatic.
- Presentations range from a lump +/− pain to acute strangulation/obstruction.
- Discomfort can be worse at the end of day/after prolonged standing.
- Classic indirect takes a few hours to present.
- Classic direct presents on standing.

DIFFERENTIAL DIAGNOSIS

- Femoral hernia
- Lymphadenopathy/lymphoma
- Metastatic lymphadenopathy
- Hydrocele
- Testicular torsion
- Femoral artery aneurysm
- Undescended testicle

INVESTIGATIONS

- **Bedside: Clinical examination** is often diagnostic.
  - Right:left incidence = 2:1.
  - Bulge is often better appreciated on *standing*/cough/Valsalva.
  - Incarcerated hernias with visible/palpable lump will persist upon lying down.
  - **NB:** Be sure to examine the scrotum.
  - Direct/indirect differentiation is often intraoperative.
- **Bloods**
  - Routine bloods including WBC, CRP, U&E, lactate.
- **Imaging: US/CT**
  - Groin US−may be useful if occult hernia or obstruction is suspected.

MANAGEMENT

- **Emergency**
  - **Strangulated/Obstructed** hernias should undergo surgical repair within 6–8 hours *from onset* to prevent bowel loss.

- **Conservative**
  - Watchful waiting is an option in some cases.
    - Elderly patients or significant co-morbidity.
    - Uncomplicated, mild symptoms (future elective repair).
  - Annual risk of incarceration 0.3% per year.
- **Surgical**
  - Symptomatic inguinal hernias in adults should be repaired.
    - Groin pain with exertion.
    - Inability to perform ADLs.
    - Chronic incarcerated hernia.
  - **Open mesh (tension-free) or non-mesh (tissue approximation) repair**
    - Utilises a patch of non-absorbable mesh to strengthen the posterior wall of the inguinal canal/deep ring.
    - NB: Mesh cannot be used in presence of infection.
    - Can be done under local anaesthesia plus sedation.
  - **Laparoscopic herniorrhaphy**
    - Cannot be used if:
      - Infection or contamination, ascites, can't tolerate GA, previous surgery involving preperitoneum (i.e. laparotomy, LSCS, TAH).
    - Main indications: Bilateral hernia, recurrent hernia.
    - Totally extraperitoneal (TEP) repair and transabdominal preperitoneal patch (TAPP) repair, both are considered tension-free repairs and use a mesh.

COMPLICATIONS OF INGUINAL HERNIA REPAIR

- Scrotal haematoma/seroma
- Wound infection
- Urinary retention
- Chronic pain/paraesthesia in the scrotum (or labia majora in females) from damage to the ilioinguinal nerve (5–10%)
- Testicular atrophy caused by damage to the testicular artery (<1%)
- Recurrence (<5%)
  - **NB:** Infection is the most important risk factor.
  - Poor operative technique.
  - Chronic cough, constipation or bladder outlet obstruction.
- Avoid heavy lifting for 6–8 weeks post-procedure

FEMORAL HERNIA

EPIDEMIOLOGY

- Female > male
- ~30% of all hernia repairs in women, <1% of all hernia repairs in men
- More common in later life (>70 years old)

SURGICAL ANATOMY

Table 2.3 Boundaries of the Femoral Triangle

Superior	Inguinal ligament
Lateral	Medial border of sartorius muscle
Medial	Medial border of adductor longus
Floor	Iliacus, psoas major, pectineus, adductor longus
Roof	Superficial fascia and great saphenous vein
Contents of the Femoral Triangle	
From medial to lateral	Canal, vein artery, nerve (CVAN)

Table 2.4 Boundaries of the Femoral Canal

Anterior	Inguinal ligament
Lateral	Femoral vein
Medial	Lacunar ligament
Posterior	Pectineal ligament
Contents of the Femoral Canal	
Lymphatics (Cloquet's node) and fat	

CLINICAL FEATURES

- Classically, a lump felt inferolateral to the pubic tubercle.
- 40% present as emergencies due to the narrow neck–more likely to strangulate.
- Cough impulse is rarely detected for the same reason.

DIFFERENTIAL DIAGNOSIS

- Femoral canal lipoma
- Saphena varix (SFJ varices)
- Lymphadenopathy
- Femoral artery aneurysm
- Femoral artery pseudoaneurysm (post-angiography)
- Sarcoma (leio/rhabdomyosarcoma)

MANAGEMENT

- All femoral hernias should be surgically repaired (high risk of complication).

Top tip: If a patient has saphena varix, ask them to lie flat and it should disappear; you should feel a thrill on coughing. The patient will likely have varicose veins elsewhere.

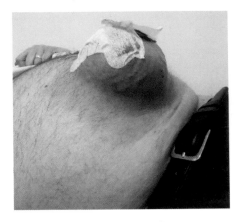

Figure 2.4   Umbilical hernia. Courtesy of Dr Jaclyn Croyle

UMBILICAL HERNIA

AETIOLOGY
- Female:male = 3:1.
- Risk factors: Pregnancy, obesity.
- Up to 50% prevalence in screened patients.

TYPES OF UMBILICAL HERNIA
- **True**
  - Always congenital.
  - Through umbilical cicatrix.
  - May close spontaneously by 3 years of age.
- **Periumbilical**
  - Always acquired.
  - Not through the umbilicus itself.
  - Common in obese patients and multiparous women.

MANAGEMENT
- Most are asymptomatic and can be managed conservatively.
- True umbilical hernias should be surgically repaired after 3 years of age.

INCISIONAL HERNIA

AETIOLOGY
- Up to 70% of laparotomy incisions eventually herniate in a lifetime
- Risk factors
  - Post-operative wound infection
  - Abdominal obesity

- Poor muscle quality (smoking, anaemia)
- Multiple operations through the same incision
- Poor choice of incision
- Inadequate closure technique

CLINICAL PRESENTATION

- Lump and defect: Vary from small (more dangerous) to complete defects.
- May be asymptomatic but tend to progressively enlarge.
- Rarely cause strangulation.

MANAGEMENT

- Repair is usually indicated if symptomatic/strangulated.
- Mesh used for larger defects (>4 cm).

SPIGELIAN HERNIA

KEY POINTS

- Defect between lateral border of the rectus abdominis and linea semilunaris.
- The hernial sac comes to lie between the layers of internal oblique, external oblique, and transversus abdominis.
- Hernial sac is found lateral to the rectus sheath, directly behind external oblique.
- Difficult to diagnose clinically.

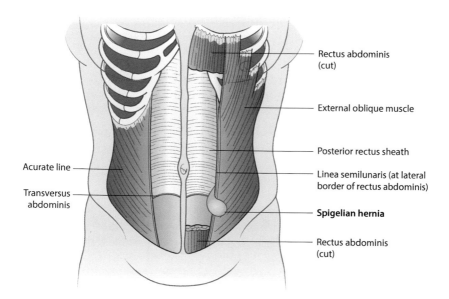

Figure 2.5   Spigelian hernia.

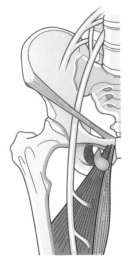

Obturator hernia
(through defect in obturator canal)

Obturator nerve supplies
• Hip adductor
• Sensation to upper medial thigh
• Sensation to knee joint

Figure 2.6   Obturator hernia.

- Usually requires imaging (US/CT).
- Direct surgical repair indicated.

OBTURATOR HERNIA

KEY POINTS

- Defect through the obturator canal (lateral pelvis into thigh).
- Causes medial thigh pain in cutaneous distribution of the obturator nerve.
- Very challenging diagnosis–CT usually required.
- High risk of incarceration/obstruction.

MCQs FOR SELF-ASSESSMENT

Chapter 3

UPPER GASTROINTESTINAL SURGERY

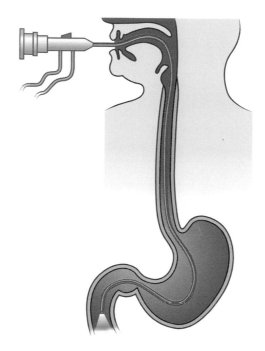

DOI: 10.1201/9781003207184-3

CONTENTS

Benign Oesophageal Disorders	45
Gastro-Oesophageal Reflux Disease (GORD)	45
Barrett's Oesophagus	46
Hiatus Hernia	47
Peptic Ulcer Disease	50
Upper Gastrointestinal Bleeding	53
Dysphagia and Odynophagia	55
Oesophageal Motility Disorders	57
Achalasia	57
Diffuse Oesophageal Spasm	59
Chagas Disease	59
Scleroderma and Oesophageal Dysmotility	60
Oesophageal Cancer	60
Gastric Cancer	63
Consent for Oesophago-Gastro-Duodenoscopy	66

BENIGN OESOPHAGEAL DISORDERS

GASTRO-OESOPHAGEAL REFLUX DISEASE (GORD)

DEFINITION

- A condition describing excessive reflux of gastric contents (acid, bile and pancreatic enzymes) into the oesophagus, through a defective lower oesophageal sphincter (LOS).
- Thus, causing symptoms and/or oesophageal mucosal injury.

KEY FACTS

- At endoscopy there may be erosive and non-erosive disease.
- An abnormal DeMeester score on pH monitoring confirms the diagnosis.
  - A composite score of number and duration of episodes when pH < 4.

EPIDEMIOLOGY

- GORD is the most frequently diagnosed upper GI disorder.
- Most commonly found in middle-aged adults.
- About 25–40% of healthy adult Americans experience symptomatic GORD.

RISK FACTORS

- Family history of GORD
- Elevated BMI
- Heavy alcohol use
- Smoking
- Pregnancy

PATHOPHYSIOLOGY

- Poor/inefficient oesophageal motility.
- Reduced LOS tone.
- Increased intragastric pressure and delayed gastric emptying.

CLINICAL FEATURES

- Retrosternal discomfort or heartburn.
- Acid reflux into pharynx.
- Commonly worse at night and after large meals.
- Dysphagia may occur if there is associated ulceration or a stricture.
- Globus: Feeling of a lump in throat.
- Pulmonary aspiration (nocturnal coughing; hoarse voice).
- Commonly associated with hiatus hernia.

INVESTIGATIONS

- Routine laboratory investigations.
- Reflux can be confirmed by 24 hours continuous pH monitoring–peaks of pH change must correspond to symptoms.

- Oesophageal manometry.
- Oesophago-gastro-duodenoscopy (OGD) should be performed in all new cases over the age of 45 to exclude malignancy.

Top tip: Patients with progressive dysphagia, especially if there is weight loss, need an urgent OGD to exclude malignancy.

MANAGEMENT

- **Lifestyle modification**
  - Smaller meals at frequent intervals.
  - Avoid late-night food intake.
  - Avoid gastric irritants like coffee, chocolate and spicy food.
  - Smoking cessation and moderation in alcohol intake.
- **Medical treatment**
  - Counteract acid secretion: Proton pump inhibitors (PPIs).
  - Symptomatic relief with antacids e.g. Gaviscon.
- **Surgical treatment**
  - Nissen's fundoplication: Wrapping the fundus of the stomach totally around the intra-abdominal oesophagus to augment the high-pressure zone
  - Dor fundoplication: Anterior wrapping of fundus around the cardia high-pressure zone
  - Toupet fundoplication: Posterior wrapping of fundus around the cardia high-pressure zone
- **Indications for surgery**
  - Persistent symptoms despite maximal medical therapy must rule out functional bowel disorder in this cohort.
  - Large volume reflux with risk of aspiration pneumonia.
  - Complications of reflux include stricture and severe ulceration.
  - Barrett's oesophagus.
  - Young patients with uncontrolled symptoms.

COMPLICATIONS

- Oesophagitis and ulceration.
- Peptic stricture.
- Barrett's oesophagus: Intestinal metaplasia (goblet cells)
- Increased risk of oesophageal adenocarcinoma.

BARRETT'S OESOPHAGUS

DEFINITION

- The **metaplastic** change of stratified squamous epithelium of the distal oesophagus to columnar epithelium. Figure 3.1
- It is classified into long segment (>3 cm) and short segment (<3 cm).

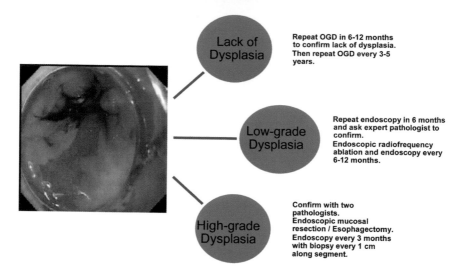

Lack of Dysplasia

Repeat OGD in 6-12 months to confirm lack of dysplasia. Then repeat OGD every 3-5 years.

Low-grade Dysplasia

Repeat endoscopy in 6 months and ask expert pathologist to confirm.
Endoscopic radiofrequency ablation and endoscopy every 6-12 months.

High-grade Dysplasia

Confirm with two pathologists.
Endoscopic mucosal resection / Esophagectomy.
Endoscopy every 3 months with biopsy every 1 cm along segment.

Figure 3.1   OGD of Barrett's oesophagus. Courtesy of Mr William Robb

AETIOLOGY

- A consequence of prolonged severe GORD.
- Most commonly found in obese patients with GORD.
- Totally 1% of individuals with Barrett's per year develop adenocarcinoma.
- Male:female = 2:1.
- Average age group is 55–65 years.

MANAGEMENT

- Lifestyle modifications, especially smoking, alcohol and maintaining a healthy weight.
- Anti-reflux medications.
- Eradication therapy for patients with *Helicobacter pylori*.
- Radiofrequency ablation and OGD surveillance.
- Mucosal endoscopic resection.
- Oesophagectomy.

Top tip: In a Barrett's segment, biopsies should be taken every 1 cm along the segment from all four quadrants of the oesophageal wall.

HIATUS HERNIA

DEFINITION

- The prolapse of the gastro-oesophageal junction (GOJ) and part or all of the stomach into the thoracic cavity through the oesophageal diaphragmatic hiatus. Table 3.1

Table 3.1   Types of Hiatus Hernias

Type I Sliding	• Most common type. • Associated with GORD. • GOJ slides up into the chest which can cause LOS to become less competent. Figure 3.2
Type II Paraoesophageal	• May result in volvulus or become incarcerated and cause obstruction. • The gastric fundus is in the chest while the GOJ is in situ. Figure 3.3
Type III Combined	• The fundus and GOJ are in the chest.
Type IV Complex	• Another organ is in the chest e.g. small bowel, colon.

KEY FACTS

- More commonly found in Western countries.
- Incidence increases with age, 10% in <40 years and 70% in >70 years.
- Majority are asymptomatic or have GORD.

INVESTIGATIONS

- CXR–lateral chest shows an air-fluid level in posterior mediastinum.
- Barium swallow–best diagnostic test.
- OGD–visualises mucosa but cannot exclude hiatus hernia.
- CT scan.

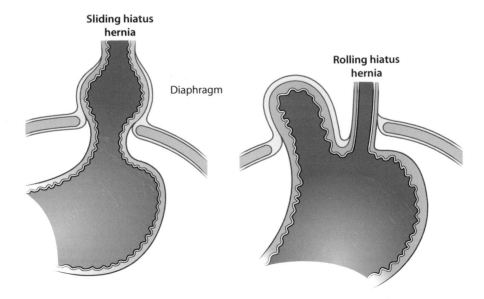

Sliding hiatus hernia

Rolling hiatus hernia

Diaphragm

Figure 3.2   Sliding and rolling hiatus hernia.

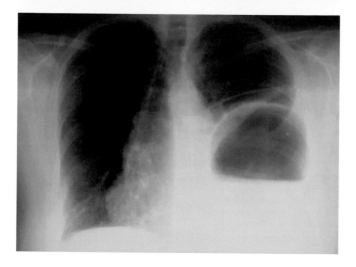

Figure 3.3   Paraoesophageal hernia with the stomach within the chest. Courtesy of Prof Tom Walsh

MANAGEMENT

- **Conservative/medical**
    - Reduce acid production: Stop smoking, lose weight, reduce alcohol.
    - Counteract acid secretion: PPIs, antacids, mucosal protectants.
    - Prokinetic agents, little effect on symptoms or oesophageal pH, e.g. pro-motil-iants (e.g. metoclopramide).
- **Surgical**
    - Indicated if persistent symptoms despite maximal medical therapy (must rule out functional bowel disorder).
    - Elective procedure of choice is laparoscopic/robotic reduction of the hernia, excision of the sac and gastric fixation (gastropexy)–Nissen fundoplication.

Top tip: Follow-up CXR post-operatively to assess the position of the stomach and assess for recurrence/re-herniation.

COMPLICATIONS OF HIATUS HERNIA

- **Oesophageal**
    - Inflammation
    - Ulceration
    - Bleeding
    - Iron deficiency anaemia
- **Non-oesophageal**
    - Gastric volvulus in paraesophageal hernia presenting with vomiting, severe acute chest pain and collapse.
    - May lead to gastric ischemia and infarction.

PEPTIC ULCER DISEASE

DEFINITION

- Injury leading to breakdown of the mucosal layer of the lower oesophagus, stomach or duodenum. Mainly occurs secondary to excessive acid production or damaged barrier mechanisms.

KEY FACTS

- The lifetime prevalence is approximately 11–14% in men and 8–11% in women.
- Most common sites: First part of the duodenum, gastric antrum and lesser curve of the stomach.
- Incidence is declining, likely due to the widespread use of antisecretory medications and treatment of *H. pylori*.
- Role of surgery is limited to emergency management of perforated or bleeding ulcers.

H. pylori accounts for 90% of duodenal ulcers and 70–80% of gastric ulcers.

AETIOLOGY

- *H. pylori* and the use of NSAIDs or aspirin are the main risk factors for both gastric and duodenal ulcers.
- *H. pylori*'s role is poorly understood, but likely that the inflammation it induces is sustained by the effect of acid and pepsin on the mucosa.
- **Other risk factors:**
  - Smoking, alcohol, psychosocial stress, steroids.
- **Gastrinoma:**
  - These are neuroendocrine tumours (NETs) that secrete gastrin and are usually found in the pancreas or duodenal wall.
  - Gastrin hypersecretion causes a clinical syndrome called Zollinger-Ellison syndrome, which results in acid hypersecretion and severe Peptic Ulcer Disease (PUD).
  - Patients get multiple gastric, duodenal and jejunal ulcers.
  - Majority are sporadic but may occur in multiple endocrine neoplasia syndrome type 1 (MEN1).

CLINICAL FEATURES

- Often nonspecific symptoms, dyspepsia, nausea, epigastric pain.
- Heartburn and acute chest pain.
- Hematemesis/melaena if a bleeding ulcer.
- Anaemia symptoms (fatigue, dizziness, lethargy).
- **Duodenal ulceration**
  - Hunger pains, nocturnal pain/early morning hours.
  - Relieved by food; pain is often cyclical.

- **Gastric ulceration**
  - Post-prandial pain, often triggered by food.
  - Associated with weight loss and anorexia.
  - Pain is less cyclical.

> Anterior duodenal ulcers, found in the first part of the duodenum, tend to perforate, while posterior duodenal ulcers bleed by eroding into the gastroduodenal artery.

INVESTIGATIONS

- **H. pylori investigations:**
  - Urease test: To assess for presence of *H. pylori*, can be performed on antral biopsies from gastroscopy or as a CO_2 breath test.
  - Urea breath test (UBT).
  - Stool antigen testing.
  - Serology (non-specific).
- Fasting serum gastrin levels: If hypergastrinemia suspected.
- **OGD**
  - Biopsy urease test (CLO test [*Campylobacter*-like organism]).
  - Gastric antral mucosal histology
  - Less commonly bacterial culture.

> Gastric ulcers should always be biopsied to rule out malignancy and repeat endoscopy to confirm healing.

MANAGEMENT

- **Control of predisposing factors**
  - Eliminate proven *H. pylori* infection by **triple therapy:**
    - 1–2 weeks course of *two antibiotics* (e.g. amoxicillin 1g BD and clarithromycin 500 mg BD).
    - PPI, BD for 1–2 weeks, then continued OD for 4–6 weeks.
- **Diminish irritant effects of acid-pepsin**
  - Achieved with antacid drugs or alginate preparations.
- **The use of mucosal protective agents**
  - E.g. sucralfate.
- **Reduction of acid secretion**
  - PPIs (omeprazole).
  - H_2 receptor-blocking drugs (cimetidine).

COMPLICATIONS

- Bleeding
  - Acute upper GI bleeding.
  - Iron deficiency anaemia due to chronic low-level bleeding.
- Perforation and sepsis

- Gastric outlet obstruction
  - Chronic scarring around pylorus.
  - Always consider gastric malignancy as a cause of outlet obstruction.

MANAGING COMPLICATIONS OF PEPTIC ULCER DISEASE

- Haemorrhage
  - Apply the ABC protocol.
  - Resuscitate with IV fluids, transfusion, PPI infusion and tranexamic acid.
  - Actively bleeding lesions which are identified by OGD can be treated by:
    - Adrenaline injection
    - Thermo-coagulation
    - Clipping
    - Haemostatic nano-powder spray
    - If these measures fail to achieve haemostasis then surgical intervention with laparotomy, gastrotomy and oversewing of the ulcer or artery
- Perforation
  - Declining incidence with advances in medical management.
  - Duodenal perforation is twice as common as gastric ulcer perforation.
  - Patients present with sudden severe abdominal pain and peritonitis.
  - Diagnosis made by the presence of pneumoperitoneum on an erect CXR.
  - Treatment:
    - ABC + resuscitation
    - Broad-spectrum antibiotics (co-amoxiclav/piperacillin-tazobactam and metronidazole/gentamicin)
    - NGT and urinary catheter
    - Laparoscopic/Open Graham patch repair
    - Performed by closure of the ulcer followed by an omental patch and fixation
- **Gastric outlet obstruction**
  - The pylorus/pre-pyloric area are common sites of chronic ulceration.
  - Healing with fibrosis leads to stricture formation and pyloric stenosis.
  - Patients present with episodic and projectile vomiting unrelated to eating.
  - On examination patients are dehydrated and undernourished.
  - Abdominal examination reveals a succussion splash.
  - Biochemical analysis reveals a hypochloremic alkalosis.
  - PFA may demonstrate a hugely dilated stomach.
  - Management involves:
    - Initial aggressive resuscitation.
    - Nutritional support through TPN, nasojejunal or jejunostomy feed.
  - Surgeries:
    - Gastrojejunostomy +/– truncal vagotomy and pyloroplasty.

Gastric malignancy should be ruled out prior to bypassing a gastric outlet obstruction.

UPPER GASTROINTESTINAL BLEEDING

DEFINITION
- Bleeding from oesophagus, stomach or duodenum (above the ligament of Treitz).

KEY FACTS
- Hematemesis: Vomiting of blood proximal to the duodenojejunal junction.
- Melaena: Black "tarry" stools due to digestion of Hb by intestinal bacteria.
- PUD is the most common cause (35–50%).
- Variceal bleeding should always be considered, as it accounts for up to 9% of upper GI bleeds and can be rapidly fatal.

CLINICAL PRESENTATION
- Haematemesis and melaena.
- Hematochezia in 15% (brisk upper GI bleed).
- Abdominal pain (relieved by food suggests PUD/gastritis).
- Heartburn, reflux, dyspepsia suggests oesophagitis/ulceration.
- Dysphagia, weight loss (upper GI malignancy).
- Features of chronic liver disease e.g. jaundice (oesophageal varices).
- Features of anaemia (fatigue, syncope, dyspnoea, chest pain).
- Background of PUD, chronic liver disease, varices, GI malignancy.
- Previous endoscopy, retrieve records.
- Medications: Aspirin/Plavix, warfarin/NOAC, NSAIDs, steroids.

PHYSICAL EXAM
- Vitals: Tachycardia, hypotension, tachypnoea, reduced urine output.
- Reduced cap refill, cool extremities, reduced JVP, reduced Glasgow Coma Scale score (GCS).
- Visible active bleeding (haematemesis/melaena).
- Features of chronic liver disease.
  - Ascites, jaundice, spider naevi, gynecomastia, caput medusae, hepatomegaly.
- Abdominal exam
  - Tenderness? Guarding? Masses?
- PR exam
  - Masses? Fresh blood? FOB positive?

Table 3.2 Differential Diagnosis of upper gastrointestinal bleeding

Oesophageal	Gastric	Duodenal
Varices	Varices	Ulcer
Malignancy	Malignancy	Malignancy
Ulcer	Ulcer	Vascular malformation (such as aorto-enteric fistula)
Oesophagitis	Gastritis	
Mallory-Weiss tear	Dieulafoy lesion	

INVESTIGATIONS

- **Bedside:**
  - ECG
  - NGT aspirate: Helps determine if upper or lower GI bleed.
- **Bloods:**
  - FBC: Check Hb and platelets.
  - U&E: Disproportionately raised urea:creatinine ratio.
  - Coagulation screen: Check for underlying coagulopathy/International Normalised Ratio (INR)
  - LFTs:
    - Evidence of chronic liver disease or liver metastases
    - Derangement resulting in coagulopathy
  - Group and crossmatch 4 units
  - ABG
- **Imaging:**
  - Erect CXR
  - OGD
  - CT angiography/angiography

MANAGEMENT OF UNSTABLE UPPER GI BLEED

- Airway
  - Protect airway, high flow O_2.
  - Intubate if vomiting or low GCS, to avoid aspiration.
  - Keep NPO.
- Breathing
  - Assess O_2 saturation.
- Circulation
  - 2 large bore IV cannulas.
  - Send full bloods as above (including group and crossmatch)
  - IV fluids (crystalloids: Hartmann's/normal saline)
  - Bolus 10–20 ml/kg if hypotensive (1 L over 30 minutes for up to 2 L then transfuse)
  - Start the transfusion as part of the resuscitation
    - Maintain Hb > 8 g/dL (10 if cardiovascular disease)
    - Consider O negative blood if unable to wait for type-specific blood
    - Activate Major Transfusion Protocol if >4 units.
  - Urinary catheter: Monitor hourly ins/outs.
- Medications
  - Correct clotting abnormalities: Consider vitamin K, FFP, PCC if high INR
  - IV PPI infusion: 80 mg omeprazole stat followed by 8 mg/hr for 72 hr
  - IV 1 g tranexamic acid TDS
  - IV octreotide/vasopressin if variceal bleed suspected:
    - Reduces portal pressures in variceal bleed
    - Sengstaken-Blakemore tube may be required in massive variceal bleed
- Inform the following:
  - Endoscopy
  - Surgical on-call
  - Senior colleague

- Anaesthetics
- HDU/ICU
- Operating theatre
- Urgent OGD for diagnostic and therapeutic purposes
  - Therapeutic options include:
    - Adrenaline injection
    - Heater probe coagulation
    - Sclerotherapy
    - Banding of varices
- Surgery may be required if:
  - Massive haemorrhage requiring ongoing resuscitation
  - Failed endoscopic management
  - Rebleeding

Massive transfusion protocol is activated when transfusion >4 units in 1 hour, >10 units in 24 hours or replacement of 50% of total body weight within 3 hours.
Rapid administration of blood products with the ratio of 1 RBC: 1 Platelet : 1 FFP.

ROCKALL SCORE

- To estimate the risk of rebleeding or death in an upper GI bleed
- Risk of mortality post-GI bleed:
  - <3 = Good prognosis
  - >8 = Poor prognosis

Table 3.3   Rockall Scoring System

	0	1	2	3
(A) Age	<60	60–79	80+	
(B) Shock	Nil	HR > 100	SBP < 100	
(C) Comorbidity	Nil major	–	IHD/CCF, major morbidity	Renal/liver failure
(D) Diagnosis	Mallory-Weiss tear	All other Dx	GI malignancy	
(E) Evidence of Bleeding	None	–	Blood, spurting vessel, adherent clot	

DYSPHAGIA AND ODYNOPHAGIA

DEFINITION

- Dysphagia is defined as difficulty swallowing
- Odynophagia is painful swallowing

CAUSES OF DYSPHAGIA

- **Congenital:**
  - Oesophageal atresia

- **Acquired:**
  - Luminal: Bolus, foreign body and bezoar.
  - Oesophageal wall: Oesophageal web, Plummer-Vinson syndrome, carcinoma, stricture, achalasia, GORD, oesophagitis, oesophageal dysmotility disorder, scleroderma.
  - Extramural: Hilar lymphadenopathy, pharyngeal pouch, retrosternal goitre, lung carcinoma.
  - Neurological: Stroke, myasthenia gravis, motor neuron disease.

CAUSES OF ODYNOPHAGIA

- Trauma: Radiation, oesophageal burn, Mallory-Weiss tear, oesophageal rupture.
- Foreign body: Oropharyngeal or oesophageal.
- GORD: Oesophagitis, oesophageal ulceration.
- Infective: Pharyngitis, tonsillitis, oesophagitis (Herpes Simplex Virus [HSV]/ Cytomegalovirus [CMV]/*Candida*), abscess.
- Neoplasia: Pharyngeal/laryngeal/oesophageal carcinoma.
- Motility-related: Achalasia, oesophageal dysmotility disorders.
- Other: Scleroderma.

Table 3.4   Taking a Dysphagia History

Key Questions in Dysphagia History	
Symptoms	**Considerations**
Degree of dysphagia	• Solids, liquids or both • Complete inability to swallow liquids is a medical emergency and requires hospital admission
Onset and duration of dysphagia	• Progressive dysphagia is suspicious for malignancy • Sudden onset while eating suggests bolus obstruction
Long history of dyspepsia, reflux and progressive dysphagia	• Benign stricture formation due to reflux
Weight loss	• Malignancy or poor feeding
Nocturnal cough	• Pharyngeal pouch, Achalasia, severe GORD
Haematemesis	• Bleeding oesophageal lesion • Peptic ulcer may cause oesophageal stricture
Fatigue (due to anaemia)	• Anaemia is associated with Plummer-Vinson syndrome, where it is linked with presence of oesophageal web • Anaemia could result from acute or chronic blood loss
Breathlessness	• Bronchogenic carcinoma • Symptom of anaemia • Recurrent aspiration pneumonia • Metastatic lung disease
Neurological symptoms	• Oesophageal motility disorder • Polio • Myasthenia gravis • Bulbar palsy • Syringomyelia

Table 3.5 Investigations for Dysphagia

Investigation	Consideration
Bloods	FBC (anaemia), U&E (dehydration)
Upper GI Endoscopy (+/– biopsy)	First-line investigation
Barium swallow	Used to diagnose dysmotility disorders ("Bird's beak" or "rat's tail" appearance in achalasia)
Manometry	Used to assess coordination and strength of peristaltic movement in the oesophagus and also the sphincter pressures.
pH studies	Naso-oesophageal wire containing pH probe placed in lower oesophagus for 24 hours Used to diagnose GORD DeMeester score is a composite measure of reflux episodes and length of occasions that pH is measured <4
CXR	Primary lung cancer Mediastinal mass Large retrosternal goitre Air-fluid level in the mediastinal shadow, which is often suggestive of the dilated oesophagus seen in achalasia Aspiration pneumonia
CT TAP	Staging of oesophageal tumours
Endoscopic US	Staging of oesophageal tumours and detecting submucosal disease

OESOPHAGEAL MOTILITY DISORDERS

PRIMARY
- Achalasia
- Diffuse oesophageal spasm

SECONDARY
- Autoimmune rheumatic disorder (e.g. scleroderma)
- Chagas disease
- Diabetes mellitus
- Amyloid
- Intestinal pseudo-obstruction
- Myasthenia gravis

ACHALASIA

DEFINITION
- Characterised by a loss of oesophageal peristalsis, increased lower oesophageal sphincter tone and failure to relax.

KEY FACTS

- Characterised by progressive dysphagia equal to solids and liquids.
- Other complications include retrosternal chest pain and recurrent aspiration.

EPIDEMIOLOGY

- Usually affects people aged 25–60 years old.
- 5% in childhood.
- Prevalence of 10 cases per 100,000.

PATHOGENESIS AND AETIOLOGY

- Unknown, but there is a definite neurological defect involving Auerbach's myenteric plexus, with loss of inhibitory interneurons and the vagi nerves showing axonal degeneration of the dorsal motor nucleus and nucleus ambiguous.

INVESTIGATIONS

- Upper GI endoscopy
- Barium swallow
  - Produces a false negative in 1/3 of patients.
  - Narrow oesophago-gastric junction with a "bird-beak" appearance caused by the persistently contracted lower oesophageal sphincter.
  - Aperistalsis.
  - Poor emptying of barium.
- Manometry
  - Absence of peristaltic waves in oesophagus.
  - High resting intra-oesophageal pressure, impaired relaxation.
  - Normal resting pressure is 0–30 mmHg.

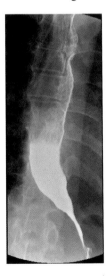

Figure 3.4 Barium swallow demonstrating the bird-beak appearance of the lower oesophagus, dilatation of the oesophagus and stasis of barium in the oesophagus. Courtesy of Dr Mark Given

COMPLICATIONS

- Nocturnal aspiration.
- Bronchiectasis.
- Lung abscess.
- Carcinoma in 3%. Squamous cell carcinoma type in mid-oesophagus.

MANAGEMENT

- Balloon dilatation
  - Successful in 70–80%, 5% risk of perforation.
- Injection of botulinum toxin
  - Injection into Lower Oesophageal Sphincter (LOS), limited long-term success.
- Peroral endoscopic myotomy.
- **Heller's cardiomyotomy**
  - Involves incision into the circular musculature of the oesophagus. Extends from 5 cm above to 3 cm below the cardia.
  - Coupled with anterior fundoplication.
  - Successful in 85–95% with 20% risk of post-op reflux.

> About 3–5% of achalasia patients develop oesophageal Squamous Cell Carcinoma (SCC).

DIFFUSE OESOPHAGEAL SPASM

PRESENTATION

- Dysphagia for solids and liquids
- Atypical chest pain (may mimic angina-like chest pain)

INVESTIGATIONS

- Difficult, but manometry may reveal "nutcracker" or "corkscrew" oesophagus with high-amplitude peristalsis of long duration.

MANAGEMENT

- Nifedipine and reassurance.

CHAGAS DISEASE

DEFINITION

- Chronic infection with *Trypanosoma cruzi*, a parasite native to Brazil.

KEY FACTS

- Causes destruction of intramuscular ganglion cells.
- Clinical picture is very similar to achalasia.
- It is also associated with cardiomyopathy, megacolon, megaduodenum and megaureter.

SCLERODERMA AND OESOPHAGEAL DYSMOTILITY

KEY POINTS

- Totally, 80% have oesophageal involvement.
- Oesophagitis is seen in CREST (calcinosis, Raynaud's, oesophagitis, scleroderma and telangiectasia) syndrome.
- Adynamic oesophagus and reflux cause stricture.
- The lower oesophageal sphincter is found to be hypotensive on manometry, unlike achalasia.
- Management: Medical or a partial fundoplication.

OESOPHAGEAL CANCER

KEY FACTS

- Sixth most common cause of death worldwide.
- The principal histologic types of oesophageal cancer are SCC and adenocarcinoma.
- SCC is the most common histology in Eastern Europe and Asia, while adenocarcinoma is most common in North America and Western Europe.
- Less than 25% are suitable for curative treatment.
- Overall 5-year survival is poor, at <15%.

ADENOCARCINOMA

- Rapidly increasing incidence in Europe, North America and Australia.
- **Pathogenesis**
  - Acid and bile reflux leading to metaplasia and dysplasia
- Most commonly occurs in the lower third of the oesophagus
- **Management**
  - Multidisciplinary treatment (chemotherapy, radiotherapy and surgery) is the mainstay of treatment
    - 25% undergoing neoadjuvant treatment have a complete response

SCC

- Most common histological subtype globally, most common in Japan, Northern China, and South Africa.
- Mostly found in the upper and middle parts of the oesophagus.
- **Pathogenesis**
  - Direct mucosal damage by carcinogens found in alcohol, smoking and nitrosamines (found in processed meat)
  - Also associated diet poor in fresh fruit and vegetables, chronic achalasia, chronic caustic strictures
- **Management**
  - Squamous cell carcinomas are sensitive to radiotherapy and may be treated with either radiotherapy or surgery
  - 50% undergoing neoadjuvant treatment have a complete response

Table 3.6 Risk Factors for Oesophageal Cancer

Adenocarcinoma	Squamous Cell Carcinoma
• Barrett's oesophagus • GORD • Obesity • High fat intake • Cigarette smoking • High alcohol intake	• High alcohol intake • Cigarette smoking • Nitrosamines in diet • Vitamin A, C deficiency • Coeliac disease • Strictures and webs • Achalasia • Peptic ulcer disease

CLINICAL FEATURES

- **Dysphagia with weight loss**
  - Any new symptoms of dysphagia, especially in those over the age of 45, require urgent referral for endoscopy.
- **Haematemesis**
  - Rarely the presenting symptom.
- **Incidental/Screening**
  - Occasionally identified as a result of follow-up/screening for Barrett's metaplasia, achalasia, or GORD.
  - High-grade dysplasia in Barrett's is associated with occult adenocarcinoma in 30%.
- **Features of disseminated disease**
  - Cervical lymphadenopathy (including Virchow's node).
  - Hepatomegaly due to metastases.
  - Epigastric mass due to para-aortic lymphadenopathy.
- **Symptoms of local invasion**
  - Hoarseness in recurrent laryngeal nerve palsy.
  - Cough and haemoptysis in tracheal invasion.
  - Neck swelling in superior vena cava (SVC) obstruction.
  - Horner's syndrome if sympathetic chain invasion.

INVESTIGATIONS

- OGD and biopsies
- **Local staging**
  - Endoluminal ultrasound scan to assess depth of invasion and paraesophageal lymph nodes.
- **Regional staging**
  - CT Thorax Abdomen Pelvis (TAP) to evaluate local invasion, locoregional lymph-adenopathy, liver disease.
  - Laparoscopy to assess for peritoneal disease in adenocarcinoma.
- **Disseminated disease**
  - PET scan is used to exclude metastases

MANAGEMENT

- **Multidisciplinary team discussion is essential**
- **Endoscopic treatment**
  - Endoscopic radiofrequency ablation for high-grade dysplasia.
  - Endoscopic mucosal resections can be used in high-grade dysplasia and pT1a tumours <2 cm.
- **Surgical treatment**
  - Surgery can be a single modality treatment for early disease without nodal involvement (≤T2N0), and for failed endoscopic treatments.
  - Surgery is combined with neoadjuvant therapy for more advanced oesophageal cancer.
  - Surgical resection is by oesophagectomy, which involves removal of most of the oesophagus, as well as the cardia, and lesser curve of the stomach.
  - Jejunostomy tube insertion is performed for nutritional support.
- **Common procedures**
  - **Ivor Lewis Procedure (2-stage oesophagectomy)**
    - Performed for distal tumours.
    - An abdominal stage and a thoracic stage, which can use open or minimally invasive approaches.
    - E.g. Laparoscopic mobilisation of the stomach and distal oesophagus, followed by thoracotomy, thoracic lymphadenectomy and intra-thoracic anastomosis.
  - **McKeown Procedure (3-stage oesophagectomy)**
    - Preferred for tumours proximal to the carina.
    - Three stages: Abdomen, thorax and neck.
  - **Transhiatal resection**
    - Abdomen to neck opened.

Ivor Lewis procedure

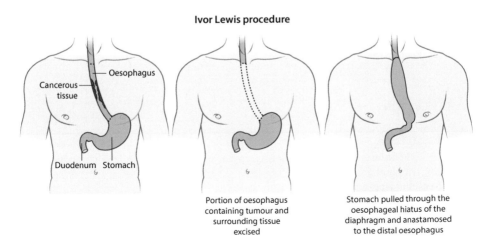

| Oesophagus | Portion of oesophagus containing tumour and surrounding tissue excised | Stomach pulled through the oesophageal hiatus of the diaphragm and anastamosed to the distal oesophagus |

Cancerous tissue

Duodenum Stomach

Figure 3.5   Ivor Lewis oesophagectomy.

- **Chemoradiotherapy**
  - Neoadjuvant chemoradiotherapy.
  - In locally advanced disease (T3-T4), or in tumours with nodal involvement (N1-N3), chemotherapy or chemoradiotherapy is required in addition to surgery.
  - Palliative chemoradiotherapy in metastatic disease
    - Improves survival compared to supportive management.
    - Must weigh against side effects and quality of life.
- **Radiotherapy**
  - Both adenocarcinoma and SCC respond to radiotherapy, but SCC response is better.
  - May cause strictures or fistulation
- **Palliative**
  - For inoperable disease, symptom control and improvement of dysphagia is the mainstay of treatment.
  - Self-expanding metal stenting (SEMS) give best relief of dysphagia.
  - Risks include: Perforation, tumour ingrowth and stent migration.

Patients are followed up with surveillance OGDs and CT TAP at intervals for up to 5 years post-operatively.

GASTRIC CANCER

KEY FACTS

- Sixth most common cancer and the third most common cause of cancer-related deaths in the world.
- Most patients present with advanced disease due to lack of screening.
- About 40% occur in the distal part of the stomach, 40% in the middle and 15% in the upper part.
- Overall 5-year survival is 31%.
- OGJ tumours are classified through the Siewert classification.

CLASSIFICATION AND AETIOLOGY

- Gastric adenocarcinoma
- Adenocarcinoma of the GOJ
- Gastrointestinal stromal tumours (GISTs)
- Neuroendocrine tumours (carcinoid tumours)
- Lymphoma (associated with *H. pylori*)

PATHOPHYSIOLOGY

- May arise from the tissues of the following:
  - **Mucosa (adenocarcinoma)**
    - Most common tumour type
    - Age of incidence >50 years

- Subclassified: Tubular, papillary, mucinous or signet-ring cells.
- May also be classified into two types, intestinal and diffuse, using the Lauren classification.
- Linitis plastica represents diffusely infiltrative disease with poor prognosis.
- **Connective tissue** of the stomach wall (previously known as leiomyoma or leiomyosarcoma, but part of the spectrum of disease called gastrointestinal stromal tumours [**GISTs**]).
- Neuroendocrine tissue (**carcinoid tumours**).
- Lymphoid tissue (**lymphomas**).

RISK FACTORS FOR ADENOCARCINOMA

- Chronic gastric ulceration related to *H. pylori*.
- Diet rich in nitrosamines (smoked or fresh fish, pickled fruit).
- Epstein-Barr virus (EBV)
- Family history of gastric cancer
- Blood type A

Table 3.7   Taking an Adenocarcinoma History

Symptoms
• Dyspepsia (new onset of dyspepsia >45 is adenocarcinoma until proven otherwise).
• Weight loss, anorexia and lethargy.
• Hematemesis, melena and occasionally acute upper GI bleeding.
• Dysphagia uncommon unless involving the proximal fundus and OGJ.
• Gastric outlet obstruction and projectile vomiting.
Signs
• Anaemia (iron deficiency due to chronic blood loss).
• Palpable epigastric mass.
• Palpable supraclavicular (Virchow's) lymph node (Troisier's sign). Suggests disseminated disease.
• Malignant pleural effusion and ascites.
• Hepatomegaly and jaundice.

INVESTIGATIONS

- Diagnosis usually by gastroscopy and biopsy.
- Staging investigations include:
    - CT TAP to assess for distant metastases and local lymphadenopathy.
    - Endoluminal US to assess for local disease.
    - Diagnostic laparoscopy to exclude small volume peritoneal metastases.
    - PET scan for distant metastases.

MANAGEMENT

- Overall patient fitness as well as tumour stage (according to Tumour Node Metastasis [TNM]) determine suitability for surgery.

Partial gastrectomy

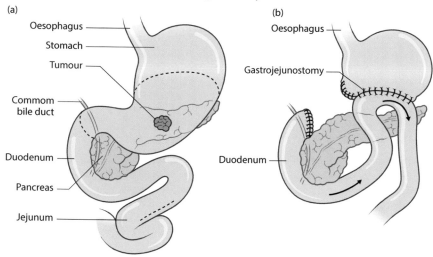

Figure 3.6 Partial gastrectomy.

- Gastrectomy (partial vs total vs extended) with D2 lymph node dissection. Figure 3.6
- Subtotal gastrectomy usually for pyloric and antral lesions.
- Diffused pathology warrants a total gastrectomy.
- Neoadjuvant chemotherapy regimens: FLOT/MAGIC.
- Palliation may be achieved with limited radiation therapy.
  - Palliative gastrojejunostomy may provide good symptom control.

PARTIAL/TOTAL GASTRECTOMY COMPLICATIONS

- **Early**
  - Haemorrhage.
  - Acute pancreatitis.
  - Anastomotic leak.
  - Duodenal stump disruption.
  - Respiratory compromise.
- **Late**
  - Dumping syndrome
    - General weakness, light-headedness, sweating.
    - Early dumping: Hyperosmolar solutions in the gut cause rapid shift, like blood loss.
    - Late dumping: Glucose surge causes insulin surge, causing hypoglycemia.
  - Bile reflux and vomiting.
  - Diarrhoea.
  - Recurrent stomal ulceration.
  - Metabolic abnormalities
    - Iron deficiency
    - Vitamin B12 deficiency.

PROGNOSIS

- Overall prognosis remains poor.
- Five-year survival for stage I disease (limited to mucosa) is 66%.
- Five-year survival for stage III disease (regional lymph node involvement) is 10%.

CONSENT FOR OESOPHAGO-GASTRO-DUODENOSCOPY

EXPLAIN TO PATIENT WHAT THE PROCEDURE INVOLVES

- Inspection of the upper GI tract (oesophagus, stomach and upper intestine) with a flexible endoscope (a tube smaller than the size of your little finger with a camera in it). Figure 3.7
- The team will be able to take photographs, make videos and take samples of the tissues, this is painless. These samples will be investigated and the photographs can be filed with your permanent records.
- Tell the patients to assume that they will be in the endoscopy department from 1 to 3 hours (emergencies will have priority).
- Explain to the patient they can opt to be sedated or they can opt not to have sedation and instead have a local anaesthetic throat spray and remain awake for the procedure.

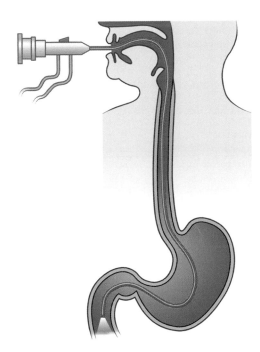

Figure 3.7 Oesophago-gastro-duodenoscopy.

INTRAVENOUS SEDATION USED

- Typically given IV midazolam (a benzodiazepine) as sedation.
- Be cautious for benzodiazepine overdose.
- Always have flumazenil (benzodiazepine antagonist) available
- They will be slightly drowsy and relaxed but not unconscious; they may not be able to remember the procedure.
- They can breathe normally throughout the procedure through their nose.
- If you opt for sedation you should not operate machinery, drive, consume alcohol or sign legally binding documents for 24 hours after receiving the medication, and you need someone to accompany you home.

PREPARATION FOR THE OGD

- The stomach must be empty, therefore no eating for 6 hours before the endoscopy. Small amounts of water are safe up to 2 hours before endoscopy.
- Routine medications may be taken; however, if they are currently on medications to reduce acid in the stomach please stop these 2 weeks before the scheduled endoscopy.
- Ask the patient to inform the staff if they are taking any blood-thinning agents like aspirin, warfarin, NOACs, or clopidogrel.
- Also inform of any allergies to latex or sedative drugs.

RISKS ASSOCIATED WITH OGD

- Note: these are extremely rare (1 in 2000 cases)
- Perforation of the oesophagus or lining of stomach
- Bleeding
- Damage to teeth
- Risks associated with sedation
- Aspiration
- Numbness, risk of scalds
- Sore throat

MCQs FOR SELF-ASSESSMENT

Chapter 4

HEPATOBILIARY SURGERY

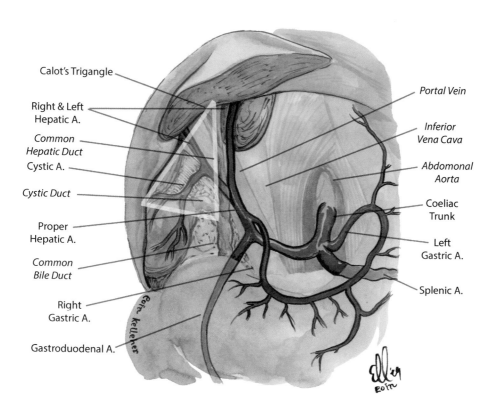

Calot's Triangle

Right & Left Hepatic A.

Common Hepatic Duct

Cystic A.

Cystic Duct

Proper Hepatic A.

Common Bile Duct

Right Gastric A.

Gastroduodenal A.

Portal Vein

Inferior Vena Cava

Abdomonal Aorta

Coeliac Trunk

Left Gastric A.

Splenic A.

DOI: 10.1201/9781003207184-4

CONTENTS

Jaundice	71
Gallstone Disease	76
Asymptomatic Gallstones	78
Biliary Colic	78
Acute Cholecystitis	79
Gallbladder Empyema	81
Gangrene of the Gallbladder	82
Perforated Gallbladder	82
Chronic Cholecystitis	83
Mucocoele	83
Gallstone Ileus	84
Obstructive Jaundice	84
Ascending Cholangitis	85
Acute Pancreatitis	87
Chronic Pancreatitis	92
Pancreatic Cancer	95

JAUNDICE

DEFINITION
- Jaundice is the result of accumulation of bilirubin in the bloodstream and subsequent deposition in the skin, sclera and mucous membranes.

Normal serum bilirubin is 3–17 mmol/L.
  Jaundice is clinically present at >40 mmol/L.

AETIOLOGY
- Jaundice is categorised based on the site of the underlying cause/disease.
- It can be divided into three main types of jaundice:
  1. Pre-hepatic
  2. Hepatocellular
  3. Post-hepatic
- **Pre-hepatic (haemolytic) jaundice**
  - Autoimmune haemolytic anaemia
  - Transfusion reactions
  - Drug toxicity
  - Congenital abnormalities of red cell structure or content
    - E.g. sickle cell disease, hereditary spherocytosis
- **Hepatocellular jaundice**
  - **Hepatic unconjugated hyperbilirubinaemia**
    - Gilbert's syndrome
    - Crigler-Najjar syndrome
  - **Hepatic conjugated hyperbilirubinaemia**
    - Viral infection–hepatitis A/B/C, EMV, CMV
    - Bacterial infection–liver abscess
    - Parasitic infection
    - Drugs–paracetamol overdose, antipsychotics, antibiotics
    - Non-infective hepatitis–chronic active hepatitis, alcohol-related
  - **Post-hepatic (obstructive) jaundice**
    - **Intraluminal abnormalities**
      - Choledocholithiasis
    - **Mural causes**
      - Biliary stricture
      - Primary sclerosing cholangitis
    - **Extrinsic compression of the bile ducts**
      - Pancreatic cancer
      - Mirizzi's syndrome

PATHOPHYSIOLOGY
- Jaundice results from high levels of bilirubin in the blood.
- Bilirubin is the normal breakdown product of the catabolism of haem, and thus, comes from the destruction of red blood cells.

- Bilirubin undergoes conjugation in the liver which makes it water soluble.
- It is then excreted in bile via the bile ducts into the duodenum.
- 10% of the unconjugated bilirubin is reduced to urobilinogen by small intestinal bacteria, reabsorbed into the ileum then excreted in the urine. **This is enterohepatic circulation.**
- The majority is converted by colonic bacteria to stercobilinogen and excreted in the faeces.
- When this pathway is disrupted jaundice occurs. Table 4.1

Unconjugated bilirubin is not water soluble.
Conjugated bilirubin is water soluble.

Table 4.1   Types for Jaundice

Pre-hepatic	• Excessive red cell breakdown which overwhelms the liver's ability to conjugate bilirubin. • This results in unconjugated hyperbilirubinemia as unconjugated bilirubin remains in the bloodstream resulting in jaundice. • Any bilirubin that manages to become conjugated will be excreted normally.
Hepatic	• Dysfunction of the hepatic cells results in the liver losing its ability to conjugate bilirubin. • If the liver becomes cirrhotic the intra-hepatic portions of the biliary tree become compressed also causing a degree of obstruction. • This can lead to a 'mixed picture' resulting in both unconjugated and conjugated bilirubin in the blood.
Post-hepatic	• Obstruction of biliary drainage occurs. • Bilirubin will have been conjugated by the liver resulting in an unconjugated hyperbilirubinemia.

Table 4.2   Symptoms and Signs of Jaundice

Symptoms	Signs
Itching due to bile salts Abdominal pain RUQ–viral hepatitis, cholestatic jaundice Intermittent–CBD stones Lethargy and general malaise	Fever/rigors–infective hepatitis, ascending cholangitis Jaundice–may be painless Scleral icterus Dark urine Pale/clay-coloured stool

Courvoisier's Law: A painless, palpable gallbladder in a patient with jaundice is unlikely to be due to gallstone disease and may suggest malignant obstruction of the ducts.

DIFFERENTIAL DIAGNOSIS

- Alcoholic liver disease
- Choledocholithiasis
- Drug induced liver injury
- Ascending cholangitis
- Pancreatic carcinoma
- Haemolytic anaemia
- Hepatitis A, B, C, E, D
- Gilbert syndrome
- Primary sclerosing cholangitis

Acute cholecystitis does not cause jaundice.
Gallstones must cause blockage of bile (e.g. ascending cholangitis, Mirizzi syndrome, choledocholithiasis, etc.) for jaundice to occur in gallstone disease.

Table 4.3 Liver Function Tests in Jaundice

LFTs in Jaundice	Significance	Haemolytic	Hepatocellular	Obstructive
Unconjugated bilirubin	Quantifies the degree of suspected jaundice	↑	↑	Normal
Alkaline phosphatase (ALP)	Raised in biliary obstruction	Normal	Normal	↑↑
Gamma GT (GGT)	More specific for biliary obstruction than ALP	Normal	↑	↑↑
Transaminases (AST, ALT)	Markers of hepatocellular injury	Normal	↑	Normal
Lactate dehydrogenase		Normal	↑	Normal
Albumin	Marker of liver synthesising function			

↑Indicates increased
↑↑Indicates significantly increased

INVESTIGATIONS

- **Bedside**
  - Urine dipstick for bilirubin
- **Blood tests**
  - FBC
    - Elevated WCC in acute cholecystitis and cholangitis.
    - Anaemia, raised MCV and thrombocytopenia seen in liver disease.
  - LFTs
    - As detailed in the table above Table 4.3

- Urea, creatinine and electrolytes
  - To assess hydration and guide fluid resuscitation.
  - Hepatorenal syndrome.
- Coagulation profile
  - PT/aPTT are markers of liver function.
  - Vitamin K deficiency with obstructive jaundice impairs function of clotting factors II, VII, IX, X causing an increased PT.
- Amylase
  - Acute or chronic pancreatitis due to lower CBD stone.
- Liver screen
  - Can be performed for patients where no initial cause for liver dysfunction found. Table 4.4
- **Imaging**
- **US abdomen**
  - First-line to identify any obstructive pathology or gross liver pathology.
  - Cholelithiasis.
  - Dilated biliary ducts (intra- and extrahepatic) associated with obstruction.
  - Architectural disturbances of the liver itself associated with liver parenchymal disease.
  - Pancreatic masses.
- **Magnetic resonance cholangiopancreatography (MRCP)**
  - Used to visualise the biliary tree, usually performed if the jaundice is obstructive, and US abdomen was inconclusive or limited, or as further workup for surgical intervention.
  - For suspected extrahepatic obstruction with no cause seen on US.
- **Endoscopic retrograde cholangiopancreatography (ERCP)**
  - Allows for therapeutic intervention. Figure 4.1
- **Contrast-enhanced CT**
  - Preferable to ultrasound if neoplastic obstruction is suspected.
  - Better definition of mass lesions and general location of CBD obstruction.
  - Detailed pancreatic imaging.
- **Liver biopsy**
  - When no extrahepatic cause of jaundice is found (i.e. no duct dilatation, no evidence of haemolysis).
  - May indicate the cause of liver dysfunction or provide histological proof of metastatic disease.

Table 4.4   Liver Screen

Liver Screen	Viral Serology	Non-Infective Markers
Acute Liver Injury	• Hepatitis screen: • A, B, C and E • CMV and EBV	• Paracetamol level • Caeruloplasmin • ANA and IgG
Chronic Liver Injury	• Hepatitis screen: • B and C	• Caeruloplasmin • Ferritin and transferrin saturation • Tissue transglutaminase (TTG) antibody • Alpha-1-antitrypsin (A1AT) • Autoantibodies (autoimmune liver conditions) • AMA, anti-SMA, ANA

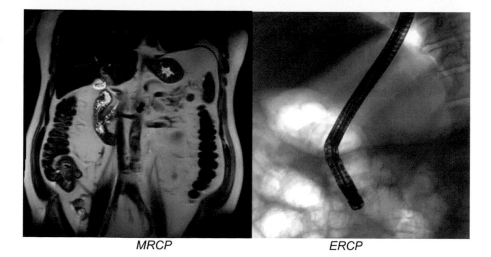

MRCP   ERCP

Figure 4.1 Magnetic resonance cholangiopancreatography (MRCP) and endoscopic retrograde cholangiopancreatography (ERCP). Courtesy of Dr Anthony Hoban

MANAGEMENT

- **Conservative**
  - Correct dehydration.
  - Monitor urinary output.
  - Monitor for coagulopathy
    - Vitamin K should be administered if PT is prolonged
    - Or FFP if any evidence of bleeding or rapid coagulopathy
  - Ensure adequate nutrition
    - Dietitian review
    - Enteral feeding
    - Rarely surgical gastrostomy or jejunostomy tube
- **Symptomatic treatment**
  - For itching caused by hyperbilirubinemia
    - An obstructive cause may be treated by cholestyramine
    - Other causes: Antihistamines
- **Specific treatment**
  - **Acute presentation**
    - ERCP +/− sphincterotomy +/− stent insertion
    - Percutaneous transhepatic cholangiogram
    - Surgical drainage
  - **Elective presentation**
    - Haemolytic jaundice
    - Steroids for autoimmune cases
    - Splenectomy
  - **Obstructive jaundice**
    - ERCP for asymptomatic uncomplicated stones.
    - Surgical drainage.

    – Cholecystojejunostomy for failed interventional treatment.
    – Surgical resection.
        – Whipple's pancreaticoduodenectomy for pancreatic tumours.
- **Hepatic jaundice**
  - Treat the causative agent and support liver function.
  - Transplantation in specific circumstances.

PROGNOSIS

- Adverse risk factors include:
- Age > 65 years
- Elevated plasma urea
- Elevated plasma bilirubin (>200 g/L)
- Uncontrolled sepsis and multiple organ dysfunction
- Underlying malignant disease

GALLSTONE DISEASE

KEY FACTS

- Gallstones present in 10% of people >50 years of age
- Gallstone disease may present with a spectrum of manifestations from asymptomatic to biliary colic to pancreatitis, to gallstone bowel obstruction, depending on where the gallstone is and what it is doing

AETIOLOGY

- Increasing age
- Female
- Obesity
- Multiparity
- Chronic haemolytic disorders
- Long-term parenteral disorders
- Rapid weight loss
- Previous surgery: Vagotomy results in GB stasis, resection of terminal ileum

PATHOPHYSIOLOGY OF GALLSTONES

- **Bile has three major components:**
  - Bile pigments (products of haemoglobin metabolism)
  - Phospholipids
  - Cholesterol
- Bile is stored in the gallbladder (GB) and secreted into the duodenum secondary to food induced cholecystokinin (CCK) stimulation.
- Gallstones form as a result of supersaturation of the bile.
- **Types of gallstones:**
  1. Pure cholesterol 10%
     - Linked to poor diet, obesity and cholesterol stones

2. Pure pigment (bile salts)10%
   - From excess bile pigments production
   - Commonly seen in haemolytic anaemia
3. Mixed 80%
   - Cholesterol and bile pigments

RISK FACTORS FOR CHOLESTEROL STONES–THE 5F'S

- Fat
- Female
- Fertile
- Forty
- Family history

Table 4.5 Common Presentations of Gallstone Disease

Asymptomatic gallstones	• The majority of gallstones are asymptomatic. • The current practice is to operate only on symptomatic patients.
Biliary/gallstone colic	• A gallstone may become impacted in Hartmann's pouch or the cystic duct and contraction of the GB may cause intermittent severe epigastric pain. • Most resolve in a few hours.
Acute cholecystitis	• If a gallstone becomes impacted in Hartmann's pouch or the cystic duct (80% of cases)–the resulting pressure can cause a chemical or bacterial inflammation (cholecystitis) which can progress or resolve.
Empyema (pus) of the GB	• If the infection/inflammation progresses the patient with a purulent GB infection may become very sick and require emergency intervention.
Gangrene of the GB	• If the infection progresses further, intraluminal pressure in the GB may cause end vessel occlusion and patchy gangrene of the fundus of the GB.
Perforation of the GB	• If the pressure is not relieved, the gangrenous wall may perforate. • Sometimes, before this occurs, the omentum–'the abdominal policeman'–wraps around the GB containing the bile leakage. • Sometimes the bile escapes causing biliary peritonitis.
Chronic cholecystitis	• The acute inflammation may settle and recur from time to time, as a mild recurring problem, not troublesome enough to warrant admission or investigations–until one day it does.
Mucocoele	• If a stone remains lodged in the neck of the GB bile can no longer enter and any bile in the GB becomes absorbed. But mucus secretion continues, producing a large tense RUQ globular mass.
Gallstone 'ileus'	• A gallstone in a contracted GB may cause chronic inflammation and erode into the duodenum. If big enough the stone can cause intestinal obstruction, anywhere up to the terminal ileum.

(continued)

Table 4.5 Common Presentations of Gallstone Disease (*continued*)

Ascending cholangitis	• A stone that enters the common bile duct (CBD) can injure the mucosa and obstruct the duct causing intermittent pain, pyrexia and jaundice–the classical **Charcot's triad** of symptoms of ascending cholangitis.
Obstructive jaundice	• If the stone obstructs the CBD lumen it can cause jaundice. In this case the GB will not be palpable (GB distension takes time). • A stone in Hartman's pouch can compress the adjacent CBD (Mirizzi syndrome). This is a very rare presentation.
Pancreatitis	• If the stone occludes the sphincter of Oddi, temporarily while exiting, or becomes impacted, the pressure may cause bile to reflux up the pancreatic duct triggering the cytokine cascade of pancreatitis.

ASYMPTOMATIC GALLSTONES

KEY POINTS

- The majority of gallstones are asymptomatic. The current practice is to operate only on symptomatic patients.
- Patients presenting with non-specific symptoms (esp. functional bowel disorder) may have gallstones diagnosed on US and be referred for cholecystectomy.
  - These patients will continue to have symptoms post-operatively and may even attribute further symptoms to their cholecystectomy.
  - The term post-cholecystectomy syndrome, which is now rarely used, described persistent symptoms despite cholecystectomy.
- It is essential to take a good history, which must include the **Rome criteria**, to exclude functional bowel disorder and if in doubt to record that the patient has been warned that symptoms may persist or progress.

BILIARY COLIC

PATHOGENESIS

- Gallstone transiently impacted in Hartmann's pouch or the cystic duct.

CLINICAL FEATURES

- **Symptoms**
  - Severe, steady dull pain in epigastrium or RUQ.
    - Pain lasts for minutes to hours
    - Typically occurring after at night or after a fatty meal
    - Pain may radiate to right scapula
  - Nausea, vomiting

- **Signs**
  - No clinical signs of acute abdomen
  - No systemic signs/no sepsis

INVESTIGATIONS

- **Bedside**
  - **Urinalysis**–to rule out pregnancy.
- **Blood**
  - **FBC**–WCC elevation to rule out cholecystitis.
  - **CRP**–elevation to rule out cholecystitis.
  - **LFTs**
    - Biliary colic and acute cholecystitis are likely to show raised ALP (ductal occlusion).
    - ALT and bilirubin should remain within normal range.
  - **Amylase**–to rule out pancreatitis.
- **Imaging**
  - **Abdominal US**
    - First-line investigation for gallstone pathology.
    - Shows cholelithiasis.
    - May show stone in cystic duct.
  - **MRCP**
    - Can show defects in the biliary tree.

ULTRASOUND FINDINGS IN GALLSTONE DISEASE

- Presence of gallstones of sludge
- GB wall thickness
- Bile duct dilation

MANAGEMENT

- **Conservative**
  - Pain management.
  - Rehydration.
  - Lifestyle advice–low fat diet, weight loss and exercise.
- **Surgical**
  - Elective cholecystectomy.

ACUTE CHOLECYSTITIS

DEFINITION

- Inflammation of GB which may begin as a chemical cholecystitis but can become secondarily infected.

PATHOPHYSIOLOGY

- Stone or sludge may block the cystic duct or erode the GB mucosa resulting in chemical and/or bacterial inflammation
- No cholelithiasis in 5%

CLINICAL PRESENTATION

- **Symptoms**
  - Severe abdominal pain
    - Epigastric or RUQ
    - Pain radiating to right scapula/shoulder
  - Fever
  - Loss of appetite
  - Nausea and vomiting
- **Signs**
  - Local peritonism in RUQ
    - Murphy's sign–pressure in RUQ causes 'catch' of breath on inspiration
  - Palpable, tender GB
  - Tachycardia
  - Jaundice

Murphy's Sign: Patient will experience pain and 'catch their breath' on inspiration when pressure is placed under the costal margin in the mid-clavicular line. A positive Murphy's sign suggests acute cholecystitis.

INVESTIGATIONS

- **Bloods**
  - FBC–elevated WCC
  - LFTs–elevated bilirubin, AST, ALT, ALP
  - Amylase–to rule out pancreatitis
- **Imaging**
  - Abdominal US
    - Look for stones and their 'acoustic shadows'. Figure 4.2
    - GB wall thickening or fluid suggests cholecystitis
    - Check for duct dilation–suggesting stone in CBD

MANAGEMENT

- **Conservative**
  - Pain management
  - Fluid resuscitation
  - Antibiotics
- **Surgical—cholecystectomy**
  - Can be performed during admission if no serious co-morbidities or electively when inflammation has settled.
    - The patient can be treated with antibiotics and supportive care and elective cholecystectomy can be performed after ~6 weeks when inflammation has settled

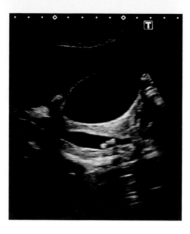

Figure 4.2 Gallbladder US showing a stone in a dilated CBD (choledocholithiasis). Courtesy of Dr Frank McGrath

- Routinely laparoscopic and often as a day case.
- Indications:
  - Symptomatic gallstones
  - Asymptomatic patients at risk of complications (diabetes, history of pancreatitis, long-term immunosuppression)
- **Risks of laparoscopic cholecystectomy**
  - Conversion to open operation, >5%
  - Bile duct injury, <1%
  - Bleeding, 2%
  - Bile leak, 1%
- **Contraindications to laparoscopic cholecystectomy**
  - Generalized abdominal sepsis
  - Major bleeding disorders
  - Late pregnancy
  - Intra-abdominal malignancy

GALLBLADDER EMPYEMA

DEFINITION

- This is when the GB bile becomes purulent.

PRESENTATION

- Patients may have a similar presentation to acute cholecystitis but usually more septic.

INVESTIGATIONS

- It may be suspected by the severity of sepsis and CRP levels
- Diagnosis is by US or CT scan

MANAGEMENT

- On admission the patient is treated with fluid, oxygen resuscitation and antibiotics.
- If the patient is young and fit, perform laparoscopic cholecystectomy.
- Manage with intraoperative drainage alone if GB is gangrenous and patient is elderly with co-morbidities.
- Percutaneous drainage of GB bile/pus by interventional radiology +/– leaving a drainage catheter (percutaneous cholecystostomy) in situ if unfit.
- Elective, planned laparoscopic cholecystectomy can be scheduled if the patient is fit.
- Patient can be followed up if unfit or has co-morbidities.

GANGRENE OF THE GALLBLADDER

PRESENTATION

- Similar to acute cholecystitis.
- Patient may be diabetic with end-vessel disease.

DIAGNOSIS

- Patchy gangrene of the GB.
- May be diagnosed pre-operatively by air in the GB wall on US.
- Usually diagnosed at laparoscopic cholecystectomy.

MANAGEMENT

- Antibiotics, fluids and oxygen if the patient presents acutely.
- **Laparoscopic cholecystectomy**–removal may be difficult as will tend to disintegrate spilling stones and bile.
- Difficulty of the procedure depends on the duration of the inflammation.
- Laparoscopic needle aspiration is an alternative option.
- If bile/stones spilled a sub-hepatic vacuum drain will guide as to the degree of contamination.
- If laparoscopic cholecystectomy avoided/abandoned, then elective cholecystectomy may be planned for after 6 weeks.

PERFORATED GALLBLADDER

CLINICAL PRESENTATION

- Patients tend to be sicker with more severe RUQ symptoms compared to acute cholecystitis.
- RUQ tenderness and guarding.
- May have generalised tenderness, guarding and rigidity.
- Bowel sounds may be absent.

INVESTIGATIONS

- US will reveal a fluid collection around the GB +/– a disrupted wall, and stones within or without the GB.
- Fluid may be contained by an omental reaction or there may be communication with peritoneal cavity.

MANAGEMENT

- IV fluids, oxygen and antibiotics.
- Percutaneous GB/collection drainage by pigtail catheter.
- Laparoscopic cholecystectomy and drainage or tube cholecystostomy alone.

CHRONIC CHOLECYSTITIS

PRESENTATION

- Patients will typically have a history of recurrent or subclinical cholecystitis resulting in chronic inflammation of the GB wall.
- May experience ongoing or recurrent RUQ or epigastric pain associated with nausea and vomiting.
- May be mild RUQ tenderness.

INVESTIGATIONS

- Diagnosis typically by US or CT.
- May be an incidental finding.

MANAGEMENT

- Management in uncomplicated cases is elective cholecystectomy.

COMPLICATIONS

- Biliary-enteric fistula–gallstone ileus.
- GB carcinoma (rare).

MUCOCOELE

AETIOLOGY

- A mucocele occurs when a stone become impacted in the cystic duct.
- The patient may have gone on to have biliary colic or acute cholecystitis, either of which may have resolved on conservative management.
- The impacted stone prevents bile from entering and prevents mucous from leaving the GB.
- Eventually, the bile in the GB becomes re-absorbed leaving only mucous.

PRESENTATION

- This is usually an incidental finding at laparoscopic cholecystectomy.
- The GB will be tense and will need to be aspirated to be able to grasp it properly.
- The patient may present with chronic RUQ discomfort, especially after meals.
- Examination may reveal a globular mass but as there is no jaundice, Courvoisier's law doesn't apply.

MANAGEMENT

- Laparoscopic cholecystectomy is curative.

GALLSTONE ILEUS

AETIOLOGY

- A gallstone in a contracted GB may erode through GB wall and into contiguous duodenum–**Cholecysto-duodenal fistula.**
- Typically occurs in the elderly.
- This gallstone, if large enough, can result in bowel obstruction with the stone impacting in the
  - Duodenum (Bouveret's syndrome)
  - Terminal ileum (causing a small bowel obstruction)

CLINICAL PRESENTATION

- Patient presents with intestinal obstruction
- The obstruction may be intermittent as the stone rolls through the small bowel intermittently getting stuck and rolling forward
- There will be no RUQ signs because the inflammation is chronic and deep

DIAGNOSIS

- A plain film of abdomen (PFA) may show air in the biliary tree and dilated loops of small bowel–this is diagnostic
- A large stone, usually in the RIF
- **CT will confirm**

TREATMENT

- Laparoscopic or open removal of obstructing stone
- The cholecystodoudenal fistula is not disturbed

OBSTRUCTIVE JAUNDICE

PATHOPHYSIOLOGY

- The most common cause is when a stone obstructs the CBD.
- A rarer cause is when a large stone in Hartmann's pouch or in the cystic duct, compresses the adjacent common hepatic duct (Mirizzi's syndrome)

CLINICAL PRESENTATION

- Obstructive jaundice due to stone in CBD is painful
- RUQ tenderness
- The GB will <u>not</u> be palpable as it does not have time to distend–unlike jaundice due to malignant obstruction where the build-up of pressure is gradual (Courvoisier's law)

DIAGNOSIS

- Diagnosis is suggested by US which may identify **a dilated CBD and stones in the GB**.
- Diagnosis is confirmed by MRCP.
- Mirizzi mass may mimic malignancy.

MANAGEMENT

- **ERCP is both diagnostic and therapeutic,** by dilating the sphincter of Oddi, or performing a sphincterotomy, a stone in the CBD may be removed by a basket or balloon.
- If stone removal difficult a stent can be inserted to relieve the jaundice, and ERCP can be attempted again later.
- **If stone impossible to remove by ERCP,** due to previous gastric surgery or duodenal diverticulum, a stone may be removed by exploring the CBD at laparoscopy and stone retrieval.
- A T-shaped tube is used to drain the CBD after laparoscopic drainage to decompress the duct.
- A rubber T tube will excite a reaction allowing early tube removal, but a silicon T tube, which is inert, should be retained much longer to avoid bile leakage after removal.
- Mirizzi's syndrome can be managed laparoscopically–cholecystectomy is hazardous as the CBD may be inflamed and adherent and easily damaged.
- Open surgery may be occasionally required for both scenarios.

ASCENDING CHOLANGITIS

DEFINITION

- Inflammation of the bile duct (cholangitis) caused by bacterial infection of the biliary tract, secondary to mucosal erosion by gallstone and raised biliary pressure.

AETIOLOGY

- **Common causes:** Choledocholithiasis, biliary stricture, neoplasm.
- **Less common causes:** Chronic pancreatitis/pseudocyst, ampullary stenosis.
- **Choledocholithiasis**
  - ~15% of patients with stones in the GB have stones in the bile ducts.
  - It is not uncommon for patients with cholangitis due to stones to have had a previous cholecystectomy, where the CBD stone was overlooked.

PATHOPHYSIOLOGY

- Biliary outflow obstruction and mucosal erosion results in biliary infection.
- During an obstruction, stasis of fluid combined with elevated intraluminal pressure allows bacterial colonisation of the biliary tree to become pathological.

CLINICAL PRESENTATION

- **Symptoms:**
  - RUQ pain–constant and severe
  - Pruritus
- **Signs:**
  - RUQ tenderness
  - Fever, rigors (one of the few causes of rigors)
  - Jaundice
  - Dark urine common (NB: Pale stools rare nowadays as most patients present early, or the obstruction is only partial)
  - Low blood pressure
  - Altered mental status

Charcot's Triad: The presence of the following suggests Ascending Cholangitis: 1. Constant severe right upper quadrant pain, 2. Obstructive jaundice, 3. Fever

Reynold's Pentad: Charcot's triad with hypotension and altered mental status.

INVESTIGATIONS

- **Bedside**
  - Urine dipstick for bilirubin
- **Bloods**
  - FBC to check for raised WCC
  - LFT to check for an increased ALP and bilirubin
  - Blood cultures
- **Imaging**
  - **Abdominal US** will show CBD dilatation and may show stone(s) in the CBD (but not usually because it is obscured by duodenal/intestinal gas).
  - **MRCP is usually diagnostic.** Contrast not needed as static fluids like bile are white on MRCP and a stone will show as a filling defect.
  - **Endoscopic US** occasionally needed to identify a tiny stone.
  - **ERCP** is both diagnostic and therapeutic.
  - **Percutaneous cholangiography** where an ERCP unsuccessful.

TREATMENT

- **Conservative–initial management**
  - IV fluid resuscitation
  - Pain management
  - IV antibiotics–broad spectrum

- **Medical**
  - ERCP and endoscopic sphincterotomy: Identifying and removing the stone through the ampulla.
  - Can use a stent to decompress the biliary tree if the stone is too large to be removed.
  - Unlikely to be successful in patients with large stones (>2 cm).
- **Surgical**
  - Choledochotomy and exploration of the CBD.
    - A T tube is usually left in the duct. This (now uncommon) technique allows for repeat cholangiograms and extractions of residual stones.

PROGNOSIS

- Good with effective drainage and antibiotics in mild to moderate cases.
- High mortality in patients with Reynold's Pentad.

ACUTE PANCREATITIS

DEFINITION

- Acute pancreatitis refers to inflammation of the pancreas.

KEY FACTS

- Severity can vary from a mild attack to developing into full-blown SIRS (systemic inflammatory response syndrome).
- Repeated episodes of acute pancreatitis can eventually lead to chronic pancreatitis.
- It can be distinguished from chronic pancreatitis by its limited damage to the secretory function of the gland, and no structural damage.

AETIOLOGY

- Majority of acute pancreatitis occurs secondary to gallstone disease or excess alcohol consumption.
- No cause will be found in 10–20% of patients with acute pancreatitis.
- **Causes:**
  - *'I GET SMASHED' mnemonic*
  - Idiopathic
  - Gallstones (60%)
  - Ethanol (30%)
  - Trauma (ERCP, post-surgery)
  - Steroids
  - Mumps
  - Autoimmune disease
  - Scorpion venom

- Hypercalcaemia
- Endoscopic retrograde cholangiopancreatography (ERCP)
- Drugs
  - NSAIDs
  - Azathioprine
  - Thiazides

PATHOPHYSIOLOGY

- Causes listed above trigger a premature and exaggerated activation of the digestive enzymes within the pancreas.
- The resulting systemic inflammatory response causes an increase in vascular permeability and subsequent fluid shifts (third spacing).
- Enzymes are released from the pancreas into systemic circulation causing:
  - Auto-digestion of fats (resulting in 'fat necrosis')
  - Blood vessels (can lead to haemorrhage into **retroperitoneal space**)
- Fat necrosis can result in the release of free fatty acids, which react with serum calcium forming chalky deposits in fatty tissue, resulting in hypocalcaemia
- Necrosis of the peri-pancreatic fat and fat in the mesentery can cause spiking of temperature and may need necrosectomy, or drainage when it liquefies

CLINICAL PRESENTATION

- **Symptoms**
  - Rapid onset of severe epigastric pain
    - Can radiate through to the back
    - May improve when leaning forward
  - Nausea and vomiting
- **Signs**
  - Epigastric tenderness–with or without guarding
  - Fever
  - Bruising
    - **Cullen's sign:** Bruising around the umbilicus (representing retroperitoneal haemorrhage).
    - **Grey Turner's sign:** Bruising in the flanks (representing retroperitoneal haemorrhage).
  - Obstructive jaundice (if a gallstone aetiology)
  - Hypocalcaemia–may result in tetany
  - **In severe cases:** Haemodynamic instability, tachycardia, hypotension, dehydration–due to third spacing.
  - Severe hyperglycaemia from islet of Langerhans failure.

DIFFERENTIAL DIAGNOSIS

- Cholecystitis
- Peptic ulcer disease
- Abdominal aortic aneurysm rupture
- Renal colic
- Chronic pancreatitis

INVESTIGATIONS

- **Bedside:**
  - ECG
  - Urine dipstick
  - Urinary amylase and lipase
- **Bloods:**
  - Ensure that the Glasgow score can be calculated
  - **FBC**–raised WCC
  - **CRP**–daily CRP monitoring to evaluate and anticipate
  - **LFTs**–for any concurrent cholestatic element to the clinical picture
  - **U&Es**–especially urea and albumin
  - **Coagulation profile**–monitor for DIC
  - **Calcium**–if low, infuse calcium in HDU, ICU or CCU
  - **Glucose**–hyperglycaemia reflecting islet function
  - **Serum amylase**
    - Three times normal range supports diagnosis
    - Amylase level is not an indicator of severity
    - If it is normal, check urinary amylase which persists longer
  - **Serum lipase**–more accurate for acute pancreatitis (remains elevated for longer than amylase) but not routinely performed in every hospital
  - **Blood cultures**–if signs of sepsis, it will guide antibiotic choice
  - **Arterial blood gases:** pH, PO_2, lactate
- **Imaging**
  - Abdominal US
    - If underlying cause unknown
    - To identify gallstones, and duct dilation
  - CXR
    - Pleural effusion
    - Signs of ARDS
    - Exclude air under diaphragm
  - Abdominal X-ray
    - Not routinely performed
    - Can show a 'sentinel loop sign' adjacent to the pancreas
  - Contrast-enhanced CT
    - If initial assessment and investigations prove inconclusive
    - To evaluate disease severity 6–10 days after admission if inflammatory response persistent or organ failure
    - Can show pancreatic swelling and/or peri-pancreatic or pancreatic necrosis
- **Fine needle aspiration (FNA)**
  - If suspected infected pancreatic necrosis
  - IR drainage of liquefied necrosis or pseudocyst

RISK SCORING

- Modified Glasgow criteria
- APACHE II
- Ranson's criteria
- Balthazar score (CT scoring system)

MODIFIED GLASGOW CRITERIA

Three or more positive criteria within 48 hours of admission = severe attack and high-dependency care referral is warranted
(Mnemonic: **PANCREAS**)

- **P**aO$_2$ < 8 kPA
- **A**ge > 55 yrs
- **N**eutrophils/WCC > 15,000 × 109/L
- **C**orrected calcium < 2 mmol/L
- **R**aised blood urea > 16 mmol/L
- **E**nzymes elevated, AST > 200 U/L, LDH > 600 U/L
- **A**lbumin < 32 g/L
- **S**ugar, blood glucose > 10 mmol/L

RANSON CRITERIA

Three or more positive criteria indicate a severe attack of pancreatitis with considerable mortality
On admission:

- WCC > 16 k
- Age > 55
- Glucose > 200 mg/dL (>10 mmol/L)
- AST > 250
- LDH > 350

48 hours into admission:

- Haematocrit drop > 10% from admission
- BUN increase > 5 mg/ dL (>1.79 mmol/L) from admission
- Ca < 8 mg/dL (<2 mmol/L) within 48 hours
- Base deficit (24–HCO$_3$) > 4 mg/ dL within 48 hours
- Fluid needs > 6 L within 48 hours

COMPLICATIONS

- **Systemic** (tend to occur within days of initial onset)
  - Disseminated intravascular coagulation (DIC)
  - SIRS
  - Acute respiratory distress syndrome (ARDS)
  - Hypocalcaemia
    - Fat necrosis from released lipases, results in the release of free fatty acids, which react with serum calcium to form chalky deposits in fatty tissue.
  - Hyperglycaemia
    - Secondary to islets cell dysfunction and disturbances of insulin metabolism.

- **Local complications**
  - Peri-pancreatic necrosis
    - Ongoing inflammation eventually leads to ischaemic infarction of the peri-pancreatic fatty tissue around the pancreas and between the leaves of the mesentery.
    - Suspect in patients with evidence of persistent systemic inflammation >7–10 days after the onset of pancreatitis.
    - The peri-pancreatic necrotic tissue is prone to infection and should be suspected in patients with clinical deterioration, raised CRP and positive blood cultures.
    - Necrosis of the pancreas itself can also occur, leading to impairment of pancreatic function (rare).
  - Pancreatic abscess
    - Circumscribed intra-abdominal collection of pus arising in close proximity to the pancreas.
    - But containing little or no pancreatic necrosis.
  - Pancreatic pseudocyst
    - A fluid collection of pancreatic enzymes, blood and necrotic tissue–lack an epithelial lining, therefore named pseudocyst.
    - Fluid commonly collects in the lesser sac.
    - Typically occurs weeks after the initial acute episode.
    - Prone to haemorrhage or rupture, and can become infected.
    - 50% will resolve spontaneously, thus conservative management is the initial treatment of choice.
    - If present >6 weeks unlikely to resolve spontaneously.

MANAGEMENT

- **Essential to assess severity** of the attack of all pancreatitis cases by the Glasgow Imrie criteria.
  - Clinical assessment never enough–cannot assess oxygen, calcium, glucose, etc. on clinical criteria.
- **If severe pancreatitis, transfer to** high dependency unit (HDU) or ICU
- No curative management for acute pancreatitis
- Treat any underlying cause
- **Supportive measures** are the mainstay of treatment
  - IV fluid resuscitation–this may need to be aggressive and must be closely monitored based on urinary output and vital signs.
  - O_2 therapy as required to maintain oxygen saturation >94%
  - NGT if patient is vomiting
  - If patient can eat, encourage oral intake as tolerated
  - Nutritional support
    - Enteral feed preferable to prevent translocation of gut bacteria and secondary septic complications, sometimes nasojejunal tube required.
    - Total parenteral nutrition (TPN) required if enteral feed not tolerated.
  - Proton pump inhibitors–reduce risk of stress ulceration
  - Urinary catheterisation
    - To monitor output: **Aim for >0.5 ml/kg/hr**
    - Fluid balance chart

- Opioid analgesia
- Antithrombotic prophylaxis
- Close monitoring
- **Medical**
  - Antibiotic therapy–only if/when blood culture positive
  - ERCP and stone extraction for proven bile duct stones
    - ERCP indicated if causing obstruction and pancreatitis
- **Surgical**
  - Endoscopic drainage of pancreatic pseudocyst.
  - Laparoscopic pancreatic necrosectomy of per-pancreatic necrosis.

PROGNOSIS

- Mortality is associated with pancreatic necrosis and the presence of sepsis.

CHRONIC PANCREATITIS

DEFINITION

- Chronic pancreatitis is a chronic fibro-inflammatory disease of the pancreas, resulting in progressive and irreversible damage to pancreatic parenchyma

KEY FACTS

- Chronic pancreatitis is characterized by recurrent or persistent abdominal pain and pancreatitis
- May arise following one or more episodes of acute pancreatitis
- Often associated with exocrine or endocrine pancreatic insufficiency
- Chronic inflammation causes:
  - Glandular atrophy
  - Duct ectasia
  - Microcalcification
  - Intraductal stone formation with cystic changes secondary to duct obstruction

AETIOLOGY

- Main causes of chronic pancreatitis:
  - **Chronic alcohol abuse (60%)**
  - **Idiopathic (30%)**
- Less common causes:
  - **Metabolic**
    - Hyperlipidaemia
    - Hypercalcaemia
  - **Infection**
    - Viral: HIV, mumps, Coxsackie
    - Bacterial: Echinococcus
  - **Hereditary**
    - Cystic fibrosis

- **Autoimmune**
  - Autoimmune pancreatitis
  - Systemic lupus erythematosus (SLE)
  - Primary biliary cirrhosis
  - Primary sclerosing cholangitis
- **Anatomical**
  - Malignancy
  - Stricture formation
- **Congenital anomalies**
  - Pancreas divisum
  - Annular pancreas

PATHOPHYSIOLOGY

- The process may affect the whole gland or part of the gland (focal)
- Features seen in acute pancreatitis can occur
  - Oedema
  - Acute inflammatory infiltrate
  - Focal necrosis
  - Intraparenchymal haemorrhage
- Chronic inflammatory changes cause progressive disorganization of the pancreas
  - Glandular atrophy and duct ectasia.
  - Microcalcification and intraductal stone formation with cystic changes secondary to duct occlusion.

Table 4.6 Symptoms and Signs of Chronic Pancreatitis

Symptoms	Signs

• Recurrent or chronic abdominal pain is the major symptom
• Typically, epigastric pain radiating to the back, worse after food and alcohol
• Nausea and vomiting
• Weight loss
• Diarrhoea–pale and bulky if exocrine failure
	• Endocrine insufficiency
	  • Impaired glucose regulation
	  • Diabetes mellitus
	• Exocrine insufficiency
	  • Malabsorption
	  • Fat soluble vitamin deficiency (ADEK) and protein
	  • Steatorrhoea and diarrhoea

DIFFERENTIAL DIAGNOSIS

- Peptic ulcer disease
- Reflux disease (GORD)
- Abdominal aortic aneurysm
- Biliary colic
- Chronic mesenteric ischemia

INVESTIGATIONS

- **Bedside**
  - Urine dipstick
  - Glucose (deranged secondary to exocrine dysfunction)

- **Bloods**
  - FBC
  - CRP
  - LFTs (to ensure no concurrent obstructive jaundice)
  - Albumin: Malabsorption
  - Serum amylase (should not be raised in chronic pancreatitis)
  - Serum lipase (should not be raised in chronic pancreatitis)
  - HbA1c
  - Fat-soluble vitamins: If exocrine insufficiency/malabsorption
- **Imaging**
  - CT Pancreas protocol to identify:
    - Pancreatic atrophy or calcification
    - Pseudocysts
    - Underlying causes for chronic pancreatitis: e.g. malignancy or congenital abnormality
  - US abdomen–cystic changes and pancreatic duct dilation
  - MRCP–ductal abnormalities
  - ERCP–pancreatic duct strictures, calculi, dilated segments
    - Sometimes involvement of pancreatic head can lead to CBD stricture and obstructive pattern of LFTs.
  - Endoscopic US (EUS) combined with aspiration cytology/biopsies to differentiate chronic pancreatitis from tumours and other pathologies.
  - Abdominal X-ray–may show calcification.
- **Faecal elastase**
  - Usually low in chronic pancreatitis with exocrine insufficiency

MANAGEMENT

- **Conservative**
  - Prevention of cause: Stop alcohol
  - Dietary modifications: Reduced fat diet, adequate carbohydrates and protein
- **Medical**
  - Pancreatic exocrine supplements: Creon.
  - Fat soluble vitamins: ADEK.
  - Analgesia: Opiates may be required.
  - Control of diabetes: May require insulin.
  - Statins: If hyperlipidaemia present.
- **Surgical**
  - Only considered for patients who fail medical therapy.
  - Surgery can be performed to decompress/drain an obstructed pancreatic duct, resect the affected part or treat reversible causes like strictures, stones, tumour, etc.
  - Surgical options include:
    - Pancreaticoduodenectomy = Whipple's procedure
    - Partial or distal pancreatectomy
    - Pancreatojejunostomy

- The choice of operation depends upon the size of the pancreatic duct and the parts involved.
- ERCP can be used for diagnostic and therapeutic purposes
  - Stone removal
  - Stent placement
  - Sphincterotomy
- Endoscopic-guided celiac plexus blockade or thoracoscopic splanchnicectomy may be performed for analgesic purposes.

PROGNOSIS

- Chronic pancreatitis is associated with significant morbidity and reduced quality of life.
- May result in endocrine and exocrine insufficiencies.
- Pancreatic malignancy is a risk in those who have had the disease for 20 years or more.

PANCREATIC CANCER

KEY POINTS

- Pancreatic cancer **typically refers to ductal carcinoma of the pancreas,** comprising up to 90% of primary pancreatic malignancies.
- Remainder of pancreatic cancer is divided into:
  - Exocrine (e.g. cystic carcinoma)
  - Endocrine tumours (islet cells of pancreas)
- High mortality rate.
- 80% occur between 60 and 80 years.
- 80% are unresectable at diagnosis.

AETIOLOGY

- Small number of clear risk factors for the development of carcinoma of the pancreas: Smoking, chronic pancreatitis, family history, late onset diabetes mellitus.

PATHOPHYSIOLOGY

- **90% are ductal adenocarcinomas**
- Rarer forms are
  - Cystic tumours
  - Ampullary cell tumours
  - Islet cell tumours
- Metastasis is common at time of diagnosis
  - Spreads by direct invasion of local structures: Typically, the spleen, transverse colon and adrenal glands.
  - Lymphatic metastasis: Typically involves regional lymph nodes, liver, lungs and peritoneum.

Table 4.7   Symptoms and Signs of Pancreatic Cancer

Symptoms	Signs
• Can be asymptomatic in the early stages • Loss of appetite • Weight loss • Nausea and vomiting • Pruritus • Pain: Epigastric, or upper left quadrant, often vague and radiates to the back	• Diabetes mellitus • Thrombophlebitis migrans • Palpable GB • Jaundice • Epigastric mass • Hepatomegaly due to metastasis

DIFFERENTIAL DIAGNOSIS

- **Causes of obstructive jaundice**
  - Gallstone disease
  - Cholangiocarcinoma
  - Benign GB stricture
- **Causes of epigastric abdominal pain**
  - Gallstones
  - Peptic ulcer disease
  - Gastric carcinoma
  - Acute coronary syndrome

INVESTIGATIONS

- **Bloods**
  - FBC: Anaemia
  - LFTs: To look for obstructive pattern (raised bilirubin, ALP, GGT)
  - Blood glucose
  - Tumour markers: **CA 19-9** (assesses response to treatment rather than initial diagnosis)
- **Imaging**
  - Transabdominal US: Pancreatic mass or dilated biliary tree.
  - CT pancreas: Using pancreatitis protocol to assess size of primary lesion, vascular invasion and metastasis.
  - Endoscopic US (EUS): For FNA biopsy for histological evaluation.
  - ERCP: For biopsy or cytology depending on location of lesion.
  - PET-CT: To differentiate neoplastic from non-neoplastic lesions and help to exclude metastatic disease.
- **Laparoscopy**
  - To out rule peritoneal disease and liver metastasis.

MANAGEMENT

- **Palliative**
  - Majority of patients are not candidates for curative surgery due to advanced disease.
  - Palliative chemotherapy can be trialled.
  - Obstructive jaundice and associated symptoms can be managed by biliary stent, via ERCP or percutaneously.
  - Pain relief: Morphine or coeliac nerve block.

- **Chemotherapy**
  - Adjuvant chemotherapy is recommended after surgery for advanced disease.
  - Chemotherapy is also recommended for metastatic disease.
- **Surgical**
  - Radical surgical resection is the only curative management option.
  - For patients with tumours at the head of the pancreas, the most common surgery is pancreaticoduodenectomy or Whipple's procedure.
  - For patients with tumours of the body or tail of pancreas, a distal pancreatectomy can be performed.

WHIPPLE'S PROCEDURE (PANCREATICODUODENECTOMY)

A Whipple's procedure involves the removal of the head of the pancreas, antrum of stomach, 1st and 2nd parts of the duodenum, the common bile duct and the gallbladder.

The tail of the pancreas and the hepatic duct are attached to the jejunum which allows bile and pancreatic juices to drain into the gut. The stomach is anastomosed with the jejunum to allow for food passage.

PROGNOSIS

- Pancreatic cancer has a high metastatic capacity.
- Prognosis remains poor, with overall 5-year survival rate of 12% in resectable disease.

 Courvoisier's Law: A palpable GB in a patient with jaundice is unlikely to be due to gallstones and suggests malignant obstruction. It is a function of time, as malignant obstruction causes gradual painless GB distention.

MCQs FOR SELF-ASSESSMENT

Chapter 5

COLORECTAL SURGERY

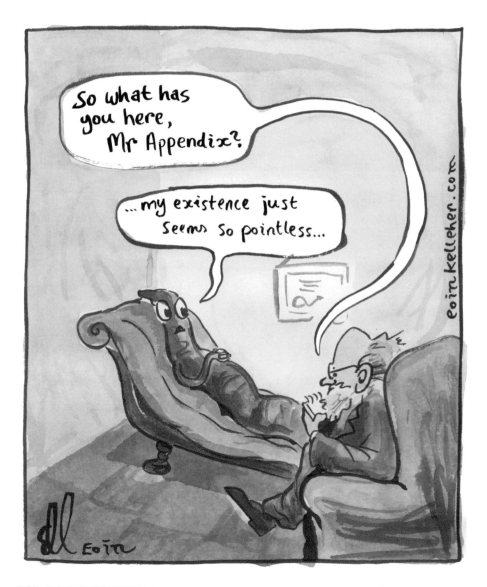

DOI: 10.1201/9781003207184-5

CONTENTS

Acute Appendicitis	101
Diverticular Disease	104
Colorectal Cancer	108
Bowel Obstruction	111
Perianal Disorders	114
Haemorrhoids	115
Anal Fissure	117
Anorectal Abscess	118
Anal Fistula	119
Pilonidal Sinus and Abscess	121
Anal Cancer	123
Stomas	124
Loop Ileostomy	124
End Ileostomy	126
End Colostomy	127
Loop Colostomy	128
Defunctioning Stoma	128
Stoma Complications	128
Stoma Stenosis	129
Stoma Retraction	129
Necrosis	130
Parastomal Hernia	130
High-Output Stoma	131
Skin Complications	132

ACUTE APPENDICITIS

KEY FACTS

- The most common cause of the acute abdomen and an indication for emergency abdominal surgery.
- The appendix is located at the base of the caecum where the taenia coli converge. Its blood supply is from the appendiceal artery, a terminal branch of the ileocolic artery.
- Has an immunological function.
- Peak age of incidence is early teens to early 20s.
- Lifetime risk is 8.6% in men and 6.7% in women.

PATHOPHYSIOLOGY

- Inflammation may be followed by localised ischemia, perforation and the development of a contained abscess or generalised peritonitis.
- Usually due to appendiceal obstruction, which is caused by:
  - Feacolith, lymphoid hyperplasia, infection, benign or malignant tumour.

CLINICAL FEATURES

- **Symptoms**
  - Abdominal pain–starts centrally and moves to the right iliac fossa.
  - Pain is exacerbated by movement.
  - Nausea, vomiting, anorexia.
  - Diarrhoea.

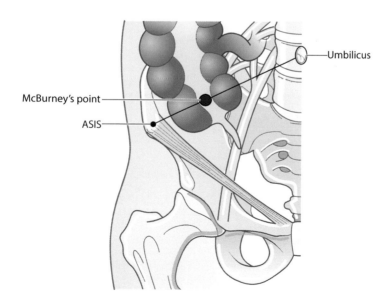

Figure 5.1   McBurney's point is two-thirds along a line from the umbilicus to the ASIS.

- **Signs**
  - Low grade pyrexia
  - Tachycardia
  - Abdominal tenderness and guarding
  - Tenderness maximally over McBurney's point
- The initial visceral pain is through the autonomic system, which can only distinguish foregut (epigastric), midgut (peri-umbilical) and hindgut (suprapubic) pain.
- Initial periumbilical pain moves to the right iliac fossa where the peritoneum gets inflamed. This has somatic innervation (T10-T12) and so produces tenderness and guarding.
- Pelvic and rectal examination (not commonly done) may be very useful especially when diagnosis is unclear.
- Inflamed appendix may be retrocaecal, pelvic, retro-ileal or retro-colic.

SPECIAL TESTS

- **Rovsing's sign:**
  - Palpation of LIF causes pain to worsen in the RIF.
- **Psoas sign:**
  - Discomfort upon hyperextension of the right hip, indicating an inflamed retro-peritoneal or retrocaecal appendix.
- **Obturator sign:**
  - Pain in RIF as a result of flexing and internally rotating the right hip, usually seen in a pelvic appendix.

DIFFERENTIAL DIAGNOSIS

- **Terminal ileal pathology:**
  - Crohn's ileitis, TB, Meckel's diverticulitis, gastroenteritis.
- **Retroperitoneal pathology:**
  - Renal colic, pancreatitis.
- **Gynaecological pathology:**
  - Ovarian cyst, ectopic, PID, ovarian torsion.
- **Special populations to consider**
  - Children–mesenteric adenitis.
  - Older adults–caecal tumour.

INVESTIGATIONS

- Acute appendicitis is a **clinical diagnosis**.
- **Bedside**
  - Midstream specimen of urine (MSU): Dipstick, culture and sensitivity.
  - β-hCG.
- **Bloods**
  - FBC: Leucocytosis
  - CRP
  - β-hCG
- **Imaging**
  - Pelvic US if there is concern over ovarian pathology
  - CT abdomen/pelvis where there is a question over the diagnosis or pathology

APPENDICITIS SCORING SYSTEM–ALVARADO SCORE

- This score is best employed as a tool for **excluding** appendicitis
- Interpretation:
  - **0–3:** Low risk of appendicitis
  - **4–6:** Observe patient, they may need intervention
  - **7–10 male:** Proceed to appendectomy
  - **7–10 female:** Diagnostic laparoscopy

Table 5.1   Alvarado Scoring System

Symptoms	Score	Signs	Score	Lab Values	Score
Abdominal pain	1	RIF tenderness	2	Leucocytosis >10,000	2
Anorexia	1	Rebound tenderness	1	Neutrophils >75%	1
Nausea / Vomiting	1	Temperature > 37.5°C	1		

MANAGEMENT

- **Resuscitation**
  - IV access and IV fluids
  - Analgesia
  - Antibiotics (IV or PO) according to local guidelines
  - DVT prophylaxis
- **Definitive management of acute appendicitis**
  - Open or laparoscopic appendectomy
  - Up to 15% of appendectomies can be negative for appendicitis
  - IV antibiotics on induction
  - Continued antibiotics only indicated for perforation
- **Definitive management of an appendix mass or appendix abscess**
  - IV antibiotics
  - If symptoms settle, scan patient again after 6 weeks with US or CT
  - Only 20% will need an appendectomy
  - If symptoms fail to settle, may need urgent appendectomy
  - Appendix abscess may be amenable to CT-guided drainage
- **Antibiotics alone for the management for uncomplicated appendicitis**
  - This is an area of much interest and research.
  - At present antibiotics are not recommended for routine use.
  - This is due to many unanswered questions.
  - Patient selection, recurrent attacks, missed neoplasm (Salminen, 2011).
  - Antibiotics are an option for those unfit for surgery.
- **Principles of appendicectomy are as follows:**
  - **Open:** Gridiron incision centred at McBurney's point (mostly in children <30 kg), or Lanz incision
  - **Laparoscopic approach:** Umbilical port, port in LIF, suprapubic port (this is considered the gold standard).
    1. Appendix is carefully located.
    2. The mesentery of the appendix is divided and ligated.
    3. The appendix is clamped and tied at the base and excised.
    4. Conversion to open appendicectomy in 10%.

COMPLICATIONS OF ACUTE APPENDICITIS

- **Perforation**–localised or generalised.
- **RIF 'appendix' mass**–usually appendicitis with densely adherent caecum and omentum, forming a 'mass'.
- **RIF abscess**–usually due to perforated retrocaecal appendicitis.
- **Pelvic abscess**–usually due to perforated pelvic appendicitis.

CARCINOID TUMOUR OF THE APPENDIX

- Most common tumour of the appendix.
- Arise from argentaffin cells (Kulchitsky cells)
- 70% occur in the appendix and mostly in the tip
- Metastasises in 4% of cases
- Discovered intraoperatively during appendectomy or during histopathological examination
- Metastases produce symptoms due to entering of serotonin into circulation
  - This release of serotonin can lead to **carcinoid syndrome.**
  - Bouts of diarrhoea, flushing and bronchospasm.
- Treatment is according to the size
  - <2 cm → appendectomy
  - >2 cm → right hemicolectomy

DIVERTICULAR DISEASE

DEFINITION

- **Diverticula:** Acquired outpouchings of sac-like mucosal projections through the colon wall.
- **Diverticulosis:** The presence of diverticula.
- **Diverticular disease:** Clinically significant diverticulosis, e.g. bleeding, infection, perforation.

KEY FACTS

- Typically affects the sigmoid colon but may affect any part of the GI tract.
- Rectum is very rarely affected.

EPIDEMIOLOGY

- Male:female = 1:1.
- 50% of diverticular disease is in the population over 50 years.
- Becoming more prevalent in younger populations.
- Approximately 4–15% of patients with diverticular disease will develop diverticulitis.

AETIOLOGY

- Low fibre diet increases intraluminal colonic pressure resulting in herniation of the mucosa through the muscularis layer.
- This herniation typically occurs at the entry point of nutrient arterioles between taenia coli (a weak spot).
- No muscle layer is involved in acquired diverticula.
- Whereas in congenital diverticula, all three colonic muscle layers are involved.

CLINICAL PRESENTATION

- **Asymptomatic diverticulosis**
  - Majority are found incidentally at colonoscopy or barium enema.
- **Symptomatic diverticulosis**
  - Intermittent LIF pain, constipation, diarrhoea.
- **Acute diverticulitis**
  - *"Left sided appendicitis"*
  - **Symptoms:** LIF pain, diarrhoea/constipation, nausea.
  - **Signs:** Fever, tachycardia, tender LIF, guarding/rebound.
  - **Labs:** Neutrophilia, elevated WCC, elevated CRP.
- **Diverticular bleeding**
  - Painless PR bleeding.
  - Spontaneous with no prodromal symptoms.
  - Large volume, bright rectal bleeding due to rupture of a peridiverticular submucosal vessel.

COMPLICATIONS

PERICOLIC/PARACOLIC ABSCESS

- Suppurative process, due to persistent colonic inflammation and micro-perforations, which lead to pericolic abscess
- Extension to paracolic space causes a paracolic abscess
- **Symptoms**
  - Commonly LIF pain that is unresolving.
  - Nausea and vomiting.
  - Systemically unwell: Weight loss, night sweats.
- **Signs**
  - Spiking/swinging fever.
  - Sepsis.
- **Treatment**
  - Antibiotics.
  - Radiologically guided percutaneous or open drainage and washout +/− resection of diseased segment of bowel.

PERITONITIS

- **Purulent peritonitis:** Due to perforation of a paracolic/pericolic abscess.
- **Faeculent peritonitis:** Due to free perforation of the diverticular segment.

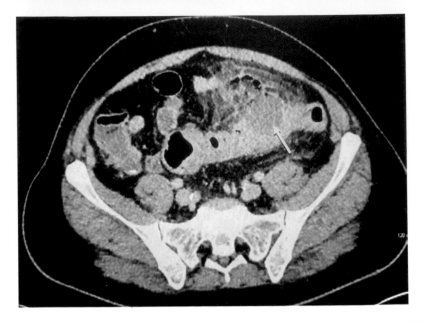

Figure 5.2 CT Abdomen and pelvis showing a diverticular abscess (arrow). Courtesy of Prof Arnold Hill

DIVERTICULAR FISTULA

- Chronically inflamed segment of colon or pericolic abscess perforates into adjacent structure.
- Typically, posterior vaginal vault (colovaginal) or bladder (colovesical).
- Colovesical fistula presents with recurrent UTIs, pneumaturia and debris in urine.

STRICTURE FORMATION

- Chronic inflammation causes luminal narrowing.
- May lead to bowel obstruction.

INVESTIGATIONS FOR ACUTE DIVERTICULITIS

- **Bloods**
  - FBC: WCC and neutrophil elevation.
  - U&E: Pre-renal failure, electrolyte disturbance from diarrhoea.
  - CRP: Monitor response to treatment.
  - Blood cultures: If sepsis suspected.
- **Imaging**
  - Erect CXR: If perforation suspected, however a negative CXR does not exclude perforation.
  - PFA: If bowel obstruction suspected (rarely done).
  - CT scan with IV contrast: Identify complications.
  - CT scan with oral or rectal contrast: **Not for acute diverticulitis or perforation**.
  - CT angiography with selective vessel embolisation: If rectal bleeding.

- **Colonoscopy**
  - Usually not done in acute diverticulitis due to risk of perforation.
  - Should be considered in 6–8 weeks to exclude underlying malignancy or to detect complications, e.g. stricture.

CLASSIFICATION OF DIVERTICULAR DISEASE

Table 5.2   Hinchey Classification of Diverticular Disease

1A	Paracolic phlegmon
1B	Pericolic/mesenteric abscess
II	Diverticulitis with walled-off abscess
III	Purulent peritonitis (perforated abscess cavity)
IV	Faeculent peritonitis

MANAGEMENT

- **Medical**
  - Uncomplicated diverticulitis, Hinchey classification I/II/III.
  - IV antibiotics.
  - Bowel rest, supportive management with IV fluid, therapy and analgesia.
  - Radiologically guided drainage of an abscess.
- **Surgical**
  - Indications:
    - Free perforation
    - Fistula
    - Refractory to medical treatment
    - Undrainable abscess
    - Hinchey III/IV
  - Laparoscopy and washout.
  - Resection of the diseased segment of bowel (Hartmann's procedure).
- **Diverticular abscess**
  - Conservative management if small.
  - CT-/US-guided drainage if possible.
  - If purulent perform laparoscopic washout +/– laparotomy.
- **Bleeding diverticulitis**
  - Usually conservative
  - CT angiography and embolisation of the feeding vessel
  - Colectomy if other methods fail
- **Diverticular stricture**
  - Endoscopic dilatation
  - Elective sigmoid colectomy
- **Chronic diverticulitis**
  - Colectomy after proper preparation
- **Colovesical or colovaginal fistula**
  - Repair of the fistula
  - Resection of the effected segment

COLORECTAL CANCER

KEY FACTS

- Colorectal cancer is the 3rd most common form of cancer.
- Most common GI malignancy.
- Male:female = 3:1.
- Peak age of incidence 55–75 years.

RISK FACTORS

- Polyposis syndromes (FAP, HNPCC, juvenile polyposis), most cases are sporadic rather than inherited.
- Strong family history of colorectal carcinoma.
- Chronic ulcerative colitis or colonic Crohn's disease.
- Diet poor in fruit and vegetables.
- Diet rich in red meat, processed meats, animal fat.
- Obesity.
- Smoking, heavy alcohol use, T2DM.

PATHOPHYSIOLOGY

- The predominant type is **adenocarcinoma**.
- Classification:
  - Well, moderately or poorly differentiated.
- Spread:
  - Colorectal carcinomas metastasize via the lymphatics.
  - Haematogenous spread is predominantly to the liver.
- Most colorectal carcinomas arise from **pre-existing adenomas**.
- Adenomatous polyps
  - Localised lesion protruding from the bowel wall into the lumen
  - Histologically there are three types of adenomas
    1. Tubular adenomas (70%)
    2. Villous adenomas (10%)
    3. Tubulo-villous adenomas (20%)
  - Villous adenomas have the greatest potential for malignant transformation, this potential is proportional to the size of the lesion
- Serrated adenomas also predispose to colorectal cancer and can look like hyperplastic polyps.
  - **Therefore, all polyps that look hyperplastic must be biopsied.**

MORPHOLOGY

- **Colorectal cancer may occur as:**
  - Polypoid
  - Ulcerating
  - Stenosing
  - Infiltrative tumour mass

- **Distribution:**
  - Rectum (30%)
  - Descending and sigmoid (45%)
  - Transverse (5%)
  - Right sided (20%)
- Synchronous carcinoma at time of diagnosis in 3–5%.

CLINICAL PRESENTATION

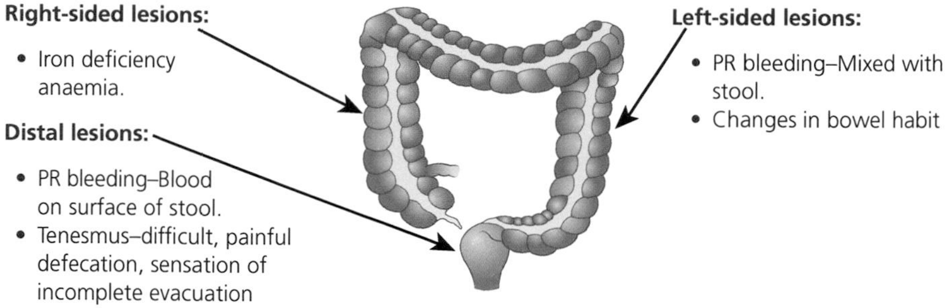

Right-sided lesions:

- Iron deficiency anaemia.

Distal lesions:

- PR bleeding–Blood on surface of stool.
- Tenesmus–difficult, painful defecation, sensation of incomplete evacuation

Left-sided lesions:

- PR bleeding–Mixed with stool.
- Changes in bowel habit

Figure 5.3   Image of the colon.

EMERGENCY PRESENTATIONS

- 40% of colorectal carcinomas will present as emergencies
- Commonly large bowel obstruction.
- Perforation with peritonitis.
- Acute PR bleeding.

INVESTIGATIONS

- **Elective**
  - PR examination or rigid sigmoidoscopy and biopsy
  - Colonoscopy and biopsy: important to visualise as far as the caecum to exclude synchronous lesions (present in 3–5%)
  - CT colonography if colonoscopy not possible
- **Emergency:** CT scan with oral and IV contrast

STAGING

- **Local extent**
  - Colon cancer–CT scan.
  - Rectal cancer–Pelvic MRI +/– endoanal US to assess T-stage (TNM).
- **Presence of metastases**
  - CT TAP is gold standard.
  - PET scan may be used to evaluate equivocal lesions.
- **Synchronous tumours**–colonoscopy or CT colonography.
- **Tumour marker (CEA)**
  - Of no use for diagnosis or staging but can be used to monitor disease relapse
  - Check CEA before and after surgery
  - If elevated, it should disappear after surgery

PATHOLOGICAL STAGING

- **Duke's classification**
  - A–confined to bowel wall only
  - B–through bowel wall
  - C–positive lymph nodes
  - D–metastases
- **TNM staging**

Table 5.3   **T**umour, **N**ode, **M**etastasis (TNM) Staging

TNM Staging for Colorectal Cancer		
T: bowel wall	T1	Invades submucosa
	T2	Invades muscularis propria
	T3	Invades through muscularis propria to sub serosa or adjacent organs
	T4	Invades visceral peritoneum
N: lymph nodes	N0	No lymph node invasion
	N1	1–3 nodes involved
	N2	4 or more nodes involved
M: distant metastasis	M0	No distant metastasis
	M1	Distant metastasis present

MANAGEMENT
POTENTIALLY CURATIVE TREATMENT

- Suitable for up to 80% of cancers and is indicated for resectable tumours with no evidence of metastases.
- The goal of surgery with curative intent is complete removal of the:
  - Tumour
  - Major vascular pedicle
  - Lymphatic drainage basin of the affected colonic segment

SURGICAL OPTIONS BASED ON TUMOUR LOCATION

- <u>Right or transverse colon</u>: right/extended hemicolectomy
- <u>Left colon</u>: left hemicolectomy
- <u>Sigmoid or upper rectum</u>: high anterior resection
- <u>Lower rectum</u>: low anterior resection or abdominoperineal resection (APR)
  - APR is usually for lesions <5 cm from the anal verge
  - APR involves removing the anal canal and sphincter complex, while leaving a permanent **end colostomy in the LIF**
- Anorectal: APR

CHEMOTHERAPY

- <u>Pre-operative (neoadjuvant) chemoradiotherapy</u>
  - For rectal cancer, reduces local recurrence.
  - For colon cancer, its role is not fully understood, and its use is decided on a case by case basis with MDT involvement.

- Adjuvant chemotherapy
  - Offered for tumours with positive lymph nodes or evidence of vascular invasion, with the goal of eradicating micro-metastases.
  - A course of oxaliplatin-containing agents is generally used.
- Hepatic or lung resection may be offered to patients with resectable metastases and resectable primary tumour. Note that a laparoscopic approach to colonic resection is now standard in many centres.

PALLIATIVE TREATMENT

- For unresectable metastases or unresectable tumours.
- Chemotherapy.
- Endoluminal stents with self-expanding metal stents for obstructing colon tumours.
- Transanal ablation of rectal obstructing tumours.
- Surgery for untreatable obstruction, bleeding or severe symptoms.
- Options include a defunctioning colostomy or ileostomy, or internal bypass.

FOLLOW-UP

1. Outpatient review–history and examination, PR, CEA.
2. Colonoscopy at 1 year, every 3 to 5 years thereafter (ESMO Guidelines).
3. CT scans annually for 3 years.

BOWEL OBSTRUCTION

DEFINITION

- Mechanical blockage arising from a structural abnormality that presents a physical barrier to the progression of gut content.
- Ileus is the hypomobility of the GI tract in the absence of a mechanical obstruction. Commonly seen in post-operative patients.

CLASSIFICATION

- Small bowel obstruction (SBO) or large bowel obstruction (LBO).
- Complete (nothing passes through) or incomplete (partial, when gas and liquid stool may pass distally) obstruction.
- May present in an acute or sub-acute manner.

OBSTRUCTION CAN BE COMPLICATED OR UNCOMPLICATED

- Uncomplicated obstruction: can often be managed conservatively with close observation.
- Complicated bowel obstruction presents as:
  - Complete obstruction, closed loop obstruction, bowel ischaemia, necrosis or perforation.
  - Often requires surgery.

- Closed loop obstruction is when the intestine is obstructed at two ends (usually the small bowel or the large bowel with competent ileocecal valve). Can rapidly progress to ischaemia, necrosis, and perforation (within 4–6 hours).
- Urgent diagnosis and treatment of closed loop obstruction is crucial.

CLINICAL PRESENTATION

Table 5.4 Clinical Presentation of Bowel Obstruction

Symptoms	Signs
Abdominal pain	Abdominal distension (pronounced and early in SBO
Constipation	Tenderness
Vomiting (bilious, SBO, faeculent, distal SBO and LBO)	High-pitched (tinkling) or absent bowel sounds
	Rigidity/guarding
Obstipation	Empty rectum on DRE

AETIOLOGY

- **SBO**
  - **Adhesions**
  - **Hernia**
  - Malignancy
  - Intussusception
  - Stricture–Crohn's disease, radiation
  - Meckel's diverticulum
- **LBO**
  - **Colon cancer** (20% of colon cancers cause LBO)
  - Hernia
  - Diverticulitis

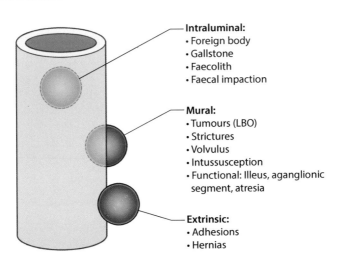

Intraluminal:
- Foreign body
- Gallstone
- Faecolith
- Faecal impaction

Mural:
- Tumours (LBO)
- Strictures
- Volvulus
- Intussusception
- Functional: Illeus, aganglionic segment, atresia

Extrinsic:
- Adhesions
- Hernias

Figure 5.4 Aetiology of bowel obstruction.

- Volvulus
- Intussusception
- Stricture
- Aetiology classified into: intraluminal, mural or extrinsic

OTHER CAUSES OF BOWEL OBSTRUCTION

- Endometriosis
- **Drugs:** antimuscarinics or opioid analgesia
- **Ogilvie syndrome/pseudo-obstruction:** post-operative obstruction without a mechanical cause
- **Superior mesenteric artery syndrome:** duodenum is compressed between the SMA and aorta, often presents with irretractable vomiting

INVESTIGATIONS

- **Erect CXR:** to rule out a coexisting perforation, 60% sensitivity.
- **PFA**
  - Dilated loops of small bowel (valvulae conniventes).
  - Dilated loops of large bowel (haustrations).
  - Air/Fluid levels.
  - **3, 6, 9 Rule:** The small bowel should be ≤3 cm, the large bowel ≤6 cm and the caecum ≤9 cm.
- **CT scan with IV or oral contrast:** To establish the cause of the obstruction.

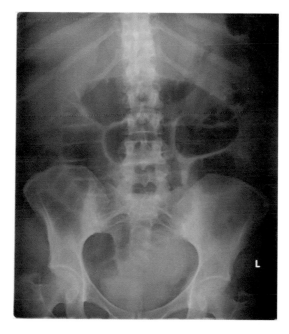

Figure 5.5   PFA of small bowel obstruction. Courtesy of Dr Niamh Adams

MANAGEMENT

- The initial approach should be conservative, as the definitive treatment will vary depending on the cause.
  - Begin IV fluids
  - Monitor fluid balance
  - Insert a wide bore NGT–decompress the stomach and then leave on free drainage
  - NPO, analgesia, urinary catheter and input/output chart
  - Electrolyte management is essential given the underlying intestinal dysfunction
- If bowel is ischaemic, it will have to be resected:
  - An end-to-end anastomosis may be possible, or the patient may require loop or end stoma.

SPECIFIC MANAGEMENT

- **Tumour:**
  - Resection, chemotherapy, radiotherapy, balloon dilation, stenting.
- **Strictures:**
  - Dilatation, resection of abnormal segment.
- **Adhesions:**
  - Adhesiolysis.
- **Hernias:**
  - Repair hernia.
- **Volvulus:**
  - Colonoscopy and pneumatic decompression.

PERIANAL DISORDERS

KEY ANATOMICAL FACTS

- **The internal sphincter** is composed of circular, non-striated involuntary muscle supplied by autonomic nerves.
- **The external sphincter** is composed of striated voluntary muscle supplied by the pudendal nerve.
- Extensions from the longitudinal muscle layer support the sphincter complex.
- The superior part of the external sphincter fuses with the puborectalis muscle, which is essential for maintaining the anorectal angle, necessary for continence.
- The upper 2/3 of the anal canal is lined by columnar epithelium. The lower 1/3 of the anal canal is lined by sensitive squamous epithelium.
- **Blood supply** to the anal canals upper 2/3 is the superior rectal artery that is from the inferior mesenteric artery. The inferior rectal artery, a branch from the internal pudendal artery, supplies the lower 1/3.
- **Lymphatic drainage** of the upper 2/3 of the anal canal drains to internal iliac lymph nodes. While lower 1/3 of the anal canal goes to inguinal lymph nodes. This is important in SCC of the anal canal.

HAEMORRHOIDS

DEFINITION

- Haemorrhoids are normal vascular and connective tissue columns that exist in three columns on the anal canal: **3, 7 and 11 o'clock** (when patient in the lithotomy position). Figure 5.6
- **Internal haemorrhoids**
  - Above the dentate line
  - Covered by mucosa
  - Painless
  - Bleed and prolapse
- **External haemorrhoids**
  - Below the dentate line
  - Covered by the anoderm
  - May thrombose and cause pain and itching

AETIOLOGY

- Hereditary factor e.g. congenital week mesenchyme.
- Poor dietary habits and constipation.
- Prolonged straining **e.g. chronic constipation.**
- Increased intra-abdominal pressure e.g. pregnancy.

FOUR DEGREES OF HAEMORRHOIDS

1. **First degree:** bleed only, no prolapse below the dentate line.
2. **Second degree:** prolapse but reduce spontaneously.
3. **Third degree:** prolapse and have to be manually reduced.
4. **Fourth degree:** permanently prolapsed may strangulate.

COMPLICATIONS

- Bleeding–chronic anaemia, acute haemorrhagic shock.
- Prolapse–can cause strangulation of vessels resulting in thrombosis if venous, gangrene if arterial.

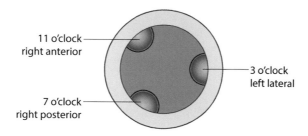

Figure 5.6   Haemorrhoids.

INVESTIGATIONS

- Exclude other causes of rectal bleeding.
- First priority is to exclude colorectal malignancy as cause of bleeding.
- Perform a digital rectal exam (DRE) to look for:
  - Prolapse
  - Skin tags
  - Assess sphincter tone
  - Exclude other anal conditions.
- If DRE is very painful, consider possibility of anal fissure or intersphincteric abscess.
- Proctoscopy.
- Consider sigmoidoscopy to rule out rectal or colonic pathology.
- Patients should be referred for colonoscopy when presenting with rectal bleeding even when symptoms strongly suggest haemorrhoids.

MANAGEMENT

- **Conservative management:**
  - Important measures to manage the clinical manifestations of haemorrhoids include:
    - Only evacuating when the natural desire to do so arises, minimise straining or lingering on the toilet.
    - The addition of stool softeners and bulking agents to ease the defecator act.
    - Increased dietary fibre and increased physical activity.
  - Topical analgesics and steroids, such as mixed hydrocortisone/lidocaine may be beneficial but should not be used for longer than a week.
  - Sitz baths: used in warm water three times a day.
  - Injection sclerotherapy: 1st and 2nd degree haemorrhoids.
  - Rubber band ligation: 2nd degree haemorrhoids.
  - Transanal haemorrhoidal dearterialisation: 2nd and 3rd degree haemorrhoids.
- **Surgical management:**
  - Indications for **haemorrhoidectomy:**
    - 3rd and 4th degree haemorrhoids.
    - 2nd degree haemorrhoids that have not been cured by non-operative treatments.
    - Fibrosed haemorrhoids.
    - Intero-external haemorrhoids when the external haemorrhoid is well defined.
  - **Types of haemorrhoidectomy:**
    - Open (Milligan-Morgan)
    - Closed (Ferguson)
    - Stapled
- **Thrombosed external haemorrhoids**
  - Can cause excruciating pain.
  - Patients will often present acutely.
  - Surgical evaluation of the haemorrhoid with excision of the skin overlying the thrombosed haemorrhoid can produce immediate relief.

ANAL FISSURE

DEFINITION
- An anal fissure (synonym: fissure-*in-ano*) is a longitudinal split in the anoderm of the distal anal canal that extends from the anal verge proximally towards, but not beyond, the dentate line.
- It is one of the most common causes of anal pain and anal bleeding.

AETIOLOGY
- **Primary**
  - Local trauma, such as passage of hard stool, prolonged diarrhoea, vaginal delivery or anal sex.
  - Usually start with a tear in the anoderm within the distal half of the anal canal. The tear then triggers cycles of recurring anal pain and bleeding.
- **Secondary**
  - Inflammatory bowel disease (e.g., Crohn's disease).
  - Granulomatous diseases (e.g. extra pulmonary tuberculosis, sarcoidosis).
  - Malignancy (e.g. squamous cell anal cancer, leukaemia).
  - Communicable diseases (e.g. HIV infection, syphilis, chlamydia).

TYPES OF ANAL FISSURE
- **Acute:**
  - <6 weeks of onset.
- **Chronic:**
  - ≥6 weeks or features on examination showing fibrosis, fibrotic edges and perianal skin tag.

CLINICAL FEATURES
- Pain is the predominant symptom, usually exacerbated by defecation.
- Occasionally bleeding or presence of perianal skin tag.
- Rarely pruritus ani.

EXAMINATION
- Anal fissures can be visualised by gentle parting or spreading of the buttocks with eversion of the anal verge.
- DRE is usually painful, and examination is precluded by spasm.
- Do not attempt if the patient is in severe pain.

ACUTE ANAL FISSURE
- Inspection:
  - The anal verge is tightly contracted, puckered anus.
  - If the two gluteal folds are gently pulled laterally, a small tear will be seen.
- DRE:
  - Better to be avoided, as it is very painful.
  - If it is essential to exclude other pathology, it should be done under general anaesthesia.

CHRONIC FISSURE

- Inspection:
  - The fissure can be seen.
  - An anal papilla or a sentinel pile may be present.
- DRE:
  - Fissure is fibrotic and indurated (buttonhole induration).
  - Sphincter is fibrosed.

MANAGEMENT

- **Best prevented by:**
  - Healthy bowel habit.
  - High fibre diet and adequate fluids.
- **Conservative management:**
  - Relief of constipation.
  - Local wound care (warm sitz baths).
  - Analgesia.
  - Chronic and secondary fissures require more extensive management and/or management of the underlying condition.
  - Topical application of pharmacological agents that relax the internal sphincter, most commonly nitric oxide donors.
    - By reducing spasm, pain is relieved, and increased vascular perfusion promotes healing (0.2% nitroglycerin and 2% diltiazem).
- **Surgical management:**
  - Lateral sphincterotomy (gold standard)
    - Closed or open
    - Chemical sphincterotomy using Botox injection to sphincter complex

ANORECTAL ABSCESS

DEFINITION

- An anorectal abscess is the acute phase manifestation of a collection of purulent material that originates from an infection arising in the crypto glandular epithelium lining the anal canal at the dentate line.

CLASSIFICATION

1. Perianal (60%)
2. Ischiorectal abscess (30%)
3. Intersphincteric abscess (5%)
4. Supralevator abscess (associated with appendicitis, Crohn's, diverticulitis)

CLINICAL FEATURES

- Severe perianal and rectal pain.
- Associated with constitutional symptoms like fever and malaise.
- Purulent discharge if the abscess spontaneously drained.

INVESTIGATIONS

- Pelvic CT or MRI if required.
- Often a clinical diagnosis.

MANAGEMENT

- Management of acute anorectal sepsis is primarily surgical, including careful examination under anaesthesia, sigmoidoscopy and proctoscopy and adequate drainage of the pus.

ANAL FISTULA

DEFINITION

- A fistula is a chronic abnormal connection between two epithelial lined surfaces.

KEY FACTS

- Usually lined with granulation tissue but may be epithelialized.
- Anorectal fistula is the chronic manifestation of the acute perirectal process that forms an anal abscess.
- When the abscess ruptures or is drained, an epithelialised track can form that connects the abscess in the anus or rectum with the perirectal skin.

AETIOLOGY

- Anorectal abscess
- Crohn's disease
- Lymph granuloma venereum
- Radiation proctitis
- Rectal foreign bodies
- Primary perianal actinomycosis

CLINICAL FEATURES

- Intermittent rectal pain.
- Chronic purulent drainage and a pustule-like lesion in the perianal or buttock area.
- Intermittent and malodorous perianal drainage and pruritus.

INVESTIGATIONS: EXAMINATION

- Perianal skin may be excoriated and inflamed.
- The external opening may be visualized or palpated as induration just below the skin.
- Proctosigmoidoscopy: Under experienced hands a fistula probe can be passed through the fistula to identify its internal opening using a proctoscope or sigmoidoscope.

CLINICAL ASSESSMENT

- Full history
- Examination under proctosigmoidoscopy is essential

TYPES OF ANAL FISTULA (PARKS' CLASSIFICATION)

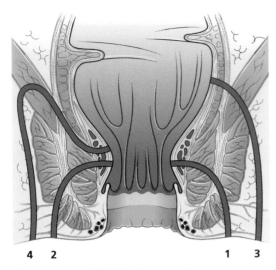

Primary track can be:

1 Intersphincteric
2 Trans-sphincteric
3 Extrasphincteric
4 Suprasphincteric

Anal fistulae can be low or high, depending on whether the internal opening is above or below the puborectalis.

Figure 5.7   Anal fistula primary tracks.

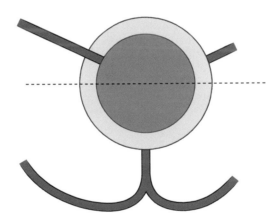

Figure 5.8   Goodsall's rule for anal fistula tracts.

Goodsall's rule: All fistula tracts with external openings within 3 cm of the anal verge and posterior to a line drawn through the ischial spines travel in a curvilinear fashion to the posterior midline. All tracks with external openings anterior to this line enter the canal in a radial fashion (Figure 5.8).

MANAGEMENT

- The goal of surgical therapy is to eradicate the fistula, while preserving faecal continence.
- Examination under anaesthesia (EUA), is part of the assessment prior to definitive treatment. Done to identify the external and internal openings.

SURGICAL MANAGEMENT OPTIONS

- **Fistulotomy:** If the fistula lies entirely below the puborectalis, with laying open of the fistulous tract. The wound then heals gradually by secondary intention.
- **Fistulectomy:** Excision of the fistula tract is another option for low anorectal fistula.
- **Seton insertion:** Either loose, tight or chemical.
    - Draining setons are used because cutting setons are too painful.
    - Setons are used for high anorectal fistula.
    - The theory is to achieve a <u>staged fistulotomy</u> by placing a seton suture that is sporadically tightened, so as to gently cut through the tract and muscle, while allowing healing and fibrosis to develop between divided muscles, thus preserving sphincteric function and faecal continence.
- **Advancement flap.**
- **Plugs and glues.**

PILONIDAL SINUS AND ABSCESS

DEFINITION

- In Latin, 'pilus' means hair and 'nidus' means nest.
- A sinus is a blind ending tract, usually lined with granulation tissue that leads from an epithelial surface into the surrounding tissue, often into an abscess cavity.
- **Intergluteal pilonidal disease** is an infection of the skin and subcutaneous tissue at or near the upper part of the natal cleft of the buttocks.

AETIOLOGY

- The theory is that it is an acquired disease rather than congenital.
- These cases have occurred in locations that would be subject to local trauma from hair, such as on the hands of barbers and animal groomers.

PATHOGENESIS

- The specific mechanism is unclear, although hair and inflammation are contributing factors.
- Loose hair tends to gather towards the natal cleft due to the anatomy and the suction of the buttocks on movement.
- This draws hair deeper into the pore, and the friction causes the hairs to form a sinus.
- Once the pore becomes infected, an acute subcutaneous abscess develops, spreads along the tract, and may discharge its contents through a pilonidal sinus in the skin cephalad to the natal cleft.
- A recurring or chronic infection can also develop in the affected area due to a retained hair or infected residue.

CLINICAL FEATURES

- May be asymptomatic.
- **Acute:** Pain, swelling and purulent discharge.
  - Fever and malaise if not drained.
- **Chronic:** A pilonidal sinus appearing after treatment of an acute pilonidal abscess or those at first presentation with or without an abscess. With recurrent or persistent pus drainage and pain.

EXAMINATION

- **Asymptomatic**
  - One or more primary pores (pits) in the midline of the natal cleft.
  - AND/OR a painless sinus opening cephalad, slightly lateral to the cleft.
- **Acute or chronic disease**
  - A tender mass or sinus draining mucoid, purulent and/or bloody fluid can be identified.
  - A hair may occasionally be seen protruding from a sinus opening.
  - Secondary tracts or pits can be identified lateral to the midline in patients with chronic or persistent complex disease.

INVESTIGATIONS

- The condition is a **clinical diagnosis,** and no imaging or laboratory tests are required.

MANAGEMENT

- Skin hygiene and hair exfoliation is important in preventing recurrence.

ACUTE

- Incision and drainage of the pilonidal abscess. Laying open of wound.
- Will usually require second operation once healed to excise remaining sinus.

DEFINITIVE

- Aims to obliterate the epithelialised sinus tract and heal the wound.
- Different debatable techniques include:
  1. **Excising the sinus tract with primary closure of the wound:** Further divided into midline closure and off-midline closure. The latter is favoured recently due to relatively lower risk of recurrence and infection.
  2. **Excising the sinus tract with laying open the wound:** To allow healing by secondary intention.
  3. **Bascom's operation:** Lateral to midline incision, to curette the deep cavity and excision of the primary midline pits. Primary closure of the midline incisions and lateral wound left to heal by secondary intention.
  4. **Karydakis procedure:** Semi lateral, 'd-shaped' incision incorporating the sinus tract down to the presacral fascia. The flap of tissue on the vertical wound side is mobilised and brought to the convex wound edge and sutured in layers over a drain.
  5. **Rotational flap procedures:** Recommended **for recurrent pilonidal sinus,** e.g. Z-plasty, modified Limberg flap.

ANAL CANCER

RISK FACTORS
- Female
- Infection with HPV (T16 and T18)
- Lifetime number of sexual partners
- History of anorectal condyloma
- Cigarette smoking
- Receptive anal intercourse
- Infection with HIV

ANAL INTRAEPITHELIAL NEOPLASIA (AIN)
- Precursor to invasive squamous anal carcinoma.
- The level of AIN (I, II, III) is dependent on the degree of cytological atypia and its depth in the epidermis.
- High proportion of AIN III (Bowen's disease) progresses to carcinomas.

ANATOMY OF THE ANAL CANAL DEFINING THE TYPES OF TUMOURS
- Two categories of tumours arise in the anal region.
- Anal canal cancers: Tumours that develop from mucosa (glandular, transitional or nonkeratinizing squamous).
- Perianal/anal margin cancers: Tumours that arise within the skin at or distal to the squamous mucocutaneous junction.

LYMPHATIC DRAINAGE
- Tumours originating above the dentate line, similar to rectal cancers, drain to the perirectal and paravertebral nodes.
- Tumours arising below the dentate line spread primarily to the superficial inguinal and femoral nodes.

TYPES OF ANAL CANAL TUMOURS
- **Squamous neoplasms**
  - Condyloma acuminatum
  - AIN
  - Bowen's disease
  - SCC
- **Adenocarcinoma**
  - Anorectal adenocarcinoma
  - Paget's disease
- Melanoma
- Neuroendocrine tumours
- Mesenchymal tumours
- Malignant lymphoma

CLINICAL FEATURES
- Rectal bleeding (approx. 45% of presentations)
- Pain
- Rectal mass

INVESTIGATIONS

- Examination of anal verge can reveal the lesion.
  - Cancer of the anal canal may not be visible, although extensive lesions may protrude to the anal verge.
  - Careful examination under anaesthesia is required to allow biopsy.
- Histology of the biopsied lesion is essential to confirm diagnosis and to determine the tissue of origin, as the treatment for SCC varies from that of adenocarcinoma.
- CT, MRI and endoanal ultrasound are useful and essential in assessing the extent of the lesion and staging the tumour.

MANAGEMENT

- It is important to detect anal cancer at an early stage, as extensive local invasion and metastatic disease are associated with a poor outcome.
- Multidisciplinary treatment of anal cancer is essential with surgeon and radiotherapist involved in assessment and treatment.
- Staging (TNM) is important for prognosis and also guides treatment approaches. Therefore, it is important to confirm lymph node involvement histologically by biopsy of accessible suspected nodes.

TREATMENT

- Wide surgical excision: For early, well-circumscribed, superficial (T1N0) carcinoma.
- Chemoradiotherapy: For anal canal and T2, T3, T4 tumours.
- Abdominoperineal resection of anus and rectum: In advanced disease, for chemoradiotherapy.
- Sphincter sparing treatment is currently being extensively investigated.

STOMAS

DEFINITION

- An ostomy (stoma) is a purposeful anastomosis between a segment of the gastrointestinal tract and the skin of the anterior abdominal wall.
- Can be temporary or permanent.

LOOP ILEOSTOMY

CLINICAL FEATURES

- Loop of ileum in the RIF may be supported by a bridge or rod.
- Two lumen present: Active proximal spouted lumen and inactive distal lumen.
- Contents: Liquid or soft effluence.

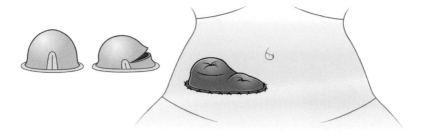

Figure 5.9 Loop ileostomy.

CLINICAL RELEVANCE

- Usually a temporary stoma.
- Usually performed to defunction bowel and protect newly formed anastomoses, e.g. in the following situations:
  - Risk of anastomotic leak
  - Sepsis
  - Patient unstable
  - Chemotherapy/radiation
  - Perianal Crohn's disease (to promote healing)

ASSOCIATED COLORECTAL SURGERY

- Low anterior resection
  - Portion of rectum and/or sigmoid colon excised, and anastomosis formed
  - Anal sphincter present
  - May require ileostomy

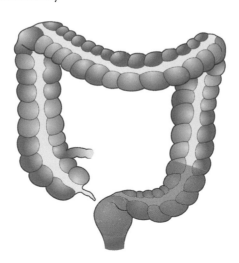

Figure 5.10 Anterior resection.

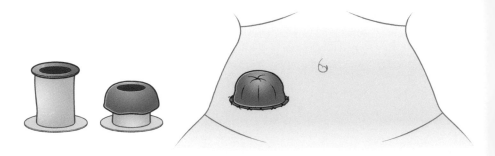

Figure 5.11   End ileostomy.

END ILEOSTOMY

CLINICAL FEATURES
- Proximal end of ileum in RIF
- Spouted
- Single lumen
- Content: Liquid/soft effluence

ASSOCIATED COLORECTAL SURGERY
1. **Panproctocolectomy**
   - Colon rectum and anus removed
   - Results in permanent end ileostomy
   - Indications: IBD, familial adenomatous polyposis (FAP)
2. **Total colectomy**
   - Surgery from caecum to rectum
   - Rectum and anus present
   - Patient can later undergo a completion proctectomy and ileo-anal J-pouch
   - Can be reversed
   - Indications: IBD emergency, LBO, colorectal cancer
3. **Ileo-anal J-pouch**
   - Ileum folded in J-shape and stapled together to make a pouch, which is then attached to the anus.
   - Temporary loop ileostomy to protect newly formed pouch.
   - Often performed after restorative proctocolectomy.
   - Pouchitis is a complication that presents with diarrhoea and pain. Treatment includes metronidazole.

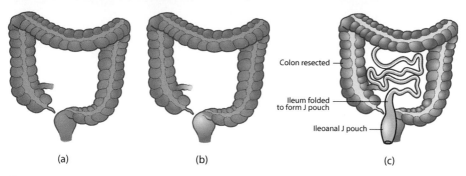

Figure 5.12 (a) Panproctocolectomy, (b) Total colectomy and (c) J-pouch.

END COLOSTOMY

CLINICAL FEATURES

- Proximal end of resected colon in the LIF.
- <u>Single lumen</u>: Flush with skin–no spout.
- <u>Content</u>: Solid effluence.

ASSOCIATED COLORECTAL SURGERIES

- Abdominoperineal (AP) resection
  - Resection of sigmoid colon, rectum and anus.
  - No anal canal.
  - Permanent end colostomy.
  - Indication: Low rectal cancer.

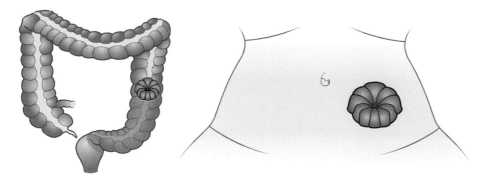

Figure 5.13 End colostomy.

- Hartmann's procedure
  - Resection of sigmoid colon and upper rectum.
  - Can also have a mucous fistula between rectum and abdominal skin. Hence this end colostomy and mucous fistula may appear like a loop colostomy.
  - This end colostomy can be reversed, i.e. be temporary.
  - Indications = emergency surgery
    - Complications of sigmoid colon cancer (perforation or obstructed).
    - Diverticular disease complications, i.e. Hinchey III or IV diverticular perforation.

LOOP COLOSTOMY

KEY POINTS
- Loop of colon in LIF or above umbilicus.
- Two lumen present: Active proximal spouted lumen and inactive distal lumen.
- Contents: Solid effluence.
- Usually temporary stoma.
- Indications: Same as loop ileostomy, therefore, loop colostomy rarely done.

DEFUNCTIONING STOMA

This is a temporary stoma often used in rectal cancer surgery. It is created when anastomosis is created following intestinal resection in order to protect the anastomosis and allow for optimal healing conditions. When healing is achieved the stoma is reversed and normal bowel continuity is regained.

STOMA COMPLICATIONS

1. Stoma stenosis
2. Stoma retraction
3. Stoma necrosis
4. Parastomal hernia
5. High output stoma
6. Skin complication
7. Psychological trauma

STOMA STENOSIS

DEFINITION

- Stoma stenosis is narrowing or constriction of the stoma or its lumen.
- This condition may occur at the skin or fascial level of the stoma.

AETIOLOGY

- Causes include hyperplasia, adhesions, sepsis and radiation of the intestine before stoma surgery, local inflammation, hyperkeratosis and surgical technique.
- Stoma stenosis frequently is associated with Crohn's disease.

CLINICAL PRESENTATION

- With GI stoma stenosis, bowel obstruction frequently occurs.
- Symptoms include abdominal cramps, diarrhoea, increased flatus, explosive stool and narrow-calibre stool.
- The initial sign is increased flatus.

MANAGEMENT

- Conservative therapy includes a low-residue diet, increased fluid intake and correct use of stool softeners or laxatives for colostomies.
- Partial or complete bowel obstruction and stoma stenosis at the fascial level require surgical intervention.

STOMA RETRACTION

DEFINITION

- In stoma retraction, the stoma has receded approx. 0.5 cm below the skin surface.
- Retraction may be circumferential or may occur in only one section of the stoma.

AETIOLOGY

- Stoma retraction is most common in patients with **ileostomies**.
- The usual causes of stoma retraction are tension of the intestine or obesity.
- Stoma retraction during the immediate post-operative period relates to poor blood flow, obesity, poor nutritional status, stenosis, early removal of a supporting device with loop stomas, stoma placement in a deep skinfold or thick abdominal walls.
- Late complications usually result from weight gain or adhesions.

CLINICAL FEATURES

- A retracted stoma has a concave, bowl-shaped appearance.
- Retraction causes a poor pouching surface, leading to frequent peristomal skin complications.

MANAGEMENT

- Typical therapy is use of a convex pouching system and a stoma belt.
- If obtaining a pouch seal is a problem and the patient has recurrent peristomal skin problems from leakage, stoma revision should be considered.

NECROSIS

AETIOLOGY

- Blood flow and tissue perfusion are essential to stoma health. A stoma may be affected by both arterial and venous blood compromise.
- The cause of necrosis usually relates to the surgical procedure, such as tension or too much trimming of the mesentery, or vascular compromise.
- Other causes of vascular compromise include hypovolemia, embolus and excessive oedema.

CLINICAL FEATURES

- Stoma necrosis usually occurs within the first **5 post-operative days**.
- Discoloration may be cyanotic, black, dark red, dusky bluish-purple or brown.
- The stoma mucosa may be hard and dry or flaccid.
- The stoma may have a foul odour.
- Associated complications may include stoma retraction, mucocutaneous separation, stoma stenosis and peritonitis.

MANAGEMENT

- Superficial necrosis may resolve with necrotic tissue simply sloughing away.
- But if tissue below the fascial level is involved, surgery is necessary.
- A transparent two-piece pouching system (stoma bag) is recommended for frequent stoma assessment.
- The pouch may need to be resized often.

PARASTOMAL HERNIA

DEFINITION

- Parastomal hernias are incisional hernias in the area of the abdominal musculature that was incised to bring the intestine through the abdominal wall to form the stoma.
- The intestine or bowel extends beyond the abdominal cavity or abdominal muscles; the area around the stoma appears as a swelling or protuberance.
- They may completely surround the stoma (called circumferential hernias) or may invade only part of the stoma.

AETIOLOGY

- Parastomal hernias can occur any time after the surgical procedure but usually happen within the **first 2 years**. Figure 5.14.

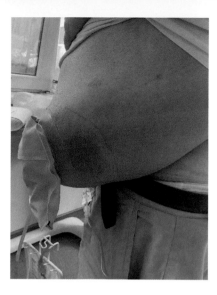

Figure 5.14 A massive parastomal hernia. Courtesy of Dr Jaclyn Croyle

- Patient-related risk factors include; obesity, poor nutritional status at the time of surgery, presurgical steroid therapy, wound sepsis and chronic cough.
- Risk factors related to technical issues include size of the surgical opening and whether surgery was done on an emergency or elective basis.
- Recurrences are common if the hernia needs to be repaired surgically.

HIGH-OUTPUT STOMA

DEFINITION

- Stoma output >1500 mls–2000 mls/24 hours (**NB: Look at stoma output chart**).

AETIOLOGY

- Surgery that results in <200 cm residual small bowel and no colon.
- Intra-abdominal sepsis.
- Intestinal obstruction (at stoma site or proximal to it). Investigate with CT scan.
- Enteric infection (e.g. *Clostridium difficile*).
- Recurrent disease in the remaining bowel.
- Radiation enteritis.
- Medication (e.g. sudden withdrawal of steroids, opiates, administration of prokinetics, laxatives).

COMPLICATIONS

- Water and sodium depletion (thirst, postural hypotension, headaches, nausea).
- Sodium depletion, therefore, kidneys trying to conserve sodium. Results in urine output <800 ml/day, renal impairment and urinary sodium <20 mmol/l.

- A urine sodium concentration can be low before serum sodium levels change.
- Hypomagnesemia: Serum magnesium <0.7 mmol/l.
- Malnutrition (due to malabsorbtion/food avoidance) with a low albumin.
- Frequent emptying of stoma bag/leakage/skin care problems. Can lead to excoriation.

MANAGEMENT

- 50% will be transient, managed with oral restriction of hypotonic liquids.
- Reduce motility with loperamide and codeine phosphate.
- Replace electrolytes (sodium, magnesium).
- Treat intra-abdominal sepsis if present.
- 30% may need TPN.

SKIN COMPLICATIONS

KEY FACTS

- Skin excoriation secondary to irritation by GIT digestive enzymes.
- More common with ileostomies than colostomies.

AETIOLOGY

- Contact dermatitis from occlusive appliances.
- Allergic responses to adhesives.
- Fungal and bacterial infections.
- Could be related to original disease (i.e. pyoderma gangrenosum in ulcerative colitis).

MANAGEMENT

- Usually skin complications are treated in conjunction with a stoma care nurse with proper adjustment of the most suitable stoma bag.
- Topical steroids in allergic dermatitis.
- Anti-fungal/anti-bacterial creams if infective dermatitis suspected.
- Proper control of IBS if skin complication is correlated.

MCQs FOR SELF-ASSESSMENT

Chapter 6

INFLAMMATORY BOWEL DISEASE

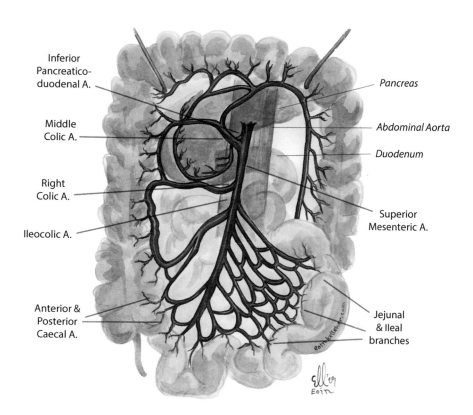

Inferior Pancreatico-duodenal A.

Middle Colic A.

Right Colic A.

Ileocolic A.

Anterior & Posterior Caecal A.

Pancreas

Abdominal Aorta

Duodenum

Superior Mesenteric A.

Jejunal & Ileal branches

DOI: 10.1201/9781003207184-6

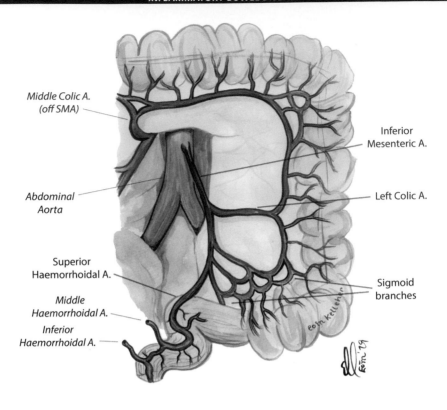

Middle Colic A.
(off SMA)

Inferior
Mesenteric A.

Abdominal
Aorta

Left Colic A.

Superior
Haemorrhoidal A.

Middle
Haemorrhoidal A.

Inferior
Haemorrhoidal A.

Sigmoid
branches

CONTENTS

Definition	135
Key Points	135
Epidemiology	135
Pathophysiology	136
Ulcerative Colitis Clinical Features	137
Crohn's Disease Clinical Features	138
Extraintestinal Manifestations	139
Surgical Management of UC	142
Surgical Management of CD	143

DEFINITION

- Inflammatory bowel disease (IBD) is a term that incorporates two major disorders: Ulcerative colitis (UC) and Crohn's disease (CD).
  - These two disorders have distinct pathology but show some clinical overlap. Table 6.1

Table 6.1   Types of Inflammatory Bowel Disease

Ulcerative Colitis	Crohn's Disease
• Inflammatory disorder of the mucosa and superficial submucosa of the colon only • Rectum always affected • May extend proximally to involve a variable amount of the large colon • Backwash ileitis–present in 20% with pancolitis; the terminal ileum may also be involved	• A chronic, non-caseating granulomatous disease • Characterised by a full-thickness inflammatory process that can affect any part of the GIT from the lips to the anal margin • Associated with several extra-intestinal disorders

KEY POINTS

- Less than 10% of patients with IBD have an extra-intestinal manifestation at initial presentation, however, ~25% of patients will develop these in their lifetime.
- The aim of treatment in IBD is firstly to induce remission and then to prevent future flare ups (i.e. maintain remission).

EPIDEMIOLOGY

- **UC**
  - Typically occurs in <u>the late teens and early 20s</u> with an equal distribution between genders.
  - 6–8% of patients have affected first-degree relative.
  - Multitude of studies examining environmental and familial risk factors but without causal association.
  - Results from poorly defined interactions between genetic and environmental factors.

- **CD**
  - Increasing incidence in Ireland (3.1–20.2/100,000)
  - Prevalence is now similar to UC (~200/100,000).
  - More common in Caucasian populations.
  - Onset in teens and twenties.
  - Smoking is a risk factor.

PATHOPHYSIOLOGY

- **UC**
  - The inflammation is usually confined to the mucosa and superficial submucosa.
    - Granular, hypervascular, oedematous mucosa.
    - Mucosal ulcers (aphthous) and crypt abscesses form.
    - Acute neutrophil infiltration occurs.
  - Residual islands of intact but oedematous mucosa may project into the bowel lumen ('pseudopolyposis').
  - Fibrosis of the mucosa and submucosa results in loss of haustration ('lead-pipe colon').
  - Long-standing disease predisposes to dysplastic changes in the epithelium and development of adenocarcinoma.
- **CD**
  - *Sites affected*:
    - Small bowel involvement in 80% (terminal ileum in particular).
    - Large bowel alone in 20%.
    - Both large and small bowel in 50%.
    - Perianal disease in over 30%.
    - Upper GIT in 5–15%.
- Chronic inflammation which is transmural i.e. it affects the entire thickness of the bowel wall.
- The wall becomes markedly thickened by oedema, but the epithelium remains remarkably intact being marked with **deep fissuring ulcers** which results in cobble-stone appearance.
- One or more discrete areas of bowel may be affected in what are termed '**skip lesions.**'
- Characterised by the presence of **non-caseating granulomas**. These contain multi-nucleated giant cells and are scattered through the bowel wall and regional lymph nodes.
- Long-standing inflammation leads to progressive fibrosis of the thickened bowel wall and elongated strictures.
- Perforation, abscesses, and fistulae are some '**fistulising**' sequelae of transmural inflammation.

ULCERATIVE COLITIS CLINICAL FEATURES

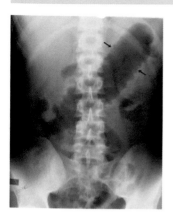

Toxic Megacolon

- Surgical emergency
- Massively dilated colon with patchy necrosis.
- Systemically ill with high fever, marked tachycardia and dehydration.
- Culminates in perforation and fatal peritonitis unless emergency colectomy is performed. Figure 6.1

Figure 6.1 Toxic megacolon. Courtesy of Dr Niamh Adams

Pancolitis

- May have backwash ileitis.
- Systemically unwell.
- **Hypokalaemia** due to impaired water and sodium absorption.
- **Hypoalbuminemia:** negative acute phase reactant from systemic response and decreased oral intake.
- **Anaemia** from blood loss and inflammatory response.

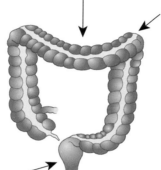

Left-sided

- To splenic flexure.
- Larger stool volume.
- Blood and mucous.
- More severe systemic complications.

Figure 6.2 Image of colon.

Proctitis

- Commonest presentation.
- Bloody diarrhoea.
- Mucus mixed with diarrhoea.
- Rectal pain and tenesmus.
- Urgency.
- Associated weight loss, anergia, loss of appetite.

CROHN'S DISEASE CLINICAL FEATURES

- **Mucosal inflammation** causes diarrhoea which, if the colon is involved, may be streaked with mucus and blood.
  - If small bowel is inflamed, diarrhoea occurs, and digestive and absorptive functions may be compromised.
  - Extensive disease results in general malabsorption causing protein-calorie malnutrition, iron and folate deficiency and anaemia.
  - In children, CD may cause marked growth retardation.
  - Excess bile salts in the faeces can cause colonic irritation (and more diarrhoea) while diminished recirculation of bile salts may result in gallstone formation.
  - Involvement of the terminal ileum may reduce vitamin B_{12} absorption, but serious deficiency usually occurs only after surgical resection.
- **Transmural inflammation**
  - CD of the terminal ileum may mimic acute appendicitis.
  - During appendicectomy, the terminal ileum is visibly inflamed and the bowel wall abnormally thick to palpation.
  - Serosal inflammation may cause a diseased segment of bowel to adhere to adjacent abdominal structures.
  - Several complications may occur if these become matted together by the inflammatory process:
    - **Adhesions:** Tough, fibrotic bands of connective tissue may cause bowel obstruction.
    - **Perforation:** Free perforation is rare, contained perforation may occur which causes localised pericolic or pelvic abscess formation.
    - **Fistula:** Develop between diseased bowel and other hollow viscera causing typical clinical phenomena.

INFLAMMATORY FEATURES OF CD

Fever
Malaise
RIF pain
Weight loss

- **Perianal problems**
  - Superficial ulcers with undermined edges are relatively painless.
  - **Fistulation** through the posterior wall of the vagina may lead to rectovaginal fistula and continuous leakage of gas and/or faeces per vagina.
  - Perianal disease is frequently associated with dense, fibrous stricturing at the anorectal junction.
  - Incontinence may develop as a result of destruction of the anal sphincter musculature because of inflammation, abscess formation, fibrotic change and repeated episodes of surgical drainage.
  - In severe cases, the perineum may become densely fibrotic, rigid and covered with multiple discharging openings (watering-can perineum).

FISTULISING FEATURES OF CD

- Ileo-enteric (ileoileal/ileocolic) presents with tender mass, fever.
- Peritonitis may occur if there is free perforation.
- Cysto-enteric fistula may present with pneumaturia.
- Entero-vaginal fistula may present with faeculent discharge.
- Entero-cutaneous may present with cutaneous discharge and cellulitis.

- **Upper GI tract**
  - The upper GI tract may be affected less frequently and may consist of oral ulceration, dysphagia with oesophageal involvement or upper abdominal pain and, perhaps, gastric outlet obstruction with gastroduodenal involvement.

STENOSING FEATURES OF CD

- Colicky abdominal pain
- Small bowel obstruction
- Weight loss ('food fear'

EXTRAINTESTINAL MANIFESTATIONS

'A PIE SAC'

A–aphthous ulcers.
P–pyoderma gangrenosum.
I (eye)–iritis, uveitis, episcleritis.
E–erythema nodosum.
S–sclerosing cholangitis/sacroilitis.
A–arthritis.
C–clubbing of the fingers.

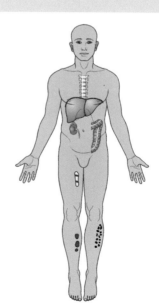

Figure 6.3   Extraintestinal manifestations of IBD.

EXTRAINTESTINAL MANIFESTATIONS OF CD AND UC

Table 6.2   Extraintestinal Manifestation of Crohn's Disease and Ulcerative Colitis

Musculoskeletal system	• Arthritis: ankylosing spondylitis, isolated joint involvement. • Hypertrophic osteoarthropathy: clubbing, periostitis. • Miscellaneous manifestations: osteoporosis, aseptic necrosis, polymyositis.
Dermatologic and oral systems	• Reactive lesions: erythema nodosum, pyoderma gangrenosum, aphthous ulcers, necrotising vasculitis. • Specific lesions: fissures, fistulas, oral Crohn's disease, drug rashes. • Nutritional deficiencies: acrodermatitis enteropathica, purpura, glossitis, hair loss, brittle nails. • Associated diseases: vitiligo, psoriasis, amyloidosis.
Hepatobiliary system	• Primary sclerosing cholangitis, bile-duct carcinoma. • Associated inflammation: autoimmune chronic active hepatitis, pericholangitis, portal fibrosis, cirrhosis, granulomatous disease. • Metabolic manifestations: fatty liver, gallstones associated with ileal Crohn's disease.
Ocular system	• Uveitis/iritis, episcleritis, scleromalacia, corneal ulcers, retinal vascular disease.
Metabolic system	• Growth retardation in children and adolescents, delayed sexual maturation.
Renal system	• Calcium oxalate stones.

INVESTIGATIONS

The investigations for UC and CD are largely similar but some differences do exist.

FOR BOTH UC AND CD

ENDOSCOPY

- **Rigid/flexible sigmoidoscopy**
  Mucosa is hyperaemic and bleeds on touch and there may be purulent exudate.

- **Colonoscopy**
  Establish extent of inflammation, distinguish between UC and Crohn's, monitor response to therapy.

BLOODS & BACTERIOLOGY

- **FBC** (low Hb due to anaemia of chronic disease or iron deficiency as a result of malnutrition)
- **ESR**
- **CRP** (may correlate with disease activity)
- **U&E**
- **Albumin** (active inflammatory disease is usually associated with a fall in serum albumin
- **Faecal calprotectin**
- **Stool culture** to eliminate the possibility of an infectious colitis:
  - *Campylobacter*
  - *Shigella*
  - *Amoebiasis*
  - *Clostridium difficile*

SPECIFIC TO CD

IMAGING

- **Small bowel enema**
  - Areas of stricturing and prestenotic dilatation.
  - Areas tend to be narrowed, irregular and when terminal ileum is involved there may be a string sign of Kantor.
- **CT with contrast**
  - Can demonstrate fistulae, intra-abdominal abscesses and bowel thickening or dilatation.
- **MR enterography**
  - Effective in showing small bowel stricturing in young patients.
  - Small bowel is examined by contrast given through a NJ tube.
- **Fistulography**
  - In patients with enterocutaneous fistulae, fistulography helps demonstrate the anatomy and complexity of fistulae and allow adequate planning for future surgery.

MANAGEMENT

- The choice of medical treatment depends on the severity of flares, disease extent, symptoms, and the risk of long-term complications. Table 6.3
- Both diseases are highly catabolic and involvement of MDT, including dieticians/nutritionists is crucial.

Table 6.3 Treatment Options for of Crohn's Disease and Ulcerative Colitis

Therapy	Indication	Used in
Local therapy (suppositories, foam or liquid enema) • Corticosteroid or 5-ASA preparations	• Used in all grades of disease severity • Ideal for proctitis • Foam enemas extend up to splenic flexure • Induce and maintain remission	• Since UC more commonly affects the rectum, this therapy is more common in UC but also used in CD
Systemic corticosteroids (oral prednisolone, budesonide, IV hydrocortisone)	• Additive to local therapy • Induce remission for moderate or severe exacerbations • Not commonly used in maintenance therapy due to side effects	• UC and CD to induce remission
Systemic therapy: Non-immunologic • 5-ASA preparations (sulfasalazine, mesalazine, or olsalazine)	• Long-term maintenance therapy to minimise relapse • Acute therapy for pancolitis	• Both UC and CD
Systemic therapy: Immunologic • Azathioprine • 6-mercaptopurine • Anti-TNF (infliximab, adalimumab, golimumab • Anti-integrin (anti-alpha-1-beta-7, vedolizumab) • Anti-interleukin (IL 12/23)	• Long-term maintenance therapy to minimise relapse • Acute therapy for pancolitis	• Both UC and CD

KEY POINTS

- Must rule out TB with CXR and Mantoux test (+/– QuantiFERON) prior to therapy with corticosteroids.
- Must rule out infective colitis prior to starting therapy.
- In prolonged courses of steroid therapy, need concomitant calcium supplementation and monitoring of bone density with DEXA scan.
- With immunologic therapy, patients are at a higher risk of skin cancers.

SURGICAL MANAGEMENT OF UC

- **Elective surgery:** If risk of malignancy or failure of medical treatment.
- **Urgent surgery:** i.e. during same hospital admission if:
  - Patients with UC develop acute fulminant colitis, characterised by:
    - >10 stools per day
    - Continuous bleeding

- Abdominal pain
- Distension
- Acute, severe toxic symptoms, including fever and anorexia.
- Patients with acute fulminant colitis require urgent surgery if they fail medical therapy.
- **Emergency surgery:** Patients with UC who develop one or more life-threatening complication require immediate surgery.
  - Complications include:
    - Colonic perforation
    - Life-threatening GI haemorrhage
    - Toxic megacolon

TYPES OF SURGERY FOR UC

- **Subtotal colectomy with ileostomy**
  - Safest operation in the emergency situation.
  - Most of the diseased colon is removed, but the patient is left with an inflamed rectal stump.
  - Months later, when the patient is well, this may be revised.
  - Alternatively, rectum may be retained and treated with local therapy plus surveillance, though cancer risk remains.
- **Restorative proctocolectomy (ileal pouch-anal anastomosis/Park's pouch):**
  - A sphincter-preserving operation avoiding permanent ileostomy.
  - Entire colon and rectal mucosa is excised and a pouch reservoir is fashioned from a loop of terminal ileum.
  - The pouch is brought into the pelvis and anastomosed to the upper anal canal.
  - A temporary ileostomy is usually retained for a few months to allow healing.
  - Many patients have excellent continence.
  - May get 'pouchitis' which is inflammation within the neo-rectum.
- **Pan-proctocolectomy with permanent ileostomy**
  - Includes removal of rectum and entire colon.
  - Generally recommended for elderly patients in whom sphincter-preserving procedures are inadvisable.

SURGICAL MANAGEMENT OF CD

- **Ileocaecal resection**
  - Most common surgical procedure for terminal ileal CD.
  - Form a primary anastomosis between the ileum and the ascending or transverse colon.
- **Segmental resection**
  - Short segmental resections of small or large bowel strictures can be performed.
  - This is usually a preferred method of treatment when there is a complication of the disease e.g. perforation or fistula formation.

- **Stricturoplasty**
  - Multiple areas of stricture formation in CD can be treated by a local widening procedure of endoscopic dilatation to avoid small bowel resection.
  - This is not commonly used for a colorectal stricture.
- **Subtotal colectomy with ileostomy**
  - Crohn's colitis accounts for 8% of such procedures for acute colonic disease.

PRE-OPERATIVE PREPARATION

- The patient's overall medical condition should be optimised by correcting any anaemia, fluid depletion, electrolyte imbalances, and malnutrition prior to surgery where possible.
- Patients with UC/CD who require surgery may be on one or more immunosuppressive drugs or biologic agents (e.g. infliximab).
- Most immunosuppressive drugs can be discontinued just before surgery without any negative effects, however this should be discussed at an MDT meeting.
- Abdominal imaging: CT enterography and MR enterography are very accurate in assessing lesions and complications (like abscess or fistula) in CD.
- Patients who undergo abdominal surgery for UC/CD are at a moderate-to-high risk for developing a VTE due to systemic inflammation. They should receive thrombo-prophylaxis.

MCQs FOR SELF-ASSESSMENT

Chapter 7

PERIPHERAL VASCULAR DISEASE

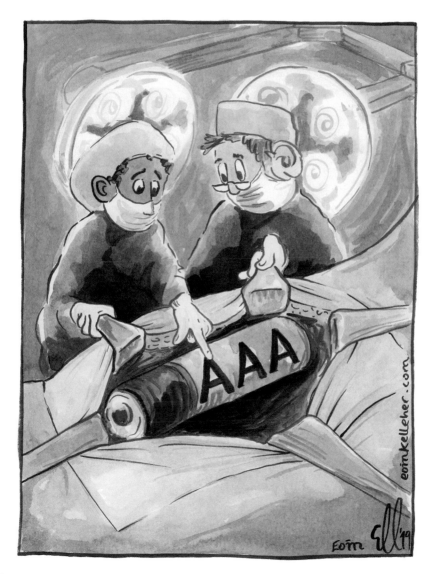

DOI: 10.1201/9781003207184-7

CONTENTS

Peripheral Arterial Disease (PAD)	147
Acute Lower Limb Ischaemia	150
Abdominal Aortic Aneurysms	151
Ruptured AAA	156
Varicose Veins	157
Deep Vein Thrombosis (DVT)	160
Carotid Artery Disease	162
Leg Ulcers	163
The Diabetic Foot	165

PERIPHERAL ARTERIAL DISEASE (PAD)

DEFINITION

- Chronic insufficiency of the arterial blood supply of the limbs (most commonly the legs) due to stenosis or occlusion of the vessels.

AETIOLOGY

- Primary pathological cause is **atherosclerosis**
- Less common causes include:
  - Fibromuscular dysplasia
  - Vasculitides (Buerger's disease, Takayasu arteritis)
  - Radiation-induced vascular injury

Table 7.1   Risk Factors for Peripheral Arterial Disease

Risk Factors	
Modifiable	Non-Modifiable
• Smoking (most important) • Hypertension • Diabetes • High cholesterol • Previous stroke/MI/angina • Hyperhomocysteinemia	• Gender: Male > female • Age > 55 • Family history

SIGNS AND SYMPTOMS

- Intermittent claudication: Muscular pain (most commonly in calves and/or buttocks) brought on by exercise and relieved by rest.
  - Caused by demand for oxygen by muscles during exertion in the context of reduced blood supply.
- Critical limb ischaemia
  - Rest pain > 2 weeks
    - Pain in the forefoot when lying flat at night, classically relieved by hanging leg over side of bed.
  - Tissue loss (ulcers, gangrene, necrosis).
- Pallor of the lower limb
- Reduced temperature of the lower limb (**remember to compare limbs**)
- No palpable pulses, i.e. femoral, popliteal, posterior tibial, dorsalis pedis
- Loss of hair
- Burning sensation, paraesthesia
- *Leriche syndrome*: Occlusion at bifurcation of aorta causing classical triad
  1. Buttock/thigh claudication
  2. Absent/reduced femoral pulses
  3. Erectile dysfunction

Table 7.2 Rutherford-Fontaine Classification for Limb Ischaemia

I	Asymptomatic
II	Intermittent claudication: • IIA (claudication distance >200 m) • IIB (claudication distance <200 m)
III	Rest pain
IV	Tissue loss (ulcers, gangrene, necrosis)

DIFFERENTIAL DIAGNOSES FOR PAD

- Spinal stenosis
- Osteoarthritis
- Nerve root entrapment (e.g. sciatica)
- Trauma

Table 7.3 Key Features on History Taking

Where is the pain? When did it begin? (Essential to distinguish between **chronic** limb ischaemia and **acute** limb ischaemia)
Is it made worse by walking?
How far can you walk before you need to stop? (**Claudication distance**)
Does the pain go away when you stop walking?
Does the pain ever occur at rest? At night? Relieved by hanging over the edge of the bed?
Noticed any change of colour or temperature of your legs?
Have you noticed any black areas or sores on your leg that do not heal? Are they painful? For how long?
PAD risk factors–are you a smoker? Do you have high cholesterol? etc. (see below)

INVESTIGATIONS

- Ankle-brachial pressure index (ABPI): Ratio of peak systolic Doppler ankle pressure to arm pressure. Table 7.4
- Duplex US
- CT angiogram/MR angiogram
- Digital subtraction angiography (DSA)

Table 7.4 ABPI Interpretation

1.1–0.9	Normal
0.9–0.5	Intermittent claudication
<0.5	Rest pain
<0.3	Tissue loss
>1.1	Calcified arteries (typically seen in diabetics, CKD, false elevation)

MANAGEMENT

- **Conservative:** Risk factor modification.
  - Smoking cessation (CRUCIAL).
  - Physical exercise, dietary modification.
- **Medical**
  - Antiplatelet therapy (aspirin, clopidogrel).
  - Statin: Lowers cholesterol, improves walking distance, reduces rate of major vascular events.
  - Control blood pressure.
  - Tight glycaemic control.
  - Cilostazol: Phosphodiesterase inhibitor which causes vasodilation–for symptom relief in intermittent claudication only.
  - Pentoxifylline (xanthine derivative)–for symptom relief in intermittent claudication only.
- **Endovascular**
  - Angioplasty (balloon +/– stenting): In many cases procedures can be performed as day case procedures. Figure 7.1
  - Procedures can also be performed under local anaesthesia.
- **Surgical**
  - Endarterectomy.
  - Bypass procedures used for disease not best managed via endovascular techniques.
  - Can use <u>synthetic graft</u> e.g. PTFE/Dacron®, or <u>vein graft</u> (the best option) e.g. great saphenous vein.
  - Examples: Fem-pop bypass, fem-distal bypass, aorto-bifem bypass, axillo-bifem bypass, fem-fem crossover.
  - Amputation if non-viable limb.

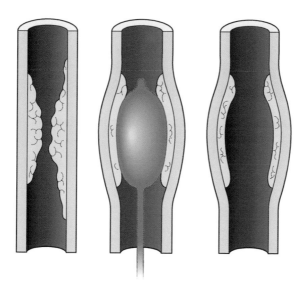

Figure 7.1   Balloon angioplasty of arterial atherosclerosis.

ACUTE LOWER LIMB ISCHAEMIA

DEFINITION
- Abrupt interruption in perfusion that threatens viability of the lower limb.

AETIOLOGY
- Acute thrombus with pre-existing atherosclerosis.
  - Acute-on-chronic ischaemia.
  - The patient often has a history of claudication.
  - Usually no obvious source of emboli.
- Embolus
  - Classically lodges at branching points of vessels.
  - Cardiac sources account for 70–80% of emboli: Mural thrombus after MI, arrhythmias, infective endocarditis, prosthetic heart valves, atrial myxoma.
  - Can occur from pre-existing atheromas or arterial aneurysms.
  - Blue toe syndrome: Atheroembolic debris resulting in distal small arterial occlusion with blueish discolouration of distal foot.
  - Paradoxical emboli can occur from intracardiac shunts (e.g. PFO) or AV malformations.
- Other causes
  - Direct arterial trauma
  - Intra-arterial drug injection
  - Aortic dissection
  - Popliteal aneurysm
  - Iatrogenic

COMPLICATIONS
- If untreated: Irreversible tissue damage within 6 hours (limb loss, mortality).

TYPES OF AMPUTATION
- Digital: Partial or full.
- Transmetatarsal: Used if several toes are gangrenous.
- Below knee amputation (BKA).
- Through knee amputation (TKA).
- Above knee amputation (AKA).

The 6 Ps

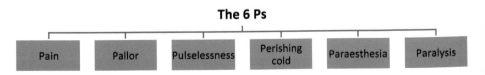

| Pain | Pallor | Pulselessness | Perishing cold | Paraesthesia | Paralysis |

Figure 7.2 Clinical features of acute limb ischaemia.

MANAGEMENT

- If clear evidence of acute ischaemia on history and exam, do not delay definitive treatment.
- Patients usually have other significant comorbidities: IHD, renal disease.
- Give oxygen.
- IV access and fluids if dehydrated (do NOT overload).
- Bloods–FBC, U&E, coagulation profile, troponin, glucose, group & save.
- CXR.
- ECG–looking for cardiac cause.
- Analgesia–morphine.
- Give unfractionated heparin.
  - Stat dose of 5000 IU then infusion of 1000 IU/hr.
  - Be sure there are no contraindications to Heparin use.
  - Check aPTT in **4–6 hours**.
  - Aim for aPTT **60–90**.
- **Definitive treatment depends on severity of ischaemia.**
  - If irreversible ischaemia (petechial haemorrhages, hard muscles): Amputation.
  - If limb is swollen or tender with loss of power or sensation–consider amputation if there are life threatening systemic complications.
  - If an obvious embolus is the cause:
    - Perform urgent embolectomy +/– fasciotomy.
    - A Fogarty catheter is used to extract the embolus.
  - If limb is viable:
    - Can continue IV heparin.
    - CT angio or perform angiography (stop Heparin 4 hours before).
    - Thrombolysis +/– angioplasty can then be performed. Be sure no contraindications to thrombolysis.

COMPLICATIONS OF REPERFUSION

- Reperfusion injury.
- Rhabdomyolysis:
  - Elevated K^+, elevated CPK, renal impairment, myoglobinuria.
  - Treat with aggressive IV fluids, diuresis with mannitol, alkalinisation of urine.
- Compartment syndrome–prevent and treat with 4-compartment fasciotomy.

ABDOMINAL AORTIC ANEURYSMS

DEFINITION

- Abnormal, localised dilatation of aorta, exceeding normal diameter by >50% or diameter >3 cm.
- **AAA is a true aneurysm: It contains all three layers of vessel wall.**
  - Transmural inflammatory change, abnormal collagen remodelling, loss of elastin and smooth muscle cells, resulting in aortic wall thinning and progressive expansion.

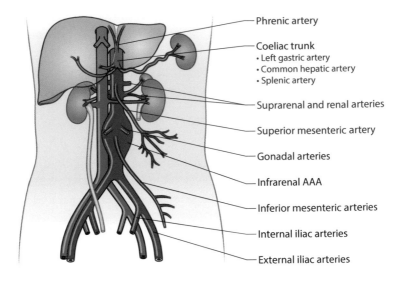

Phrenic artery

Coeliac trunk
• Left gastric artery
• Common hepatic artery
• Splenic artery

Suprarenal and renal arteries

Superior mesenteric artery

Gonadal arteries

Infrarenal AAA

Inferior mesenteric arteries

Internal iliac arteries

External iliac arteries

Figure 7.3   Infra-renal abdominal aortic aneurysm.

KEY FACTS

- Male:Female = 9:1.
- Prevalence: 4% in males >65 years.
- **95% of AAA's are infrarenal.**
- Described as either fusiform or saccular.
- >80% of patients with ruptured AAA die before reaching hospital.
- 50% of patients with ruptured AAA who arrive will not survive surgery.

RISK FACTORS

- Risk factors as for PVD
    - 10-fold increased risk in **smoking**.
    - 50% increased risk in **poorly controlled HTN**.
    - Increased expansion and rupture risk associated with smoking and uncontrolled HTN.
- Collagen and elastin defects e.g. Marfan's syndrome, Ehlers-Danlos syndrome.
- AAA diameter >5.5 cm and expansion rate >0.5 cm/6 months associated with increased risk of rupture.
- Aortitis: From bacteraemia, endocarditis, mycotic aneurysms.

SURVEILLANCE

- The rate of expansion is directly related to the size of the aneurysm.

CLINICAL FEATURES

- Most are asymptomatic: <50% detected on exam by a pulsatile and expansile mass in abdomen.

Table 7.5 Surveillance Guidelines for AAA

Surveillance (Current UK Screening/Surveillance Guidelines)	
3–4.4 cm	Annual surveillance USS
4.5–5.4 cm	3-monthly US surveillance
>5.5 cm	Surgical repair (open vs endovascular)

- **40% detected incidentally** on imaging for other reasons.
- There is an associated increased risk of peripheral aneurysms, particularly popliteal aneurysm.
- Symptoms arise from aneurysm expansion, rupture or peripheral embolism and include:
  - **Abdominal/Back/Flank pain.**
  - Distal peripheral embolisation or ischaemia.
  - Upper GI bleeding from aorto-enteric fistula.
  - Syncope or shock with large pulsatile mass, ecchymoses or death from a ruptured AAA.

DIFFERENTIAL DIAGNOSIS

- If patient presents with sudden onset abdominal/back/flank pain:
  - Ischaemic bowel
  - Perforated PUD
  - Pyelonephritis
  - Nephrolithiasis
  - Acute pancreatitis

INVESTIGATIONS: IMAGING

- **US**
  - Best initial imaging modality
  - 98% accuracy (user dependant)
  - Non-invasive
  - Does not define extent of aneurysm
  - Inadequate for planning repair
- **CT abdomen with IV contrast**
  - Highly accurate in determining size and extent of aneurysm
  - Defines relationship of AAA to renal arteries
  - Can tell if AAA is leaking
  - Determines suitability of endovascular repair

MANAGEMENT: ELECTIVE REPAIR

- **Open surgical repair**
  - Uses a synthetic (Dacron) graft to repair aneurysm.
  - Long midline incision (laparotomy).
  - Aorta clamped below renal arteries where possible to prevent renal ischaemia.
  - Graft can be straight if iliac arteries not involved or bifurcated if iliac arteries involved.
  - 3–7% mortality
- **Endovascular aneurysm repair (EVAR)**
  - Insertion of a stent over aneurysmal segment.
  - Small groin incisions (may be vertical or transverse).

- When possible can also be percutaneous.
- Does not require cross clamping of aorta.
- Procedure carried out under direct radiological guidance.
- Uses high doses of nephrotoxic contrast.
- Reduced early mortality.
- High early re-intervention rate if endoleak occurs.
- Requires lifelong surveillance post-op for endoleak.

ENDOVASCULAR ANEURYSM REPAIR (EVAR) VIDEO:

COMPLICATIONS OF AAA REPAIR

- **Early**
  - Death.
  - Haemorrhage: Uncontrolled vessels or anastomotic breakdown.
  - Myocardial ischaemia: 20% of patients.

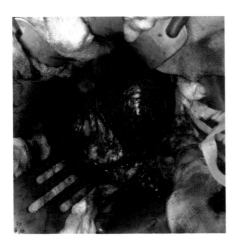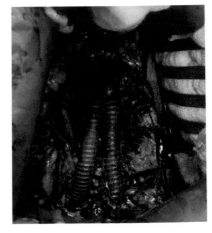

Figure 7.4   Aortobiliac aneurysm (a) pre- and (b) post-repair. Courtesy of Dr Amr Kazim

- Cardiac arrhythmias.
- Cardiac failure.
- Bowel ischaemia: May present with abdominal pain, bloody diarrhoea. Urgent laparotomy if evidence of peritonitis.
- Abdominal compartment syndrome.
- Atelectasis, ARDS, RTI.
- Endoleak (from EVAR).
- Renal dysfunction: Pre-existing renal disease, nephrotoxic contrast/antibiotics, prolonged hypotension/dehydration, use of NSAIDs.
- Limb ischaemia.
- Wound infection: Reduced by prophylactic antibiotics.
- Impaired sexual function.
- **Late**
  - Graft infection: Usually needs to be removed.
  - Graft limb occlusion: Within 30 days, may present with acute ischaemic limb.
  - Aortoenteric fistula.
  - Endoleak (from EVAR).

ENDOLEAK

- An endoleak is persistent blood flow into an aneurysmal sac after EVAR is performed.

Table 7.6   Classification of Endoleak

Type I	Leak at attachment sites of graft
Type II	Backflow of blood into aneurysmal sac by collateral vessels (IMA, lumbar)
Type III	Leak through defect in graft
Type IV	Leak through fabric of graft due to porosity
Type V	Expansion of aneurysm sac without evidence of leak on imaging

OTHER TYPES OF ANEURYSM

- **Thoraco-abdominal**
  - Often asymptomatic.
  - Can present with chest pain, back pain, acute aortic regurgitation and acute cardiac failure.
  - Widened mediastinum on CXR.
  - Rupture is rare without pre-existing symptoms.
  - 20% mortality with elective repair.
  - Endovascular repair may be used (fenestrated or branched grafts).
- **Femoral**
  - Presents with pulsatile groin swelling +/− lower limb ischaemia.
- **Popliteal**
  - Mostly asymptomatic but bilateral.
  - Can cause acute limb ischaemia.
- **Carotid**
  - Rare.
  - Pulsatile neck swelling.
  - May have neurological or pressure symptoms.
  - Diagnosed with carotid duplex US.

- **Cerebral**
  - Often asymptomatic unless ruptured.
  - Can present with headaches, visual acuity loss, facial pain.
  - Usually an incidental finding.
- **Iliac**
  - Mostly asymptomatic.
  - Rupture may be missed as acute abdomen or renal colic.
- **Visceral**
  - Splenic artery aneurysms most common.

RUPTURED AAA

CLINICAL FEATURES

- Presentation may be delayed if rupture is contained within retroperitoneal space.
- A contained leak may initially be haemodynamically stable but can proceed rapidly to rupture.
- Longstanding leak causing aorto-enteric fistula can present with high output cardiac failure and GI bleed.
- Sudden onset abdominal/back/flank pain.
- Sudden collapse with hypotension.
- May have a history of AAA under surveillance.
- Pulsatile abdominal mass is *not always palpable*.

MANAGEMENT

- Airway.
- Breathing (give 15 L 100% O_2 via non-rebreather mask).

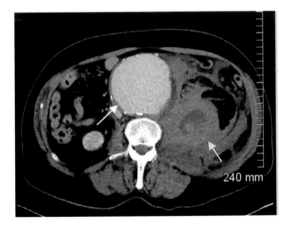

Figure 7.5 CT angiogram showing a ruptured AAA (white arrow) note the retroperitoneal hae-matoma (yellow arrow). Courtesy of Dr Mark Given

- Circulation (wide bore IV access ×2, give IV fluids).
  - Bloods (FBC, U&E, coagulation profile, group and cross-match 10 units).
  - Request platelets and FFP.
  - Urinary catheter: Monitor urinary output.
- **Do not aggressively hydrate: Allow permissive hypotension to avoid worsening a rupture.**
- Analgesia.
- Alert vascular surgeon, anaesthetist, theatre, ICU.
- Gain consent for surgery.
- If not a candidate for surgery: Analgesia and palliative care.
  - Based on age, co-morbidities, extent of aneurysm, patient's wishes, family's wishes.
- To aid diagnosis and allow planning of repair: CT angiogram.
- If a candidate for open/endovascular repair: Urgent transfer to theatre.
- ICU care post-op.

VARICOSE VEINS

DEFINITION

- Varicose veins are tortuous dilated segments of veins, associated with venous hypertension that is caused by incompetent valves.

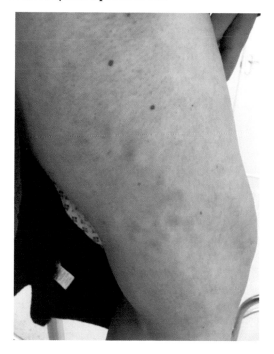

Figure 7.6 Varicose veins. Courtesy of Dr Azlena Ali Beegan

AETIOLOGY

- **The venous system of the leg is comprised of three groups:**
  1. <u>Superficial veins</u>: Great and small saphenous systems (GSV, SSV) and tributaries.
  2. <u>Deep venous system</u>: Veins running between the muscular compartments of the leg.
  3. <u>Perforators in the calf and thigh</u>: Connect superficial and deep systems.
- Blood passes from the superficial system to the deep systems via perforators.
- Backflow is prevented by **the presence of valves** in the deep and perforator veins.
- Varicose veins are tortuous dilated segments of veins associated with venous hypertension **caused by incompetent valves**.
- Typical varicose veins are superficial branches of the long and short saphenous system.
- More common in females.

Table 7.7   Risk Factors for Varicose Veins

• Advancing age • Prolonged standing • Elevated BMI • Smoking • Sedentary lifestyle	• High oestrogen states • Pregnancy • Pelvic masses • Previous DVT • Ligamentous laxity • Lower limb trauma

CLINICAL FEATURES

- Patients may present with worsening symptoms or complications or cosmetic concerns.
- **Symptoms:**
  - Achy pain
  - Heaviness of leg
  - Oedema–worse in evening, hot weather
  - Dry skin
  - Tightness
  - Itching

COMPLICATIONS

- Stasis dermatitis/Eczema.
- Phlebitis.
- Lipodermatosclerosis–fibrosing dermatitis of subcutaneous tissue.
- Skin pigmentation–due to hemosiderin deposition.
- Ulceration.
- Bleeding.

DIAGNOSIS AND INVESTIGATIONS

- Typically a clinical diagnosis.
- Always examine the abdomen to assess for an abdominal/pelvic mass.
- Trendelenburg test and Perthes test can help clinically identify point(s) of incompetence.
- **Ultrasound duplex of superficial and deep veins** is the gold standard to define anatomy and levels of incompetence.

TRENDELENBURG TEST

- Ask patient to lie supine, so that you can perform a test to examine at what level the venous valve defect is occurring.
- Raise their affected leg so that venous blood drains from the limb.
- Keep their leg elevated and place a tourniquet around their thigh.
- Ask the patient to stand and watch to see if any varicose veins reappear.
- If the varicose veins do not refill, then the defect is above the level of the tourniquet, if they do refill then the defect is at a level below the tourniquet.
- Repeat further down limb until the level of the defect is found.

TRENDELENBURG VIDEO:

MANAGEMENT

- **Conservative**
  - Leg elevation.
  - Exercise.
  - Weight loss.
- **Medical**
  - Compression stockings.
  - Topical agents for skin changes, i.e. moisturising creams.
- **Surgical**
  - Radiofrequency ablation.
  - Laser ablation.
  - Sclerotherapy (usually cosmetic).
  - Local stab avulsions.
  - Open ligation +/− great saphenous vein stripping.
- **Indications for surgery**
  - Cosmetic.
  - Symptomatic.
  - Prevent complications.

COMPLICATIONS OF SURGERY

- Nerve injury resulting in area of pain/paraesthesia/numbness.
- Deep vein thrombosis (DVT).

- Recurrence.
- Bruising/haematoma.
- Bleeding.
- Wound infection.

DEEP VEIN THROMBOSIS (DVT)

DEFINITION
- Occurs when a blood clot/thrombus forms in a deep vein.

AETIOLOGY

Table 7.8   Virchow's Triad

Virchow's Triad (Factors Contributing to Thrombosis)
1 Stasis of blood flow
2 Endothelial injury
3 Hypercoagulability

RISK FACTORS

Table 7.9   Risk Factors for Deep Vein Thrombosis

Trauma, Travel (long-distance flights)
Hormones (OCP, HRT)
Road traffic accidents (fractures)
Operations
Malignancy
Blood disorders: Factor V Leiden, protein C/S deficiency, antithrombin deficiency
Obesity, **O**ld age, **O**rthopaedic surgery
Serious illness (prolonged hospital stay)
Immobilisation, **I**nadequate hydration
Smoking

CLINICAL FEATURES
- Limb swelling.
- Pain.
- Warmth.
- Erythema.
- Homan's sign–calf pain on dorsiflexion of foot (unreliable and should not be performed due to risk of embolisation).
- May have mild pyrexia and tachycardia.
- May be asymptomatic (hence a high index of suspicion is needed).
- **Complications of DVT:**
  - PE, chronic venous insufficiency, venous gangrene.

INVESTIGATIONS

- D-dimer: Sensitive but not specific.
- **Duplex scan:** Investigation of choice for DVT.
- CTPA: Best for suspected PE.

PROPHYLAXIS

- Prophylactic low molecular weight heparin.
- Thrombo-embolic deterrent stockings (TEDS).
- Mobilisation.
- Hydration.
- Smoking cessation.
- Stop oral contraceptive pills (OCP) 4–6 weeks pre-op.

Table 7.10   Wells Probability Score for DVT

• Active malignancy (1)
• Paralysis, paresis or recent plaster immobilisation of lower limbs (1)
• Localised tenderness along deep venous system (1)
• Entire leg swollen (1)
• Calf swelling >3 cm and larger than asymptomatic side (1)
• Pitting oedema (1)
• Collateral superficial veins (1)
• Previously documented DVT (1)
• Alternative diagnosis as likely as DVT (–2)
Interpretation:
DVT likely: >2 points
DVT unlikely: <1 point

MANAGEMENT

- **Uncomplicated DVT**
  - Therapeutic LMWH then switch to warfarin for 3–6 months.
- **Complicated DVT**
  - IV unfractionated heparin or LMWH while converting to warfarin.
  - Thrombolysis or thrombectomy if severe thrombosis.
  - IVC filter
    - Inserted percutaneously via jugular/femoral vein to catch and prevent PEs.
    - Used in recurrent PE despite treatment, if contraindications to anticoagulation and if anticoagulation cannot be used during major surgery.
    - Risks of IVC filter placement–air embolism, arrhythmias, pneumo-/haemothorax, IVC obstruction, bleeding.

THROMBOLYSIS

- Agents include streptokinase, urokinase, recombinant tPA.
- Administered via catheter as a low dose intra-arterial infusion.
- **Indications**
  - Acute limb ischaemia.
  - Venous thrombosis.
  - Acute surgical graft occlusions.
  - Thrombosed popliteal artery aneurysm.

- **Contraindications**
  - Bleeding disorders.
  - Current peptic ulcer.
  - Recent haemorrhagic stroke.
  - Recent major surgery.
  - Evidence of muscle necrosis–may cause reperfusion injury.
- **Complications**
  - Allergy.
  - Catheter leak, occlusion.
  - Bruising.
  - Major bleed or stroke.

CAROTID ARTERY DISEASE

DEFINITIONS

- **Carotid artery stenosis** is narrowing of the carotid arteries. It occurs in 10% of people 80–89 years.
- **CVA:** Rapidly developing neurological deficit lasting >24 hours.
- **TIA:** Acute episode of focal neurological deficit that resolves within 24 hours.

CLINICAL FEATURES OF SYMPTOMATIC CAROTID ARTERY DISEASE

- **Cerebrovascular accident (CVA)**
  - Completed stroke.
  - Stroke in evolution–progressive neurological deficit over days and weeks.
  - FAST criteria
    - Facial droop.
    - Arms: Can they raise them and keep them elevated.
    - Speech difficulties.
    - Time: Call for help if one of these signs are present.
- **Transient ischaemic attack (TIA):** Can have a transient change in facial expression, drooping of the corner of the mouth, dribbling.
- **Amaurosis fugax:** Transient monocular visual loss, like a curtain coming down over eye.
- **Cerebral hypoperfusion.**

INVESTIGATIONS

- **Carotid duplex scan** is the screening test of choice, but can be difficult to perform if vessels are calcified.
- Carotid MR angiography.
- Cranial CT/MR angiography.
- Cardiac echo/telemetry: Useful in excluding cardiac source of embolic stroke.

MANAGEMENT

- **Medical**
  - Antiplatelet agents–aspirin, Plavix

- Anticoagulants–use in non-cardiac emboli is controversial.
- Smoking cessation.
- Blood pressure control.
- Tight glucose control.
- Statin.
- **Surgical/Endovascular**
  - Carotid endarterectomy/stent.
  - Indications
    - 50–99% stenosis with recent TIA/CVA.
    - Consideration of intervention if asymptomatic but >70% stenosis in younger patients and low interventional risk.
  - **Contraindications**
    - Severe neurological deficit after cerebral infarction.
    - Occluded carotid artery.
    - Severe comorbidities.

CAROTID ENDARTERECTOMY

- Can be performed under general or local anaesthetic.
- Incision along anterior border of sternocleidomastoid muscle.
- Shunting of carotid artery following clamping can allow for ongoing cerebral perfusion during surgery.
- Endarterectomy is carried out in a smooth plane in the media of the artery.
- A smooth tapering endpoint on the internal carotid is obtained.
- Endarterectomy is usually closed with a synthetic patch.
- **Post-op**
  - Observe for haematoma that may compromise the airway.
  - Antiplatelet therapy.
  - Monitor blood pressure post-operatively (may be labile).
- **Complications of surgical treatment**
  - CVA–increased risk in stenting vs endarterectomy. Patients also have a risk of intraoperative CVA.
  - MI–increased risk in endarterectomy vs stenting.
  - Death.
  - Wound haematoma–can cause airway obstruction.
  - Recurrent stenosis.
  - Cranial nerve injury.
    - Vagus–vocal cord paralysis, dysphagia.
    - Hypoglossal–deviation of tongue.

LEG ULCERS

DEFINITION

- An area of full thickness skin loss of the lower limb.

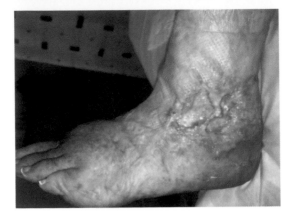

Figure 7.7   Mixed arterial and venous ulcer. Courtesy of Dr Azlena Ali Beegan

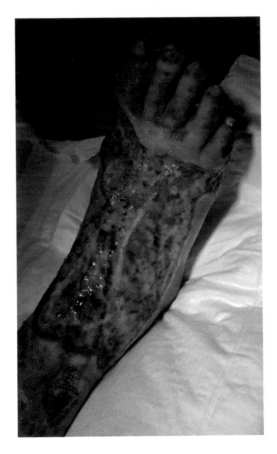

Figure 7.8   Arterial ulcer. Courtesy of Dr Amr Kazim

CAUSES

- Venous
- Arterial
- Mixed arterial and venous
- Neuropathy
- Diabetes
- Trauma
- Vasculitic–Buerger's disease, Takayasu's arteritis
- Malignancy–consider if ulcer does not heal with adequate medical management
- Infection
- Lymphedema

It is important to ask about both arterial and venous risk factors for ulceration.

Table 7.11   Clinical Features of Arterial and Venous Ulcers

	Arterial	Venous
Site	Distally, i.e. digits	Medial gaiter region
Edges	'Punched out,' well defined	Sloped
Depth	Deep	Superficial, shallow
Size	Small	Large
Base	Necrotic	Granulation tissue
Margin	Regular	Irregular
Cause	Arterial insufficiency	Venous hypertension
Surrounding features	Features of PVD (pallor, hair loss, trophic changes, onychogryphosis, cool, weak/absent pulses, prolonged cap refill)	Features of chronic venous insufficiency (oedema, haemosiderin, lipodermatosclerosis, varicose veins)
Management	As per chronic PVD in patients with critical limb ischaemia	4-layered PROFORE dressing Leg elevation Venous support stockings Skin graft Antibiotics if infection Consider varicose vein surgery if possible once ulcer healed to reduce recurrence rate

THE DIABETIC FOOT

FEATURES OF THE DIABETIC FOOT

- Ulceration
- Infection
- Sensory neuropathy
- Poorly healing wounds

AETIOLOGY

- Small and medium vessel disease.
- Sensory neuropathy resulting in unnoticed tissue damage.
- Autonomic neuropathy resulting in reduced sweating, which leads to dry, cracked skin and infection.

RISK FACTORS

- Previous ulcers
- Diabetic neuropathy:
  - Stocking distribution
  - Charcot's joints
- Associated PAD:
  - Diabetic patients usually have calcified peripheral arteries.
  - ABI may be falsely elevated.
- Calluses
- Living alone
- Evidence of other diabetic complications e.g. renal/visual impairment.

CLINICAL FEATURES

- Ulcers commonly on pressure points (toes, heels).
- Evidence of sensory loss.
- If arterial disease is present, foot may be cool with reduced/absent pulses.
- Secondary infection of ulcer +/− cellulitis.
- ABI may be falsely elevated if calcified vessels.
- Toe pressures are a useful adjunct in determining perfusion in this population.

INVESTIGATIONS

- ABIs/Toe pressures.
- Duplex US.
- CT Angio/MR Angio if co-existing arterial disease suspected.
- Check blood glucose level and HBA1c, renal function, blood pressure.

MANAGEMENT

- Best done at a specialist multidisciplinary clinic.
- Regularly inspect feet.
- Appropriately fitted footwear and avoid walking barefoot.
- Chiropodist for debriding calluses and for nail care.
- If infected ulcer:
  - Broad spectrum antibiotics.
  - +/− Debridement of dead tissue.
  - +/− Amputation of non-viable digits if adequate arterial supply for healing of amputation.
  - X-ray/MRI to rule out underlying osteomyelitis.
- Consider revascularisation if significant arterial disease.
- Consider amputation if no response to medical or other surgical treatments.

NEUROPATHIC ULCERS

- Caused by trauma unnoticed by the patient.
- Punched out appearance.
- Located over pressure points or calluses.
- Surrounded by inflammatory tissue.
- Frequently painless due to neuropathy.

MCQs FOR SELF-ASSESSMENT

Chapter 8

BREAST DISORDERS

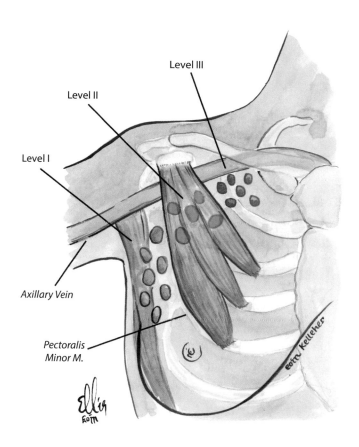

DOI: 10.1201/9781003207184-8

CONTENTS

Breast Cancer	171
Breast Cancer Screening	178
Benign Breast Disease	179

BREAST CANCER

KEY FACTS

- Most commonly occurring cancer in women.
- Commonest in Western world: 1 in 12 lifetime risk for women.
- Incidence increases with age.
- Rare before the age of 25.
- <1% occur in men.

AETIOLOGY

- Increasing age
- Genetic
  - Positive family history (particularly a first-degree relative).
  - BRCA1 and BRCA2 genes (about 70% chance of developing breast cancer before age of 80).
  - Inherited mutations in many other genes (CHEK2, PALB2, etc.).
  - Previous breast or ovarian cancer.
- Other factors related to exposure of estrogen
  - Early menarche.
  - Late menopause.
  - Nulliparity.
  - Obesity.
  - Hormone replacement therapy (HRT) for >10 years.
- Breast pathologies
  - Ductal carcinoma in situ (DCIS) and lobular carcinoma in situ (LCIS) are both associated with increased risk of developing breast cancer. DCIS is a precursor of invasiveness in the ipsilateral breast.
  - LCIS although not a pre-malignant change in itself, is regarded as a marker for development of malignant disease in either breast.
  - Atypical ductal hyperplasia (ADH) and atypical lobular hyperplasia.
  - Prior history of breast cancer.
  - Intraductal papilloma.

PATHOLOGICAL FEATURES

- Virtually all cancers of the breast are **adenocarcinoma**.
- The most common form is **invasive ductal carcinoma** (80%).
- Other forms:
  - Invasive lobular carcinoma
  - Medullary carcinoma
  - Tubular carcinoma
  - Mucinous carcinoma
  - Inflammatory breast cancer
- 70% express estrogen (ER) or progesterone (PR) receptors.

INVASIVE DUCTAL CARCINOMA

- Most common histological subtype of breast cancer
  - Accounts for 80% of all mammary tumours.
- Tumours are graded 1–3 according to the degree of nuclear atypia and tubule differentiation.

INVASIVE LOBULAR CARCINOMA

- Represents up to 15% of all breast cancers.
- Represents approximately 10% of all invasive breast cancers.
- Tend to be multicentric and can be bilateral.
- Size frequently underestimated radiologically.

DUCTAL CARCINOMA IN SITU

- Pre-malignant condition.
- 10–15% develop invasive carcinoma.
- Mammogram frequently shows microcalcifications.
- Pathologically graded: **Low, intermediate, and high grade**.
- DCIS is treated with wide local excision with clear margins.
- Mastectomy is needed for large lesions and multicentric disease.
- High-grade DCIS is treated with post-operative radiotherapy after lumpectomy (but not mastectomy).
- Axillary surgery is not needed.

CLINICAL FEATURES

- **Breast lump**
  - Most common symptom.
  - Usually painless.
  - Hard irregular lump.
  - Can be immobile, tethered or fixed (attached to chest wall).
- **Nipple abnormalities**
  - Bloody discharge.
  - Recent nipple inversion (involvement of Cooper's ligament), distortion or deviation.
- **Skin changes**
  - **Dimpling**, tethering, rash, colour change or ulceration.
  - Late presentation may be with skin ulceration or tumour ulcerating through the skin.
  - Peau d'orange: Sensation of the texture of an orange peel arises as a result of tumour invasion of the dermal lymphatics causing dermal oedema Figure 8.1.

CLASSICAL SIGNS OF BREAST CARCINOMA

- Hard irregular breast lump
- Skin tethering or dimpling
- Recent nipple inversion
- Bloody nipple discharge
- Skin ulceration
- Peau d'orange

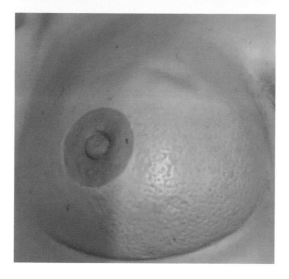

Figure 8.1   Image of Peau d'orange.

INVESTIGATIONS

- All breast lumps or suspected carcinomas are investigated with triple assessment.
- Triple assessment results must be discussed at the multidisciplinary team (MDT) meeting.

TRIPLE ASSESSMENT

- **Clinical assessment**
  - Accurate history and breast examination.

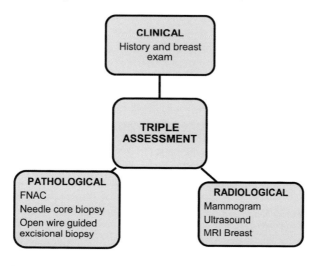

Figure 8.2   Triple assessment.

- **Radiological assessment**
  - Mammogram
    - Those over 35 years old.
    - Two-view, lateral and oblique.
    - Suspicious findings: Mass, microcalcifications, stellate/spiculated mass.
    - Overall sensitivity 77–95%.
    - For women <35 the sensitivity of mammography is low due to the high density of the breast tissue which obstructs the view.
  - US Breast
    - Used to assess lesions or lumps identified on physical exam or mammogram.
    - Also used to assess the lymph nodes.
  - MRI Breast
    - Used in lobular carcinoma to assess the extent of the disease, multicentricity, and the opposite breast.
- **Pathological assessment**
  - Fine needle aspiration cytology (FNAC)
    - Performed in the outpatient clinic, US-guided.
    - Mainly used to aspirate benign cysts.
    - Does not distinguish between invasive and non-invasive.
    - Not used very much in diagnosis.
  - Needle core biopsy
    - Performed under local anaesthetic.
    - Finds receptor status, differentiates between invasive carcinoma and in situ carcinoma.
    - Gene profile tests: Oncotype diagnosis, used to determine the clinical usefulness and patient benefit of adjuvant chemotherapy.
  - Open wire-guided excisional biopsy (if core biopsy fails)
    - Performed under general anaesthetic.
    - Wire placed under radiological guidance into the area of abnormality used as a guide for the surgeon.
- **Staging investigations** (not routinely done unless positive lymph nodes)
  - Once a diagnosis of cancer is made, staging includes:
    1. Staging CT TAP
    2. Liver US, bone scan, LFTs, serum calcium

Table 8.1   American Joint Committee on Cancer TNM Classification

AJCC TNM (Tumour, Node and Metastasis) Classification		
Stage (Simplified)	TNM	5-Year Survival
I	T1, N0	>85%
IIA IIB	T1N1, T2N0 T2N1, T3N0	>70%
IIIA IIIB IIIC	T3N1, T1-3N2 T4, peau d'orange, ulceration, satellite metastases T1-3 with any N3	<50%
IV	Distant metastasis	<20%

Table 8.2   TNM Staging

T/N/M	Stage	Description
T (Primary)	Tis	Carcinoma in situ
	T0	No primary tumour located
	T1	Tumour < 2 cm
	T2	Tumour 2–5 cm
	T3	Tumour > 5 cm
	T4	Extension into chest wall
N (Nodes)	N0	No nodal involvement
	N1	Mobile ipsilateral axillary nodes
	N2	Fixed ipsilateral axillary nodes
	N3	Ipsilateral supraclavicular nodes
M (Metastases)	M0	No metastases
	M1	Distant metastases

SURGICAL MANAGEMENT

- **Tumour resection**
  - Mainstay of non-metastatic disease.
  - **Breast-conserving therapy (BCT)–wide local excision.**
    - Most common procedure.
    - Provided breast is adequate size and tumour location is appropriate to ensure clear margins Table 8.3.
    - Usually combined with external beam radiotherapy to residual breast to reduce risk of local recurrence.

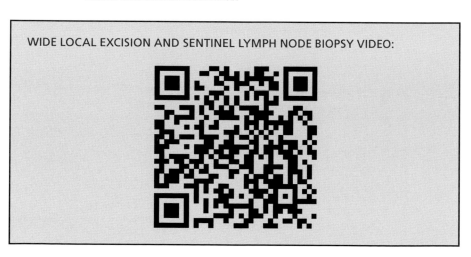

WIDE LOCAL EXCISION AND SENTINEL LYMPH NODE BIOPSY VIDEO:

- **Simple mastectomy**
  - Best local treatment and cosmetic result for:
    - Large tumours (especially in small breast)
    - Late presentation with complications such as ulceration
    - Multi-centric disease or where there is widespread disease.

Table 8.3 Contraindication for Breast-Conserving Therapy

Absolute Contraindication for BCT	Relative Contraindication for BCT
Multifocal disease	Small breast size
History of previous radiation therapy to the area of treatment	Large tumour size (>5 cm)
First or second trimester of pregnancy	Connective tissue disease
Inability to undergo radiation therapy for invasive disease	
Persistent positive margins after attempts at conservation	

- Performed with reconstruction at the same time (immediate) or later stage (delayed).
  - **Implant reconstruction**
    - Tissue expanders
    - Saline/Silicone implants
  - **Autologous Figure 8.3**
    - Free flap: Deep inferior epigastric perforator (DIEP) flap Figure 8.4
    - Pedicle flap: Latissimus dorsi (LD) flap

- **Regional lymph nodes**
  - **Sentinel node biopsy**
    - One or two nodes primarily draining tumour is identified by radioactive tracer (technetium 99) and blue dye injected around tumour.
    - Sentinel node is described as 'hot and blue' as a result of the accumulation of both the radioactive material and the blue dye due to lymphatic drainage.

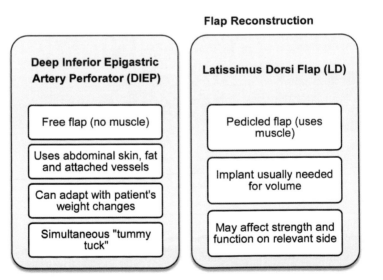

Flap Reconstruction

Figure 8.3 Flap reconstruction.

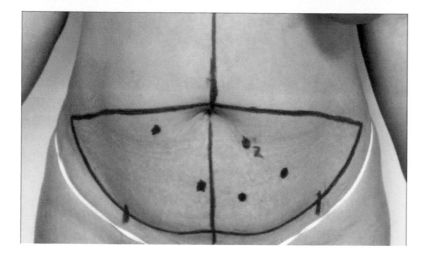

Figure 8.4 Mapping of DIEP flap for breast reconstructive surgery. Courtesy of Mr Jamie Martin-Smith

- – If positive nodes are identified, then a full axillary clearance is required.
- – Avoids major axillary surgery where not necessary.
- ● **Axillary node clearance**
  - – Involves three levels: Lateral, behind and medial to the pectoral muscles.
  - – Associated with risk of ipsilateral arm lymphoedema (20–40%) and axillary numbness (80%).
  - – Potential nerve complication:
    - – Long thoracic nerve (winging of the scapula).
    - – Thoracodorsal nerve.
- ● **Metastatic disease**
  - ● Limited for symptomatic control of local disease e.g. mastectomy for fungating tumour.

MEDICAL MANAGEMENT

- ● In non-metastatic disease, medical therapy is utilised to reduce the risk of systemic relapse, usually after primary surgery as adjuvant therapy.
- ● Occasionally used as a treatment of choice of elderly or those unfit/inappropriate for surgery.
- ● **Endocrine (hormonal) therapy**
  - ● Tamoxifen for 5–10 years
    - – Selective ER modulator antagonist.
    - – Used in ER +ve patients (**pre-menopausal**).
  - ● Anastrozole (Arimidex)
    - – Aromatase inhibitor.
    - – Used in ER +ve patients (**post-menopausal**)
    - – Caution with osteoporosis due to side effect of reduced bone density.

- **Targeted therapy**
  - Trastuzumab (Herceptin):
    - Antibody directed at HER2/neu receptors.
    - Used in HER2 receptor positive patients.
  - Lapatinib
    - Tyrosine kinase inhibitor which binds to the tyrosine kinase domains of EGFR and HER2/neu receptors, inhibiting signal transduction.
    - Used in HER2 receptor positive advanced breast cancer patients in combination with other medical treatments.
- **Chemotherapy**
  - Offered to some patients with tumours that have spread or are at high risk of spreading/recurrence.
    - +ve nodes, poor grade, large tumours, young patients, positive oncotype DX, high recurrence rate.
  - **Oncotype DX test**
    - Genomic test that analyses the activity of a group of 21 genes that can affect how a cancer is likely to behave and respond to treatment.
    - It is a *prognostic test*: Information about how likely (or unlikely) the breast cancer is to recur, and *predictive test* (likelihood of benefit from chemotherapy) in early-stage ER +ve breast cancer patients.
  - **Examples of chemotherapy agents:**
    - CMF: Cyclophosphamide, methotrexate, 5-FU
    - CA: Cyclophosphamide, anthracycline
    - Taxane based: Paclitaxel, docetaxel
- **Radiotherapy**
  - Offered to patients with:
    - Breast-conserving surgery, high grade tumour, large tumour (≥ 5 cm), 1–4 lymph nodes positive, positive surgical margins.
- **Palliative treatment in metastatic breast cancer** (for symptom management and to increase survival time).
  - Sites of metastases: Lymph nodes, lung, liver, bones, brain.
  - Endocrine therapy: As above.
  - Chemotherapy: As above.
  - Radiotherapy: To reduce pain of bony metastases or symptoms from cerebral or liver disease.

BREAST CANCER SCREENING

BREASTCHECK

- BreastCheck is an Irish government-funded programme.
- The aim is to reduce deaths from breast cancer by diagnosing and treating the disease at an early stage.
- *Women aged 50–69 are offered a free mammogram in 2-year intervals.*
- Screening mammography is used to identify features in the breast suspicious for malignancy e.g. spiculated calcification and microcalcification.

EXTRA READING:

Link to European
Guidelines on Breast Cancer
Diagnosis and Treatment:
https://tinyurl.com/y4b4sldj

BENIGN BREAST DISEASE

FIBROADENOMA
- Benign overgrowth of one lobule of the breast, epithelial and fibrous component.
- Most common under 30, but may occur at any age.
- Features: Painless, mobile, discrete lump.
- Diagnosis: Ultrasound followed by core biopsy.
- Treatment: Excision if >3 cm, for cosmesis, or symptomatic.

BREAST CYSTS
- Fluid filled cysts–may be clear, yellow, green, milky or brown in colour
- Benign.
- Features: Round symmetrical lumps, discrete or multiple, often painful.
- Diagnosis: Fine needle aspiration, triple assessment to exclude malignancy.
- Treatment: Aspiration if symptomatic.

FIBROCYSTIC DISEASE
- Non-cancerous breast lumps which can sometimes cause discomfort.
- Often periodically related to hormonal influences from the menstrual cycle.
- Occurs between 15–55 years.
- Features: Swelling, 'lumpy' breasts, multiple breast cysts.
- Diagnosis: Triple assessment to exclude malignancy.
- Treatment: Reassurance, proper fitting bra, evening primrose oil to relieve discomfort.

BREAST INFECTIONS
- Lactational infections
  - Due to staphylococcal infection.
  - Treatment with oral antimicrobial and aspiration if abscess present.
- Recurrent mastitis and duct ectasia
  - Chronic inflammation of the subareolar mammary ducts.
  - Associated with smoking.
  - Bacteria rarely found
  - Presents with recurrent greenish-yellow nipple discharge or breast abscess.
  - Treat with broad spectrum antibiotics and drainage of the abscess.

FAT NECROSIS

- Necrosis of the adipose tissue in the breast as a result of traumatic injury.

GYNAECOMASTIA

- Benign growth of the breast tissue in males usually due to imbalance in the estrogen levels compared to androgens in the breast leading to increased estrogenic activity.
- In young males: Cannabis is the most common cause.
- In elderly men: Spironolactone is the most common cause.
- Other causes:
    - Hypogonadism (Klinefelter's syndrome).
    - Hyperthyroidism.
    - Chronic liver disease.
    - Neoplasms secreting estrogens or their precursors.
    - Medications: Estrogen, cimetidine, anabolic steroids/androgens.
- Management
    - Exclude neoplasm (mammography +/− core biopsy).
    - Conservative: Tamoxifen.
    - Surgery: If symptomatic.

MCQs FOR SELF-ASSESSMENT

Chapter 9

ENDOCRINE DISORDERS

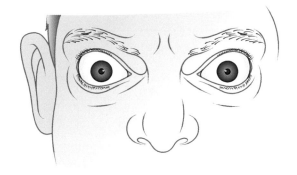

DOI: 10.1201/9781003207184-9

CONTENTS

Anatomical Review	183
Types of Thyroid Disease	185
Differential Diagnosis of Neck Swelling	186
Investigation of Thyroid Disorders	187
Thyroidectomy	189
Thyrotoxicosis	189
Graves' Disease	192
Thyroid Cancer	194
Papillary Thyroid Cancer	194
Follicular Thyroid Cancer	195
Medullary Thyroid Cancer	195
Anaplastic Thyroid Cancer	196
Primary Hyperparathyroidism	197
Secondary and Tertiary Hyperparathyroidism	199
Phaeochromocytoma	199
Cortisol Excess and Cushing's Disease	200
Conn's Syndrome (Primary Hyperaldosteronism)	202

ANATOMICAL REVIEW

THYROID GLAND

- The thyroid is formed from **two triangular lobes** (the left and right) connected by a central isthmus overlying the 2nd and 3rd tracheal rings.
- Found between the levels of **C5-T1**, invested within the pretracheal fascia Figure 9.1.

Table 9.1   Thyroid Vasculature

Arterial supply
Inferior and superior thyroid arteries
Venous drainage
Superior, middle and inferior thyroid veins
Lymphatic drainage
Prelaryngeal, pretracheal and paratracheal nodes

PARATHYROID GLANDS

- Two pairs in total, generally found on the posterior aspect of the thyroid gland, also within the pretracheal fascia.

IMPORTANT NEARBY STRUCTURES

- The **external laryngeal branch** of the superior laryngeal nerve (vagal branch) passes medial to the superior portion of the gland to innervate cricothyroid muscle.

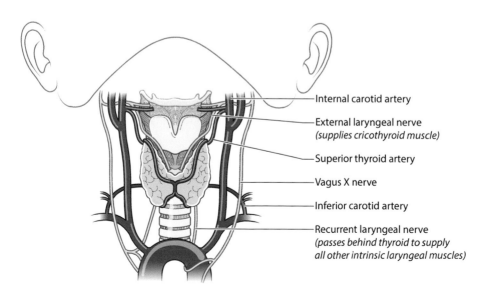

Figure 9.1   Surgical anatomy of the thyroid.

- The **recurrent laryngeal nerve** (vagal branch in root of neck/superior mediastinum) lies between the trachea and oesophagus, emerging medial to the inferior portion of the gland. Passes along the medial surface of each thyroid lobe before entering the larynx the inferior cornu of the thyroid cartilage.

 Top tip: The recurrent laryngeal nerve is very vulnerable during thyroid and parathyroid surgery!

CENTRAL CONTROL

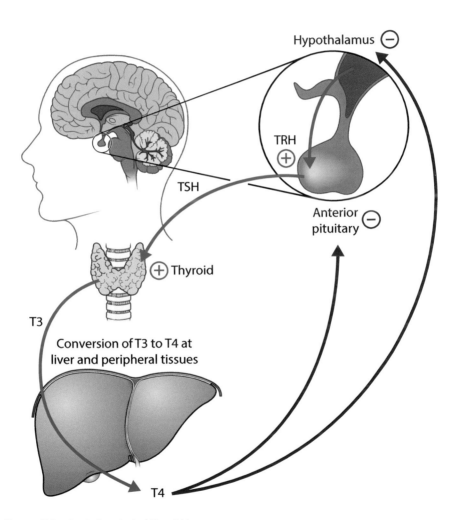

Figure 9.2   Central control of thyroid hormones.

Table 9.2   Thyroid Function Tests

Thyroid Function Tests (TFTs)	TSH	T4
Hyperthyroidism	↓	↑
Hypothyroidism	↑	↓

Table 9.3   Clinical Presentation of Hyperthyroidism

Hyperthyroidism
Behavioural: Hyperactivity/irritability/restlessness
Cardiac: Tachycardia/palpitations
Mood: Mood swings/nervousness/panic attacks
Eyes: Protruded/puffy eyes
Sleep: Insomnia
Menstrual: Irregular menstruation or short and light menstruation

Table 9.4   Clinical Presentation of Hypothyroidism

Hypothyroidism
General: Fatigue/lethargy/feeling cold/weight gain
Behavioural: Sluggishness
Cardiac: Bradycardia
Menstrual: Irregular uterine bleeding

Top tip:

Hyperthyroidism = Increased metabolism.
Hypothyroidism = Decreased metabolism.

TYPES OF THYROID DISEASE

Table 9.5   Types of Thyroid Disease

Graves' disease	Hyperthyroidism, goitre, eye disease, and pretibial/localised myxoedema.
Hashimoto's thyroiditis	Chronic autoimmune thyroiditis, female:male (7:1). High TPO and thyroglobulin antibodies. Hypothyroidism is characteristic. Surgery is rarely required.

(continued)

Table 9.5 Types of Thyroid Disease (*continued*)

Amiodarone-induced	Can cause hyper- and hypothyroidism. Amiodarone inhibits mono-deiodination of T4, blocks T3 receptors, and has a direct toxic effect that leads to follicular destruction.
Iodine deficiency	May present with a diffuse goitre. Usually painless and slow growing. Occurs in areas with low naturally occurring iodine levels and no dietary supplements.
Cystic thyroid nodule	Also known as a 'simple cyst.' May lead to thyroid pain and dysphagia (due to sudden haemorrhage or haemorrhagic infarction of cyst).
Thyroglossal cyst	Midline structures that move with protrusion of the tongue. Forms in the thyroglossal duct and may be found at any point along this structure. 40% present in adulthood. Excised using the **Sistrunk procedure**.
Thyroiditis	**Acute** suppurative thyroiditis is extremely rare and is managed with antibiotics and surgical drainage as appropriate. **Subacute** (de Quervain's): Often painful, usually a self-limiting condition that involves the enlargement of one or both lobes. Inflammatory markers may be raised. Occasionally steroids are necessary for treatment. **Chronic** (Reidels'): Mimics malignancy, presents as a woody, hard swelling. Can co-exist with sclerosing cholangitis or retroperitoneal fibrosis. Resection of the isthmus may be required in the event of a compromised airway.

DIFFERENTIAL DIAGNOSIS OF NECK SWELLING

Table 9.6 Differential Diagnosis of Neck Swelling

	Posterior Triangle	Anterior Triangle	Midline
Congenital	Cystic hygroma: Zenker's diverticulum	Branchial cleft cyst	Thyroglossal cyst
Inflammatory (most neck lumps)	Post-viral lymphadenopathy Bacterial/suppurative lymphadenopathy: • Mycobacteria • Actinomycosis • Brucellosis • HIV		-
Neoplastic	Metastatic • Lung, oesophagus, breast, SCC of the aerodigestive tract Salivary gland • 80% in parotid Lymphoma Lipoma	Thyroid Carotid body tumours/ chemodectoma	-

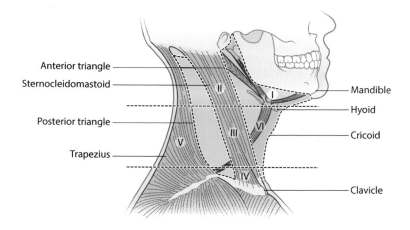

Figure 9.3   Anatomy of the neck.

Notes: I–VI = anatomical levels to describe the location of a cervical lymph node.

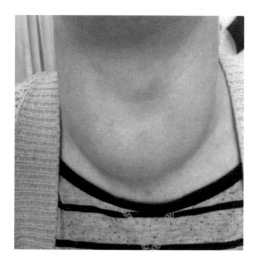

Figure 9.4   Image of a goitre. Courtesy of Prof Tom Walsh

INVESTIGATION OF THYROID DISORDERS

BLOODS

- **TFTs:** Evaluation of thyroid status using TSH and T4 is essential. It may be useful to also measure T3 Table 9.7.

Table 9.7   Thyroid Function Test

TSH	T4	Diagnosis
↓	Normal	Subclinical/sub-biochemical hyperthyroidism TSH is appropriately suppressed. Check T3 to rule out T3-thyrotoxicosis. Requires monitoring as 5% progress to clinical hyperthyroidism. Repeat TFTs in 8 weeks *Treat if:* • Atrial fibrillation • Symptomatic hyperthyroidism • Osteoporosis in postmenopausal women • Multinodular goitre
↓	↑	Hyperthyroidism
Normal	↑	**Drug related** is often a cause. Check for administration of heparin, amiodarone, propranolol and glucocorticoids. May also indicate peripheral resistance or autoimmune thyroid pathology
↑	Normal	Subclinical/sub-biochemical hypothyroidism Most common in women >60 *Treat if:* • Pregnant • Symptomatic • Hyperlipidaemia and/or atherosclerosis
↑	↓	Hypothyroidism

- **Autoantibodies:** More likely to be elevated in Graves' disease.
  - Anti-TSHR Ab: Anti-thyrotropin receptor antibodies
  - Anti-Tg Ab: Anti-thyroglobulin antibodies
  - Anti-TPO Ab: Anti-thyroid peroxidase antibodies

IMAGING

- Ultrasound (US) is the imaging of choice in thyroid pathology as it is non-invasive and does not expose the patient to radiation.

Table 9.8   Ultrasound Features of the Thyroid

Ultrasonographic Features	
More Likely Malignant	More Likely Benign
• Solid • Irregular margins • Microcalcifications • Increased vascularity • Size > 5 cm • Lymphadenopathy	• Cystic • Smooth • Macrocalcifications

- **Nuclear imaging–scintigraphy**
  - Uses technetium.
  - This form of imaging does not exclude or confirm cancer.

- 'Hot' nodules demonstrate technetium uptake. Unlikely to be cancer.
- 'Cold' nodules: No technetium uptake. 10% chance of malignancy.
- **CT Neck (non-contrast)** if there is a suspicion of malignancy or retrosternal extension.
  - Also assesses lymphadenopathy/invasion of local structures.

SURVEILLANCE OF A SINGLE NODULE

- <1 cm: Most likely no need for FNAC
- >1 cm and suspicious for malignancy: FNAC

BIOPSY

- Fine needle aspiration cytology (FNAC) under US-guidance is usually performed.
  - Graded similarly to breast cytology i.e. British Thyroid Association, Th1-Th5, or the Bethesda system (USA).
  - This will not show the gland's architecture, but a core biopsy is more risky in the thyroid gland.
- If FNAC does not demonstrate malignancy in a suspicious lesion, repeat in 6 months. If there is still no evidence of disease, malignancy is unlikely.
- Follicular cells are worrisome: 25% will have underlying malignancy.
  - FNAC cannot determine if a follicular lesion or Hurthle cell variant (the only benign thyroid tumours) is benign or not. These patients require lobectomy and the entire lesion needs to be examined histologically to exclude capsular or lymphovascular invasion (the determinants of malignancy).

THYROIDECTOMY

KEY POINT

MDT: Important in managing patients with goitre and thyroid nodules. Input is taken from surgeons, endocrinologists, histopathologists and radiologists.

Table 9.9 Indications for Thyroidectomy

Indications for Thyroidectomy (*the 4 C's*)	
Cancer	Cosmesis
Compression of adjacent structures	Carbimazole (or other medical treatment) failure

THYROTOXICOSIS

DEFINITION

- A hypermetabolic syndrome due to elevated thyroid hormone levels.

Table 9.10 Clinical Presentation of Thyrotoxicosis

Symptoms	Signs–Extremities	Signs–Face
Sweats, tremors, palpitations	Fine tremor	*Graves' Ophthalmopathy:* Proptosis, exophthalmos, chemosis, ophthalmoplegia
Weight loss despite increased appetite	Palmar erythema	
Insomnia	Acropachy	
Anxiety	Onycholysis	
Heat intolerance	Warm and diaphoretic	Any cause of hyperthyroidism: Lid lag, lid retraction, alopecia
Diarrhoea	Fast, irregular pulse	
Oligomenorrhoea	Graves' dermopathy/pretibial myxoedema. 15% of those with eye signs. Was more common, now rarer due to earlier treatment	

Table 9.11 Causes of Thyrotoxicosis

Causes
Graves' disease
Toxic multinodular goitre
Solitary toxic nodule
Thyroiditis • Hashimoto's • Postpartum • De Quervain's
Amiodarone
Complications
Increased risk of atrial fibrillation
Osteoporosis
Thyroid storm

INVESTIGATION OF THYROTOXICOSIS

- **ECG**
  - May demonstrate either sinus tachycardia or atrial fibrillation. The patient may require cardiac monitoring.
- **Biochemical**
  - TFTs–hyperthyroidism (high fT4, low TSH); TSH suppression correlates well with the severity of disease.
  - TPO–may be elevated but is a non-specific marker of autoimmune attack.
- **Ultrasound**
  - Will allow evaluation of goitre or nodules, if any are present.
- **Scintigraphy**
  - Diffuse uptake: Graves'.
  - Patchy uptake: Toxic multinodular.
  - Single area of uptake: Solitary nodule.

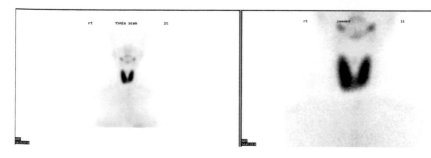

Figure 9.5 (Left and Right) Thyroid uptake scan following administration of pertechnetate. Demonstrates homogeounous tracer uptake. Courtesy of Dr Aoife McErlean

GENERAL MANAGEMENT OF THYROTOXICOSIS

- **Beta blockade:** To minimise the cardiac effects of thyrotoxicosis. Propranolol most commonly used.
- **Anticoagulation:** If atrial fibrillation is uncontrolled.
- **Carbimazole:** Can be used in an acute setting. A high initial dose may be tapered following repeat TFTs.

Top tip: Achieving euthyroid status before surgery is essential to avoid precipitating a thyroid storm.

DEFINITIVE MANAGEMENT OF THYROTOXICOSIS

Table 9.12   Management of Thyrotoxicosis

Graves' disease	**Carbimazole** for 18 months.
	• If disease is refractory, consider **radioiodine** treatment or **surgery**.
	• If thyroid orbitopathy, surgery preferable to radioiodine therapy.
Toxic multinodular (TMN) goitre	**Radioiodine** therapy is the preferred approach, followed by **surgery**, particularly in the presence of a large gland with pressure symptoms or retrosternal extension.
Solitary adenoma	**Surgery** is the preferred approach, followed by **radioiodine** treatment.
Thyroiditis	**Analgesia**, preferably NSAIDs. **Beta blockade**. **Steroids** tapered over 2 weeks.

GRAVES' DISEASE

DEFINITION

- An autoimmune syndrome that presents with hyperthyroidism, a smooth diffusely enlarged goitre (sometimes with a bruit) and other signs and symptoms, listed below.
  - Commonly occurs in women aged 20–40 years old.
  - TSH receptor antibodies.

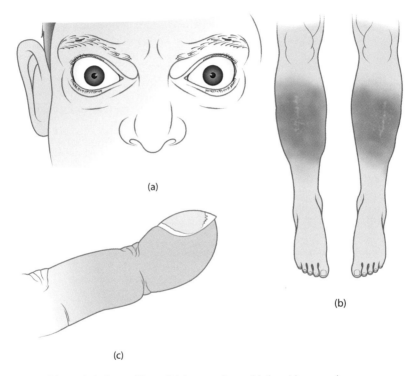

(a)

(b)

(c)

Figure 9.6   (a) Exophthalmos, (b) pretibial myxoedema, (c) thyroid acropachy.

Table 9.13   Thyroid Eye Disease

Proptosis/exophthalmos
Periorbital oedema
Conjunctival injection
Ophthalmoplegia
• Look up to stretch inferior rectus to provoke as the inferior rectus muscle becomes fibrous and tight. The same manoeuvre may be accompanied by a measurable increase in intraocular pressure).

INVESTIGATIONS OF GRAVES' DISEASE

- **TFTs**–High fT4, low TSH (TSH correlates well with the severity of disease).
- **Autoantibodies**
  - TSH receptor antibodies positive.
  - TPO antibodies: Up to 80%.
  - Thyroglobulin antibodies: Up to 70%.
- Scintigraphy will demonstrate increased uptake.

MANAGEMENT OF GRAVES' DISEASE
MEDICAL

- **Beta blocker** for symptom relief.
- **Carbimazole** acts to block the action of TPO, which prevents the formation of thyroid hormone. Requires 18 months of treatment starting with a high dose and titrating down.
- **Propylthiouracil** (PTU) (10× less potent than carbimazole). Blocks conversion of T4 to T3.
  - If someone can't tolerate carbimazole being lowered, consider moving forward with therapy.
  - At 18 months, often 50% remission.
  - If relapse, move on to surgery or radioiodine.
- Side effects of carbimazole/PTU
  - Teratogenicity (more common with carbimazole)
  - Agranulocytosis
  - Hepatotoxicity (more common with PTU)
  - Rash, urticaria, arthralgia

RADIOACTIVE IODINE

- First-line treatment in the USA. Second-line in Europe.
- Transient hyperthyroidism may occur as gland is destroyed.
- 2–5% risk of hypothyroidism per annum after treatment.
  - Need lifelong monitoring.
- Side effects of radioactive iodine treatment.
  - Hypothyroidism.
  - Transient thyroiditis.
  - Transient worsening of Graves' ophthalmopathy.

SURGERY

- **Thyroidectomy** (complete removal of thyroid gland).
- **Subtotal thyroidectomy** (risk of recurrence proportionate to the volume of gland remaining).
- Patient should be euthyroid prior to surgery (decreases vascularity of gland). Lugols iodine may help in this respect.
- **Indications**
  - Cancer.
  - Compression of adjacent structures: Thyroid mass effect.
  - Carbimazole (or other medical therapy) failure.
  - Cosmesis/severe ophthalmopathy.

- **Benefits**
  - Avoids long-term risks of radioactive iodine.
  - Provides tissue for histology.
- Children, young women and pregnant women (second trimester) are ideal candidates.
- If Graves' ophthalmopathy is present, total thyroidectomy is indicated.

THYROID CANCER

Table 9.14   Types of Thyroid Cancers

Types of Thyroid Cancers	Approximate Proportional Values
Papillary carcinoma	80%
Follicular carcinoma	10%
Medullary carcinoma	4%
Anaplastic carcinoma	<3%

PAPILLARY THYROID CANCER

Table 9.15   Epidemiology of Thyroid Cancer

Epidemiology	Risk Factors
- Incidence of 12.5 per 100,000 - Female:male = 2.5:1 - Most commonly occurs in those aged 30–50 years old	- Radiation exposure - Family history

PATHOLOGICAL FEATURES

- NOT encapsulated.
- May be partially cystic.
- Papillae consisting of one or two layers of tumour cells surround a well-defined fibro-vascular core.
- Follicles and colloid typically absent.
- Approximately one-half will contain psammoma bodies.

METASTATIC ACTIVITY

- 2–10% of patients will have metastatic disease at presentation.
- Of these, 2/3 have pulmonary disease and 1/4 have skeletal disease.
- Rarer sites include the brain, kidneys, liver and adrenals.

PROGNOSTIC FACTORS

- **Age:** Younger age at diagnosis is a positive prognostic factor.
- **Tumour size:** Smaller tumour size is a positive prognostic factor.

- **Soft tissue invasion:** Negative prognostic factor.
- **Distant metastases:** Negative prognostic factor.
- Overall, the prognosis in papillary cancer is good. One series demonstrated a 6% mortality for patients with non-metastatic disease over 16 years.

FOLLICULAR THYROID CANCER

Table 9.16   Epidemiology of Follicular Thyroid Cancer

Epidemiology	Risk Factors
• Female:male = 3:1 • Most commonly in 50–70 year olds	• Radiation exposure • Family history • Iodine deficiency

PATHOLOGICAL FEATURES

- Well-differentiated tumour of the thyroid epithelium.
- Capsulated.
- Colloid may be present and is a positive prognostic indicator.
- Hurthle cell and insular variants are somewhat more aggressive.

METASTATIC ACTIVITY

- Lymphatic involvement seen in 8–13% of cases.
- Distant metastases seen in 10–15% of patients.
- Typically spreads haematogenously to bone (lytic lesions) and lungs.
- May also involve the brain, liver, bladder and skin.
- Metastases may be hormonally active, leading to hyperthyroidism.

MEDULLARY THYROID CANCER

DEFINITION

- A neuroendocrine tumour of the parafollicular or C cells of the thyroid gland.
- The production of calcitonin is a feature. CEA may also be expressed by medullary cancers.
  - Flushing and diarrhoea will be present if calcitonin levels are high.
- TFTs usually normal.
- May be sporadic or occur as part of an inherited syndrome (MEN2).
  - Sporadic: 80% of cases with a slight female preponderance. Present with a single nodule and often cervical lymphadenopathy.
  - Familial: As part of MEN2.
- Prior to surgical treatment, patients must be evaluated for other neuroendocrine tumours.

ANAPLASTIC THYROID CANCER

DEFINITION
- Undifferentiated tumours of thyroid follicular epithelium.
- Aggressive; disease specific mortality approaching 100%.

AETIOLOGY
- Typically in older women and presents with a rapidly enlarging neck mass.
- About 20% will have synchronous differentiated cancers.

TREATMENT
- Early palliative care input important.
- Usually no indication for surgical intervention.
- Chemotherapy and radiotherapy may be used to provide symptomatic relief.

Table 9.17   Clinical Features of Anaplastic Thyroid Cancer

Thyroid Cancer Signs and Symptoms
Appearance of thyroid node/neck lump
History of rapid growth
Fixation of a thyroid node to over or underlying structures
New onset hoarseness or vocal cord paralysis
Ipsilateral cervical lymphadenopathy
May be an incidental finding on imaging

INVESTIGATIONS
- **ECG**
- **Biochemical**
  - TFTs
  - FBC, U&E, LFTs
- **Imaging**
  - US
  - Scintigraphy
  - Staging CT may be necessary
    - **NB** If you suspect cancer, do NOT use contrast (delays/interferes with radioiodine)
- **Pre-surgical workup**
  - Evaluate the patient's fitness for surgery.
  - Anaesthetic review is often indicated.
  - Patients may require an ECG.

TREATMENT
- **Multidisciplinary Team (MDT) Meeting:** Treatment is largely determined by histological type. Radiology and Endocrinology specialist input are paramount in planning treatment. Most suspected thyroid cancers are discussed at MDT.

- **Thyroidectomy**
  - Mainstay of treatment. Thyroid lobectomy in smaller cancers.
  - Modified radical neck dissection if clinical or radiological (US, CT, Radioiodine scan) evidence of metastatic disease.
- **Thyroidectomy complications**
  - Early: Strap haematoma, transient hypoparathyroidism (8%), hypocalcaemia, side effects of anaesthesia, seroma, laryngeal nerve injuries, vocal cord paresis.
  - Intermediate: Infection.
  - Late: Permanent hypoparathyroidism (2%).
- **Radiotherapy**
  - May use radioiodine following surgery and MDM to control occult disease (micro-metastases).
  - External beam radiation used in anaplastic cancer to reduce tumour size and symptoms but does not improve survival.
- **Medical Management**
  - Following total thyroidectomy, patients will require lifelong thyroid hormone replacement using a higher dose than for replacement therapy in order to suppress TSH as differentiated thyroid tumours are hormone dependent.

Top tip:

Strap Haematoma: Rare but life-threatening complication of thyroid surgery that may lead to airway obstruction!

KEY POINT

Strap Haematoma is an EMERGENCY that requires immediate decompression by opening of deep wound layers to relieve tension before taking to patient theatre to secure the bleeding vessel.

PRIMARY HYPERPARATHYROIDISM

AETIOLOGY

- 85% of cases due to a solitary adenoma.
- 10–15% of patients will have enlargement of multiple glands, sometimes in the context of MEN syndromes.
- Parathyroid cancer and ectopic adenomas are rare (occasionally intrathoracic).
- Now seen more commonly due to widespread serum auto-analysis (serendipity syndrome).
- Incidence 3/1000 general population; 21/1000 in women 55–75 years.

DIAGNOSIS

- Diagnostic:
  - High corrected calcium.

- High PTH.
- Increased 24-hour urinary calcium excretion.
  - This helps exclude familial hypocalciuric hypercalcaemia.
- Imaging of the gland responsible aids planning minimally invasive surgery and can help in cases of ectopic parathyroid glands.
  - Sestamibi
  - US

TREATMENT

- **Acute:** Correction of serum calcium is essential.
  - IV access and administer IVF. May require 5–7 L per day.
  - Monitor urine output.
  - Furosemide may be used once adequate hydration is achieved.
  - Avoid bisphosphonates if surgery is anticipated.
- **Definitive:** Parathyroidectomy
  - The four parathyroid glands are typically pea-sized and found on the posterior aspect of the thyroid gland.
  - Isolating the responsible gland prior to surgery may allow for a minimally invasive technique to be employed.
  - Intraoperative PTH measurement can provide evidence of curative surgery.
  - Serum calcium must be monitored during the post-operative period.

PRESENTATION

- Mostly asymptomatic (often an incidental finding of hypercalcaemia)

Table 9.18   Clinical Features of Primary Hyperparathyroidism

System	Symptoms and Signs	Complications
Renal	**STONES** Polyuria, polydipsia	Urinary tract stones, renal insufficiency
Psychiatric/ neurological	**MOANS** Parasthesia, reduced deep tendon reflexes	Depression, dementia, psychosis
Skeletal	**BONES** Bone pain	Arthritis (pseudogout), osteopenia/ osteoporosis/osteitis fibrosa cystica (due to bone resorption), pathological fractures
GIT	**GROANS** Abdominal pain, constipation, vomiting	Pancreatitis, PUD
Generalised	**FATIGUE OVERTONES** Fatigue, malaise, weakness, muscle cramps	–
Cardiovascular	–	Hypertension, dysrhythmias, short QT

SECONDARY AND TERTIARY HYPERPARATHYROIDISM

Table 9.19   Clinical Features of Secondary and Tertiary Hyperparathyroidism

	Secondary	Tertiary
Aetiology	Hyperplasia in all four glands due to chronic hypocalcaemia Hypocalcemia from • Chronic kidney disease • Phosphate malabsorption and vitamin D deficiency	Autonomous PTH secretion due to hyperplasia/adenomatous changes in parathyroid glands after prolonged secondary hyperparathyroidism Causes renal osteodystrophy
Biochemistry	• High PTH • Low calcium • High/normal Phosphate NB: (phosphate is usually raised in the setting of a non-parathyroid cause)	• High PTH • High calcium • Phosphate is <u>not</u> elevated
Treatment	Treat underlying cause • Phosphate binders • Diet change • Parathyroidectomy	Parathyroidectomy of 3.5 glands • Remaining ½ gland can be left in the neck or implanted into the upper arm

Malignant Hyperparathyroidism: Parathyroid hormone-related peptide (PTHrP) can be secreted by some malignant tumours: small cell carcinoma of the lung; breast carcinoma; renal cell carcinoma.

PHAEOCHROMOCYTOMA

DEFINITION

- Catecholamine-producing tumours of the neural crest.
- Arise from chromaffin cells of the adrenal medulla (phaeochromocytoma) or sympathetic ganglia (catecholamine-secreting paragangliomas).

AETIOLOGY

- Rare: Incidence of 2–8/million per year.
- Most common in the 4th and 5th decade of life.
- Phaeochromocytomas may occur as part of familial syndromes such as MEN and VHL.

Table 9.20   Rule of 10s for Phaeochromocytoma

Rule of 10s (Now a Controversial Rule, But a Useful Learning Tool)			
10% bilateral	10% extra-adrenal	10% malignant	10% recur
10% normotensive	10% calcify	10% children	10% familial

PRESENTATION

- **Classic triad:** Episodic headache, sweating and tachycardia.
- Sustained or paroxysmal hypertension (85–95% of patients).
- Headache (up to 90%).
- Generalised sweating (60–70%).
- Other: Palpitations, tremor, pallor, panic attacks, weakness and dyspnoea.
- Increased availability of imaging has led to an increase of asymptomatic presentation.

INVESTIGATIONS

- **24-hour urine collection** of fractionated catecholamines and metanephrines: The most specific (98%) and sensitive (98%) test for diagnosis.
- **Plasma fractionated metanephrines** have a high false positive rate. Only examine in patients with a high index of suspicion.
- **CT/MRI** imaging to locate the tumour.
- **MIBG scan** may be useful for metastatic or ectopic disease (paraganglioma in islets of Zukerkandl).

TREATMENT

- Mainstay of treatment is **total adrenalectomy** (partial resection is indicated in bilateral disease).
- Prior to treatment, substances known to provoke phaeochromocytoma paroxysms must be avoided (metoclopramide, glucagon and histamine).
- Alpha-adrenergic blockade 10–14 days prior to surgery to control hypertension and to encourage volume expansion.
- Beta-adrenergic blockade 2–3 days prior to surgery, once sufficient alpha-blockade is achieved.
- Laparoscopic resection is possible in approximately 90% of patients.
- Malignant tumours can only be identified by their metastatic activity, which commonly involves local organs. Distant metastases may occur up to 20 years following resection. As such, patients require long-term follow-up.

CORTISOL EXCESS AND CUSHING'S DISEASE

Table 9.21   Clinical Features of Cushing's Disease

Clinical Features
Weight gain (buffalo hump; truncal obesity)
Muscle wasting (lemon on a stick)
Striae
Facial plethora (moon facies)
Thinning of the skin, easy bruising
Mood changes: Lethargy, depression, suicidal ideation, psychosis
Menstrual irregularities
Hirsutism in women, hair loss in men
Glucose intolerance, diabetes

CAUSES

- **Iatrogenic**
- **Primary adrenal disease**
  - Unilateral: Adrenal adenoma (10%) or carcinoma.
  - Bilateral: ACTH-independent bilateral adrenal hyperplasia.
- **Secondary adrenal disease**
  - Cushing's disease: ACTH-secreting pituitary adenoma.
- **Ectopic ACTH secretion**

INVESTIGATIONS

- **Cortisol levels**
  - High (morning peak and midnight nadir pattern is lost).
  - 24-hour urinary cortisol elevated.
- **Overnight dexamethasone suppression test**
  - 1 mg dexamethasone given.
  - In normal patients, morning cortisol will be low.
- **High-dose dexamethasone suppression test**
  - 2 mg dexamethasone given QDS for 24 hours.
  - To distinguish pituitary or ectopic source of ACTH-dependant Cushing's syndrome.
  - Pituitary will still show some inhibition, ectopic will not.
  - This will not inhibit primary adrenal or ectopic disease and cortisol levels will be unaffected.
- **ACTH**
  - High in patients with pituitary adenomas and ectopic production.
  - Low in primary adrenal disease.
- **CT/MRI** in order to localise tumours.

TREATMENT

- Iatrogenic
  - Taper and stop exogenous glucocorticoids
- Adrenal adenoma
  - Surgical excision, unilateral adrenalectomy
- ACTH-independent bilateral adrenal hyperplasia
  - Bilateral adrenalectomy
- Cushing's disease
  - Trans-sphenoidal resection
- Ectopic ACTH secreting tumours
  - Excision

POST-OPERATIVE MANAGEMENT

- Following surgical resection of adrenal glands, patients will require cortisol replacement.
- Even following unilateral excision, cortisol levels may take several months to recover.
- Patients may be administered hydrocortisone in the post-operative setting and switched to oral agents such as prednisolone.

- Following <u>bilateral</u> adrenalectomy, patients will require lifelong cortisol <u>and</u> mineralocorticoid replacement.
- Patients should be counseled about the risk of an Addisonian crisis and be given suitable advice regarding illness and medical alert jewellery.

CONN'S SYNDROME (PRIMARY HYPERALDOSTERONISM)

DEFINITION

- Usually autonomous aldosterone secretion by adrenocortical tissue (zona glomerulosa).
- Commonly a single benign adenoma. Occasionally micro- or macronodular bilateral disease. Aldosterone-secreting cancer is extremely rare.

Table 9.22   Clinical Features of Conn's Syndrome

Clinical Features
Hypertension
Hypokalemia (not always)
Hypernatremia (not always)
Metabolic alkylosis (not always)
Fluid retention
Reduced plasma renin activity (PRA)

Table 9.23   Complications of Conn's Syndrome

Complications
Hypertension
Cardiac arrhythmias
Cardiac fibrosis
Increased cardiac mortality

INVESTIGATIONS

- **Biochemical:** Failure of aldosterone suppression with sodium load or fludrocortisone suppression test.
  - Plasma aldosterone: Renin ratio.
- **Imaging:** CT/MRI. Adrenal vein sampling with measurement of aldosterone cortisol and renin. This allows localisation, particularly useful when bilateral findings on CT.
- **General:** Monitor BP, electrolytes, ABG, ECG, TTE.

TREATMENT

- Classic Conn's syndrome with a solitary adenoma: Laparoscopic or retroperitoneo-scopic adrenalectomy.
  - Small lesions may allow partial adrenalectomy.
- Bilateral disease dependent on localisation studies.
  - If bilateral secretion, probably best managed by medical therapy with aldosterone agonists (spironolactone or eplerenone).

MCQs FOR SELF-ASSESSMENT

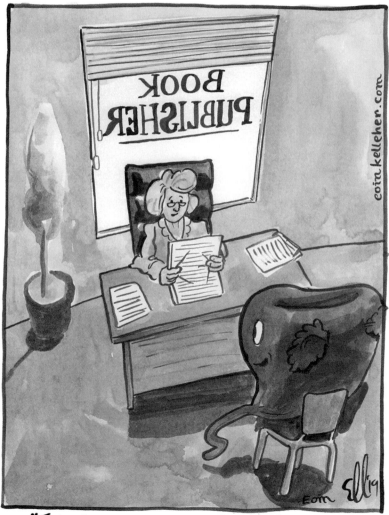

"This is a seminal work, Mr Prostate."

DOI: 10.1201/9781003207184-10

CONTENTS

Common Urological Devices	207
Acute Urinary Retention (AUR)	211
Benign Prostatic Hyperplasia	213
Urinary Tract Stones	215
Renal Cell Carcinoma	219
Bladder Cancer	221
Prostate Cancer	223
Testicular Tumours	225
Acute Testicular Pain	227
Testicular Torsion	227
Torsion of the Appendix Testis/Hydatid of Morgagni	228
Acute Epididymo-Orchitis	228
Renal Transplant	229

COMMON UROLOGICAL DEVICES

URINARY CATHETERS

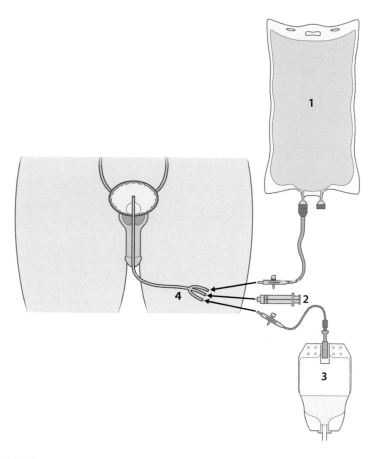

Figure 10.1 Three-way urinary catheter. (1) Irrigation fluid bag that is hung up. (2) Syringe to inflate catheter balloon within the bladder. (3) Urine collection bag. (4) The 3-way urinary catheter.

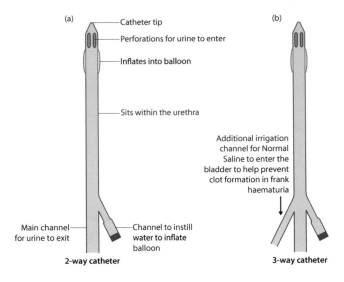

(a)
Catheter tip
Perforations for urine to enter
Inflates into balloon
Sits within the urethra

(b)
Additional irrigation channel for Normal Saline to enter the bladder to help prevent clot formation in frank haematuria

Main channel for urine to exit
Channel to instill water to inflate balloon

2-way catheter

3-way catheter

Figure 10.2   Left and right. Types of urinary catheters.

SUPRAPUBIC CATHETER

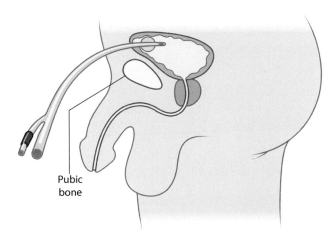

Pubic bone

Figure 10.3   Suprapubic catheter. The catheter is the same type used in urethra urinary catheters. It is inserted through a transcutaneous approach into a full distended bladder.

NEPHROSTOMY

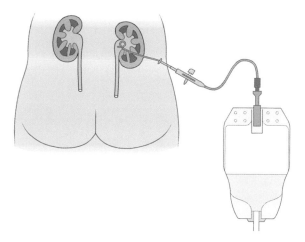

Figure 10.4 Nephrostomy. On physical exam, the wound can be found in/near the renal angle. This is inserted by an interventional radiologist in the setting of urinary tract obstruction causing hydronephrosis.

JJ URETERIC STENT

A stent may be placed within the ureter to bypass any obstruction (e.g. calculi or stricture or tumour).

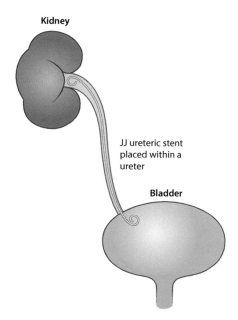

Figure 10.5 JJ ureteric stent.

The stent can be inserted anterograde via nephrostomy or retrograde via cystoscopy. The two curls on either ends of the stent hold it in place and stop it from migrating.

UROSTOMY OR ILEAL CONDUIT

The ureters are diverted into an isolated portion of small bowel that opens to the abdominal surface as a stoma. Output of the stoma into the stoma bag will be urine only. A urostomy may be formed after a procedure like radical cystectomy.

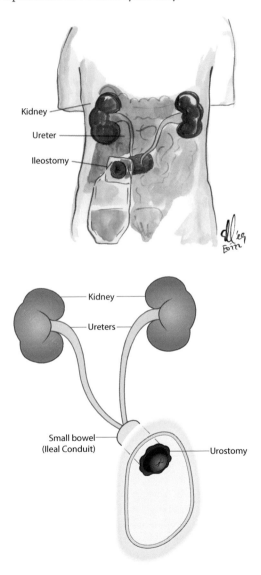

Figure 10.6 Ileostomy and Urostomy.

ACUTE URINARY RETENTION (AUR)

EPIDEMIOLOGY

- Male:female = 13:1.
- Overall incidence rate 6.8/1000.
- Increases with age: 60-year-old men have a 20% chance of developing AUR over a 20-year period.

AETIOLOGY

- **Mechanical obstruction (most common cause).**
  - Benign prostatic hyperplasia (BPH) is the most common underlying condition in men with AUR.
- Constipation.
- Haematuria causing clot retention.
- Cancer (prostate/bladder, or pelvic cancer in women).
- Urethral stricture.
- Urolithiasis.
- Infection: Cystitis, prostatitis, urethritis.
- Phimosis (especially paediatric patients)
- Prolapse in women: Cystocoele/rectocoele.
- Post-operative/post-partum.
- Medication-induced:
  - **Antimuscarinics:** Decrease bladder sensation and detrusor contractility.
  - **Sympathomimetics:** Increase muscle tone.
  - **Opioids:** Decrease bladder sensation.
- Neurologic impairment (interrupted motor/sensory neural supply):
  - Spinal cord injury: Demyelination, infarction, trauma.
  - Mass: Epidural abscess/metastasis.
  - Guillain-Barré syndrome.
  - Diabetic neuropathy.
  - Stroke.
  - Multiple sclerosis.
  - Cauda equina syndrome.
- Dyssynergia (incomplete urinary sphincter relaxation).
- Inefficient detrusor muscle
  - Most often in patients with baseline obstructive urinary symptoms.
- Trauma to pelvis, urethra, penis.

CLINICAL PRESENTATION

Table 10.1 Clinical Presentation of Acute Urinary Retention

Signs	Symptoms
Suprapubic tenderness.	Inability to pass urine despite urge.
Enlarged palpable bladder that is dull to percussion.	Lower abdominal/suprapubic discomfort.

(continued)

Table 10.1 Clinical Presentation of Acute Urinary Retention (*continued*)

Signs	Symptoms
DRE: Enlarged prostate, mass, loss of perineal sensation, decreased anal tone.	Restlessness/distress/delirium.
Pelvic exam (females): Pelvic mass.	
Neurological exam: Neurological impairment.	

KEY POINT

Acute on Chronic Urinary Retention

Patient may have a previous history of urinary retention. The bladder has a larger capacity from chronic retention and therefore less discomfort with acute retention. They tend to only feel the urge to urinate when there is a much larger volume of urine in the bladder than the average person.

INVESTIGATIONS

- **Bedside bladder scanner:** Ultrasound (US) estimate of volume in bladder. Quick and does not require formal training to use.
- **Urinary catheterisation:** Diagnostic and therapeutic–measures volume of urine output.
- **Blood tests:** WCC and CRP for infection, urea and creatinine for post-renal AKI.
  - PSA is unreliable–will be falsely elevated.
- Post-relief of retention, need to investigate cause:
  - **Urinalysis:** Urine culture and sensitivity for UTIs.
  - **Imaging:** US KUB/pelvis, functional cystogram, MRI spine/brain.
  - **Urodynamics:** Evaluates storage, flow, and voiding ability; sphincter activity and post-void residual volume.
  - **Cystoscopy:** Visualisation of possible strictures/mass.

TREATMENT

- **Urethral catheterisation**
  - Contraindications
    - Recent urological surgery: Radical prostatectomy, urethral reconstruction.
    - Pelvic fracture: Perineal bruising, blood at tip of meatus.
  - Size
    - First line: 14–18 French catheter.
    - Urethral stricture: Smaller 10–12 French catheter.
    - Enlarged prostate: Larger 20–22 French catheter.
  - Complications
    - Urge sensation from irritation (treat with antimuscarinics).
    - Leakage or blockage of catheter.
    - Urethral trauma/strictures/false channel formation.

- Infection, abscess, fistula formation.
- Bladder perforation.
- Urinary incontinence due to bladder neck.
- <u>Post-obstruction relief complications</u>
  - Transient hypotension–usually self-resolves.
  - Post-obstructive diuresis–fluid loss may need to be replaced orally or by IV.
  - Haematuria–rarely significant and usually self-resolves. Due to capillary rupture during bladder distension.
- **Self-intermittent catheterisation (SIC)**
  - Fewer complications than urethral catheterisation, increased spontaneous voiding.
  - Suitable for inpatients with expected temporary AUR.
  - Suitable for outpatients with recurrent acute-on-chronic urinary retention requiring long-term catheterisation or high post-void residual volumes.
  - Outpatients require training regarding technique and hygiene.
- **Suprapubic catheterisation**
  - For patients with contraindications to or failed urethral catheterisation or long-term catheterisation.
  - Usually inserted by urologist/surgeon via transcutaneous route when the bladder is fully distended.
  - Most patients can be managed as outpatients after bladder decompression.
  - Hospitalisation may be required if evidence of urosepsis, malignancy, clot retention or AKI.

> **Top tip:** Bladder decompression treats the symptom. Do not forget to investigate and treat the cause.

BENIGN PROSTATIC HYPERPLASIA

DEFINITION

- Benign enlargement of the prostate gland in the transition zone.

KEY FACTS

- Causes bladder outlet obstruction.
- Occurs in men over 60 years of age, with risk increasing with age.

CLINICAL PRESENTATION

> **Top tip:** Severity of symptoms does not correlate with degree of obstruction.

Table 10.2 Clinical Presentation of Benign Prostatic Hyperplasia

Symptoms	
Obstruction-related (bladder trying to overcome outlet obstruction)	Overactive-related (bladder becomes 'overactive' trying to overcome bladder obstruction)
Poor flow	Frequency
Hesitancy	Urgency
Intermittent stream	Urge incontinence
Dribbling	
Sensation of incomplete bladder emptying/double voiding	
Nocturia	
Signs	
Homogenous enlargement of the prostate on DRE	

INVESTIGATIONS

- **Bloods:** Urea and creatinine–renal function may be affected by chronic retention.
- **PSA:** Evaluate for malignancy.
- **Urine:** Dipstick/culture and sensitivity, rule out infection as a cause of symptoms.
- **Urodynamics** and post-void residual volume.
- **US KUB:** To assess presence of hydronephrosis and prostate size.
- **MRI prostate/TRUS biopsy of prostate** if evidence of prostate malignancy.
- **Cystoscopy** if there is suspicion that bladder disease may be causing the symptoms.

TREATMENT

- **Conservative: Surveillance**
  - For men with mild symptoms and reasonable flowmetry.
  - Watchful waiting until symptoms becomes significant.
  - Decreasing fluid intake at night.
  - Diet changes (i.e. avoiding caffeine and alcohol).
- **Medical**
  - Alpha-adrenergic antagonists (e.g. tamsulosin, silodosin)
    - Inhibit alpha receptors within the smooth muscles of the prostate and bladder neck.
    - Improve voiding symptoms and flow rate but may cause retrograde ejaculation.
  - 5-Alpha reductase inhibitors (e.g. finasteride, dutasteride)
    - Inhibit conversion of testosterone to dihydrotestosterone (DHT).
    - Shrink the prostate by 25–50% if used for >6 months.
    - Decrease PSA by 50% after >9 months (meaning falsely low results if monitoring for prostate cancer)
  - Type 5 phosphodiesterase (PDE5) inhibitors (only one drug approved for use in BPH i.e. tadalafil)
    - Mostly used for erectile dysfunction.

- **Surgical**
  - When medical therapy fails, and complications occur (e.g. urinary retention, recurrent UTIs, significant haematuria, bladder stone formation and renal injury secondary to BPH).
  - **Minimally invasive procedures**
    - Transurethral needle ablation
    - Transurethral microwave thermotherapy
    - UroLift.
  - **Transurethral resection of the prostate** (TURP)
    - Performed via rigid cystoscopy
    - Prostate is resected internally to 'widen the channel.'
  - **Laser therapies**
    - Holmium laser (YAG)
    - Photoselective vaporisation of the prostate (PVP)
    - GreenLight lasers.
  - Transurethral electrovaporisation of the prostate (TUVP).
  - Transurethral incision of the prostate (TUIP).
  - Open, laparoscopic or robotic radical prostatectomy.

COMPLICATIONS OF SURGERY

- Post-operative haemorrhage–most common complication.
- Failure to resolve symptoms.
- Sepsis.
- Urinary incontinence–due to damage of sphincter.
- Retrograde ejaculation and/or erectile dysfunction.
- Urethral strictures–prolonged catheterisation and recurrent instrumentation.
- Prostate cancer may be detected in the resection chips.
- Transurethral resection (TUR) syndrome
  - Due to excessive hypotonic (glycine) irrigation solution absorption during surgery, through venous sinuses of the prostate.
  - Causes dilutional hyponatraemia, hypervolaemia, hypertension and confusion.
  - Treatment includes diuresis and fluid restriction.
  - Risk is reduced when:
    - The surgery time is limited to <1 hour
    - Decreased fluid pressure/hanging height
    - Use of bipolar diathermy and therefore using saline as irrigation fluid.

URINARY TRACT STONES

AETIOLOGY

- **Dehydration/poor fluid intake** (most common)
- Anatomy: Obstruction and stasis of urine e.g. congenital PUJ obstruction
- Hypercalciuria
- Hypomagnesuria

- Hyperuricosuria
- Diet e.g. high potential renal acid load (PRAL)
- Recurrent UTIs
- Disease states:
  - Gout
  - Diabetes mellitus
  - Obesity
  - Type 2 renal tubular acidosis
  - Sarcoidosis
  - Cystinuria
  - Inflammatory bowel disease
  - Hyperparathyroidism
  - Medullary sponge kidney
  - Adult polycystic kidney disease
- Medications:
  - Vitamin C/D, protease inhibitors, furosemide, acetazolamide.

CLINICAL PRESENTATION

Table 10.3   Clinical Presentation of Urinary Tract Stones

Symptoms	Signs
Sudden onset of severe, stabbing, intermittent, radiating 'loin to groin' pain	Renal angle tenderness
May be associated with rigors/chills, fever, nausea/vomiting, and tachycardia/palpitations	Suprapubic tenderness
Urinary symptoms of UTI, e.g. frequency, urgency, dysuria	Pyrexia
	Haematuria

Table 10.4   Differential Diagnosis of Urinary Tract Stones

Differential Diagnosis
Acute appendicitis
Acute epididymitis
Acute cholecystitis
Pelvic inflammatory disease
Abdominal aortic aneurysm

Table 10.5   Types of Urinary Tract Stones

Types of Stones
Calcium oxalate (80%)
Calcium phosphate
Uric acid: Radiolucent on X-ray
Struvite (Mg, NH4, P): Most staghorn calculi; urease-forming organism e.g. *Proteus*, *Klebsiella*
Cysteine (rare)–cystinuria, Fanconi syndrome

INVESTIGATIONS

- **Blood tests:**
  - FBC–raised WCC suggests superimposed infection.
  - U&E–deranged renal function tests (urea and creatinine) indicate renal impairment.
  - CRP–inflammation marker suggesting superimposed infection.
  - Serum corrected calcium–high levels of precipitate stone formation.
  - Phosphate and uric acid levels–high levels of precipitate stone formation.
  - PTH–if clinically appropriate in investigating risk factors.
- **Urine tests:**
  - Urine dipstick showing microscopic haematuria (85% of urolithiasis) or evidence of concurrent UTI.
  - MSU for microscopy, culture and sensitivity for urine organism.
  - 24-hour urine collection for pH, volume, calcium, oxalate, citrate, uric acid, sodium, potassium and creatinine (evaluation for risks in recurrent stone formation).
- **Radiological:**
  - Plain film X-ray of the kidneys/ureters/bladder (KUB) may show the presence of the stone in approximately 80% of cases.
  - Non-contrast CT KUB is the **gold-standard** imaging for nephrolithiasis and will help determine the site and size of the stone and in assessing the presence of complications.
  - Renal US to assess for hydronephrosis (most will not see ureteric stones) and for young patients to avoid radiation where possible.
  - Contrast CT urogram or intravenous pyelogram (IVP)–to identify stones and any other causes of obstruction.

COMPLICATIONS OF UROLITHIASIS

- AKI.
- Any level of obstruction in bilateral kidneys or in patients with single kidney.
- Complete or significant obstruction.
- Urinary infection or sepsis.
- Unable to tolerate pain.
- Unable to tolerate oral intake.

MANAGEMENT OF ACUTE EPISODE

Table 10.6   Stone Width and Passage Rate

Stone Width (mm)	Approximate % of Stones Passed without Surgical Intervention
1	90%
2	85%
3	83%
4	77%
5	56%

(continued)

Table 10.6   Stone Width and Passage Rate (*continued*)

Stone Width (mm)	Approximate % of Stones Passed without Surgical Intervention
6	41%
7	30%
8	31%
9	3%

Urology 10(6):544, 1977.
Am J Roentgenol 178:101. 2002.

- For distal stones <10 mm with no complications.
- For proximal stones, discuss attempting trial of passage with the patient.
- Trial for stone passage:
  - Analgesia (NSAIDs +/− opioids).
  - Antiemetic.
  - Increased oral fluid intake.
  - Alpha-blocker (e.g. tamsulosin) to help move stone along.
  - For uric acid stones, dissolution therapy with sodium bicarbonate or potassium citrate.
  - Follow-up in 4 weeks to ensure passage of stone.

Top tip: If any complications are present, <u>urgent treatment</u> is required, and therefore, conservative treatment is not appropriate.

SURGICAL

- Ureteroscopy–device of choice is laser lithotripsy. Another option is pneumatic lithotripsy.
- Extracorporeal shock wave lithotripsy (ESWL)–non-invasive, multiple sessions, out-patient. Not good for large stone burden.
- Percutaneous nephrolithotomy (PCNL)–access via the back into the kidney. Used for large stones, proximal stones and staghorn calculi.
- Open/laparoscopic Stone surgery–if less invasive procedures fail.

EMERGENCY

- If evidence of infection or severe obstruction is present, then urgent urine diversion is required:
  - Nephrostomy insertion by interventional radiology.
  - Anterograde ureteric stent insertion via nephrostomy.
  - Retrograde ureteric stent insertion via rigid cystoscopy.

RENAL CELL CARCINOMA

Table 10.7   Classification of Renal Mass

Renal Mass	
Benign	Malignant
• Papillary adenoma • Angiomyolipoma • Simple cysts • Pseudo-tumour	• Renal cell carcinoma • Wilms' tumour: Nephroblastoma in children • Transitional cell carcinoma: Renal pelvis and collecting system • Squamous carcinoma of the renal pelvis • Lymphoma • Metastases

EPIDEMIOLOGY

- Most common age for presentation is between 60 and 80 years.
- Male:female = 2:1.
- Subtypes: Clear cell type (75%), papillary (10%) and chromophobe and collecting duct tumours.

AETIOLOGY

- Smoking
- Obesity
- Hypertension
- Horseshoe kidney
- Chronic kidney disease
- Genetic: Von Hippel–Lindau disease, tuberous sclerosis, adult polycystic kidney disease (APCKD).

CLINICAL PRESENTATION

- Largely asymptomatic.
- Most tumours are found incidentally on imaging.
- 20% of patients present with metastatic disease (most commonly lung and bone).

SYMPTOMS

- Abdominal/flank pain.

SIGNS

- Haematuria
- Scrotal varicoceles (majority left-sided)
- Abdominal mass
- Invasion into the renal vein or IVC may produce peripheral oedema, ascites and hepatic dysfunction.

PARANEOPLASTIC SYNDROMES ASSOCIATED WITH RCC

- Weight loss
- Fever/pyrexia of unknown origin

- Hypertension
- Anaemia
- Hypercalcaemia
- Hepatic dysfunction (Stauffer's syndrome)
  - High ESR, ALP, bilirubin, GGT, PT
- Polycythaemia

INVESTIGATIONS

- **Bloods**
  - FBC for Hb to check for anaemia.
  - Urea and creatinine to check renal function.
  - Serum calcium and ALP may be elevated indicating bone metastasis.
- **Imaging**
  - Renal US.
  - CT KUB with contrast (triphasic) to confirm the site and size of the mass and to exclude any local metastasis.
  - Isotope bone scan for metastasis if clinically or biochemically indicated.
  - CT TAP to stage.
  - CT brain if neurological symptoms.
- **Renal biopsy**
  - Not necessary before excision because most solid renal lesions are malignant
  - May be indicated if diagnosis uncertain on imaging
  - Used for tissue sample in metastatic disease prior to systemic treatment
  - Significant false-negative rate.

Table 10.8   TNM Staging Renal Cell Carcinoma

TNM Staging RCC	
T0	• No evidence of primary tumour
T1	• Tumour < 7 cm in greatest dimension, limited to kidney
T1a	• Tumour < 4 cm in greatest dimension, limited to kidney
T1b	• Tumour > 4 cm in greatest dimension, limited to kidney
T2	• Tumour ≤ 7 cm in greatest dimension, limited to kidney
T3	• Tumour extends into major veins or invades adrenal gland or perinephric
T3a	tissues but not beyond Gerota's fascia
T3b	• Tumour invades adrenal gland or perinephric tissues but not beyond
T3c	Gerota's fascia
T4	• Tumour grossly extends into renal vein(s) or vena cava below diaphragm
	• Tumour grossly extends into vena cava above diaphragm
	• Tumour invades beyond Gerota's fascia
NX	• Regional lymph node cannot be assessed
N0	• No regional lymph node metastasis
N1	• Metastasis in a single region lymph node
N2	• Metastasis in more than one regional lymph node
MX	• Distant metastasis cannot be assessed
M0	• No distant metastasis
M1	• Distant metastasis

Source: American Joint Committee on Cancer (AJCC) 2010.

TREATMENT

- Surveillance is an option when there is limited life expectancy.
- Risk of metastasis is 1% in 3 years when primary RCC is <3 cm in size.
- Radical or partial nephrectomy
  - Depends on tumour size and location.
- Nephron-sparing surgery
  - In situations such as solitary kidney, bilateral renal tumours or poor renal function
- Poor response to chemotherapy and radiotherapy for primary tumour.
- Chemotherapy is used for metastatic disease.
- Radiotherapy is used for brain and bone metastasis.
- Immunotherapy such as IL-2 or tyrosine kinase inhibitors or interferons is used for advanced RCC.

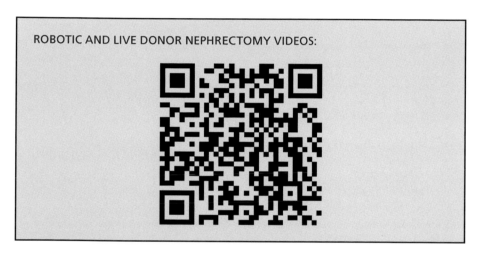

ROBOTIC AND LIVE DONOR NEPHRECTOMY VIDEOS:

BLADDER CANCER

EPIDEMIOLOGY

- Male:female = 4:1.
- Most diagnosed over 55 years old.
- Transitional cell carcinoma is the most common form of bladder cancer in the developed world.
- Squamous cell is the most common in the developing world.

AETIOLOGY

- Transitional cell carcinoma
  - Smoking
  - Aromatic hydrocarbons e.g. workers in the petrochemical, industrial dye, rubber industries and metal workers.

- Squamous cell carcinoma
    - Schistosomiasis infection
    - Chronic cystitis (e.g. long-term catheterisation).
- Adenocarcinoma

CLINICAL PRESENTATION

- **Symptoms**
    - Haematuria.
    - Irritative symptoms e.g. dysuria, frequency, urgency.
- **Signs**
    - Often no signs unless advanced disease e.g. pelvic mass, enlarged lymph nodes, cachexia.

INVESTIGATIONS

 Top tip: Painless haematuria is always cancer of the urinary system until proven otherwise.

- **Serial urine cytology** may reveal malignant cells.
- **Flexible cystoscopy** under local anaesthesia is used to visualise the bladder.
- **CT** urogram or **US** KUB.
- CT TAP for staging.
- **Pathology sample is required for staging**
    - Transurethral resection of bladder tumour (TURBT) is both diagnostic and therapeutic.
    - Staging is by TNM.

Table 10.9   Staging TNM Bladder Cancer

Staging TNM Bladder Cancer	
T0	No evidence of primary tumour
Ta	Non-invasive papillary carcinoma
Tis	Urothelial carcinoma in situ
T1	Tumour invades lamina propria (subepithelial connective tissue)
T2	Tumour invades muscularis propria
T3	Tumour invades perivesical soft tissue
T4	Extravesical tumour directly invades any of the following: Prostatic stroma, seminal vesicles, uterus, vagina, pelvic wall, abdominal wall
N0	No lymph node metastasis
N1	Single regional lymph node metastasis in the true pelvis (perivesical, obturator, internal and external iliac or sacral lymph node)
N2	Multiple regional lymph node metastasis in the true pelvis (perivesical, obturator, internal and external iliac or sacral lymph node metastasis)
N3	Lymph node metastasis to the common iliac lymph nodes
M0	No distant metastasis
M1	Distant metastasis

AJCC 8th edition.

TREATMENT

- **Carcinoma in situ (Tis)**
  - High risk for progression and recurrence.
  - TURBT if not extensive.

    AND/OR

  - Intravesical immunotherapy (via a urinary catheter) with BCG (upregulates host immune response against the tumour).
  - Repeat TURBT will assess presence of persistent cancer.
  - Options include repeating intravesical therapy or cystectomy.
- **Ta superficial transitional cell carcinoma**
  - TURBT.

    AND

  - Intravesical chemotherapy post-resection with mitomycin C as a single dose (reduces the risk of tumour recurrence but not disease progression).
- **T1 invasive transitional cell carcinoma**
  - TURBT then repeat TURBT to confirm stage and ensure complete tumour removal.

    AND

  - 6-week course of intravesical BCG.
  - If failure to eradicate cancer, cystectomy is recommended.
- **T2-4 invasive transitional cell carcinoma**
  - Curative therapy can be offered with neoadjuvant systemic chemotherapy and radical cystectomy (urinary diversion will be required via urostomy/ileal conduit).

 Top tip: Regular cystoscopy for surveillance is necessary as recurrence is common.

PROGNOSIS

- Recurrence rate is high if only TURBT performed.
  - CIS 80%, Ta 50%, T1 70%
- Poor prognosis in invasive disease.
  - 40–50% 5-year survival in muscle invasive tumour.

PROSTATE CANCER

EPIDEMIOLOGY

- Almost all are **adenocarcinomas**.
- Usually presents after 65 years old.
- Most arise in the peripheral zone (70%) of the prostate.

AETIOLOGY

- Family history.
- Age.

CLINICAL PRESENTATION

- **Symptoms**
  - Lower urinary tract symptoms (LUTSs).
  - Bone pain if metastasis present.
- **Signs**
  - Firm, irregular, 'craggy' prostate on DRE.

INVESTIGATIONS

- Serum PSA: Should not be used on its own for the detection of prostate cancer. Used as part of a multi-modal investigation.
- MRI prostate: PIRADS score predicts likelihood of prostate cancer.
- Transrectal ultrasound guided (TRUS) biopsy of prostate: Done under sedation.
- Isotope bone scan: To assess for bone metastases.
- Staging CT TAP in high-risk cases.

HISTOLOGY GRADING

- Done by **Gleason scoring**.
- Higher grade suggests worse prognosis.
- Reported as (X+Y=Z): X being the most abundant and Y the second most abundant grade detected. Z is the sum.

TREATMENT

- **Surveillance 'watchful waiting'**
  - For men with low-risk disease and life expectancy <10 years.
  - Unlikely for disease progression to occur within 10–15 years in low-risk disease.
  - Monitor symptoms and PSA, restaging biopsy may be required.
- **Localised prostate cancer**
  - Radical prostatectomy can be done open/laparoscopic/robotic (high risk of incontinence and erectile dysfunction post-op).
  - External beam radiotherapy and/or brachytherapy.
  - Androgen deprivation therapy (ADT) may be added in higher risk cancer.

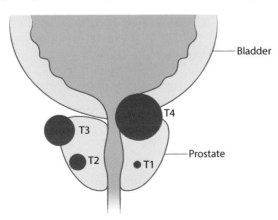

Figure 10.7   Visual representation of tumour staging of prostate cancer.

Table 10.10   Staging TNM Prostate Cancer

T0	No evidence of primary tumour
T1	Clinically inapparent tumour that is not palpable
T2	Tumour is palpable and confined within prostate
T3	Extra prostatic tumour that is not fixed or does not invade adjacent structures
T4	Tumour is fixed or invades adjacent structures other than seminal vesicles such as external sphincter, rectum, bladder, levator muscles and/or pelvic wall
N0	No positive regional nodes
N1	Metastases in regional nodes
M0	No distant metastasis
M1	Distant metastasis

AJCC 8th edition.

- **Locally advanced prostate cancer**
  - External beam radiotherapy and ADT.

    OR

  - Radical prostatectomy and lymph node dissection.
- **Metastatic disease**
  - ADT.
  - Radiotherapy for symptomatic bone metastases.
- **Medical ADT**
  - Gonadotropin-releasing hormone (GnRH) agonist–decreases luteinising hormone.
  - GnRH antagonist–binds to GnRH receptors.
  - Anti-androgen.
  - Side effects: Osteoporosis, sexual dysfunction, hot flushes, increased body fat and gynecomastia.
- **Surgical ADT**
  - Bilateral orchidectomy (cost effective and can achieve immediate decrease in testosterone).

TESTICULAR TUMOURS

EPIDEMIOLOGY

- Germ cell tumours constitute 90% of testicular cancers.
- Stromal tumours 5%.

AETIOLOGY

- Undescended testis
- Testicular dysgenesis
- HIV infection
- Family history
- Previous history of testicle cancer.

Table 10.11   Classification of Germ Cell Tumours

Seminoma	Non-seminoma Germ Cell Tumour (NSGCT)
• Peak incidence is 30–40 years of age • Lymphatic spread to retroperitoneal and intrathoracic lymph nodes is more common than haematogenous	• Peak incidence is 20–30 years of age • Lymphatic spread • Haematogenous spread most commonly to lungs, brain and liver

CLINICAL PRESENTATION

- **Symptoms**
  - Dull ache in scrotum or lower abdomen.
  - Symptoms associated with metastasis.
- **Signs**
  - Non-tender firm mass on testicle.
  - More common on right side because undescended testis is more commonly on the right.
  - Scrotal swelling (hydrocoele).
  - Endocrine manifestations (e.g. gynaecomastia).

INVESTIGATIONS

- Urgent scrotal US is mandatory for any testicular mass.
- Serum tumour markers–LDH, BHCG and AFP used for staging and monitoring response to treatment.
- CT and MRI are the most useful means of detecting spread.
- Testicular biopsy is not done due to risk of 'seeding' the scrotum.

Table 10.12   TNM Staging of Testicular Cancer

T0	No evidence of primary tumour
Tis	Germ cell neoplasia in situ
T1	Tumour limited to testis or epididymis without lymphovascular invasion
T2	Tumour limited to testis or epididymis with lymphovascular invasion
T3	Tumour directly invades spermatic cord soft tissue with or without lymphovascular invasion
T4	Tumour invades scrotum with or without lymphovascular invasion
N0	No regional lymph node metastasis
N1	Lymph node mass < 2 cm and < 5 nodes positive
N2	Lymph node mass > 2 cm but <5 cm *OR* > 5 nodes positive
N3	Lymph node mass > 5 cm
M0	No distant metastasis
M1	Distant metastases

AJCC 8th edition.

TREATMENT

- Consider sperm cryopreservation for those who want to preserve fertility.
- Orchidectomy via inguinal route is the mainstay of treatment.

- Retroperitoneal lymph node dissection may be required.
- Chemotherapy if there is spread to lymph nodes or distant metastasis.
- Abdominal external beam radiotherapy can be used for seminoma spread.

PROGNOSIS

- Resected localised disease has high 5-year survival of >98%.

ACUTE TESTICULAR PAIN

DIFFERENTIAL DIAGNOSIS

1. Testicular torsion
2. Torsion of the appendix testis/hydatid of Morgagni
3. Acute epididymo-orchitis.

TESTICULAR TORSION

EPIDEMIOLOGY

- Can occur at any age but 65% occurs between 12 and 18 years old.
- Due to inadequate fixation of the testis to the tunica vaginalis allowing increased mobility.

CLINICAL PRESENTATION

- **Symptoms**
  - Sudden onset severe unilateral testicular pain.
  - May be associated with nausea and vomiting.
  - Abdominal pain (the genitals must be examined in any boy presenting with RIF pain).
- **Signs**
  - Tender swollen testicle on palpation.
  - Oedematous erythematous scrotum.
  - High-riding testis due to shortening of cord.
  - Absent cremasteric reflex (elevation of testicle on stroking upper inner thigh).

MANAGEMENT

- Analgesia.
- Colour duplex US to assess blood flow to the testicle, if available immediately and low suspicion of torsion.
- Immediate scrotal exploration is required to salvage the testis. (6-hour window from onset of symptoms to save testicle–viability decreases with increasing time).
- A viable testicle is distorted and fixed (orchidopexy).
- A clearly non-viable testicle is excised (orchidectomy).

- The contralateral testicle is also fixed in cases of torsion to reduce the risk of a 'bell clapper' deformity.
- Manual detorsion can be attempted while awaiting surgery.

 Top tip: Do not delay scrotal exploration for ultrasound if there is suspicion of torsion. Testicular torsion is an emergency.

TORSION OF THE APPENDIX TESTIS/HYDATID OF MORGAGNI

AETIOLOGY

- Embryologic remnant of the Müllerian duct system.
- Difficult to clinically differentiate from testicular torsion.

CLINICAL PRESENTATION

- **Symptoms**
  - Similar to testicular torsion
- **Signs**
  - Non-tender testicle
  - Localised tender mass on the testis
  - 'Blue dot' sign–gangrenous appendix visible through the scrotum skin
  - Cremasteric reflex is preserved

MANAGEMENT

- Scrotal exploration if any doubt regarding testicular torsion.
- Excision of hydatid of Morgagni during scrotal exploration.
- Testicular US if no delay.
- Can be managed conservatively with analgesia and scrotal support if diagnosis established via US.

ACUTE EPIDIDYMO-ORCHITIS

DEFINITION

- Epididymitis is inflammation of the epididymis.
- Orchitis is inflammation of the testis.

AETIOLOGY

- Sexually transmitted infections: Chlamydia or gonorrhoea.
- UTIs: *Escherichia coli*.

- Viral: Mumps or Coxsackie virus.
- Non-infectious: Behcet's disease or amiodarone use.

CLINICAL PRESENTATION

- **Symptoms**
  - Gradual increased testicular pain.
  - Dysuria and frequency may be present.
  - Urethral discharge if STI causing the inflammation.
- **Signs**
  - Swelling and tenderness of testis/epididymis/cord.
  - Scrotal swelling–hydrocoele.
  - Fever.

INVESTIGATIONS

- WCC and CRP for infection.
- Urine culture and sensitivity for organism.
- STI screen.
- Ultrasound testicles to confirm diagnosis.

MANAGEMENT

- Scrotal elevation, local ice therapy and oral NSAIDs may help.
- Antibiotics therapy is prescribed according to local guidelines for STIs and non-STIs.

RENAL TRANSPLANT

KEY FACTS

- Treatment of choice in patients with end-stage renal disease (ESRD).
- Improves quality of life and reduces mortality risk compared with maintenance dialysis.
- Should be discussed with all patients with irreversible and progressive chronic kidney disease.
- Donor can be living or deceased–recipient survival higher with live-donor transplant.

AETIOLOGY

- Common causes causing ESRD requiring transplant:
  - Diabetes
  - Hypertension
  - Polycystic kidney disease
  - Chronic glomerulonephritis

CONTRAINDICATIONS TO RENAL TRANSPLANT

- Active infection
- Active malignancy

- Active substance abuse
- Reversible renal failure
- Uncontrollable psychiatric illness
- Treatment non-adherence
- Significantly shortened life expectancy

KEY POINTS

Due to the co-morbidities associated with requiring a renal transplant, careful evaluation is required when considering a patient as a candidate. This is to identify the patient's potential candidacy, perioperative risks and post-operative long-term complications.

PRE-TRANSPLANT WORKUP

- Thorough history and examination including psychosocial evaluation:
- Haematology: FBC and coagulation profile.
- Biochemistry: U&E, calcium, phosphate, albumin, LFTs.
- Endo: TFTs, PTH, HbA1C.
- Immunology: Group and HLA typing, HLA antibodies and cross-matching.
- Serology: HIV, CMV, EBV, HBV (HBsAg, HBsAb), HCV, RPR, MMR.
- Toxicology screen.
- TB: PPD/CXR, interferon-gamma release assay.
- Imaging: CXR, PFA, Doppler US aorta/renal, MRA brain (for PCKD).
- Cardiac: ECG, TTE, stress test, coronary angiogram.
- Malignancy screening.

KEY POINTS

Induction immunosuppressive therapy may include medications not usually used for maintenance. These are antilymphocyte medications such as anti-thymocyte globulin or anti-interleukin-2 receptor antibodies or anti-CD20 antibodies.

DURING HETEROTOPIC TRANSPLANT

- The donor transplant kidney is placed in a new location, usually the iliac fossa.
- The renal artery and vein are anastomosed to the external iliac artery and vein.
- The ureter is implanted to the bladder.
- The existing kidneys are not usually removed.

MAINTENANCE IMMUNOSUPPRESSIVE THERAPY

- **Most centres use triple therapy:**
  - Calcineurin inhibitor (cyclosporine or tacrolimus)
  - Anti-metabolite (azathioprine or mycophenolate)
  - Glucocorticoid (prednisone).

Table 10.13   Drugs Used in Renal Transplant

Immuno-Suppressive Medication	Side Effects
Cyclosporine	Hirsutism, gingival hyperplasia, diabetes, hypertension, hyperlipidaemia, tremor and nephrotoxicity
Tacrolimus	Diabetes, nephrotoxicity, hypertension, hyperlipidaemia, pruritis and alopecia
Mycophenolate	Diarrhoea, GI toxicity and bone marrow suppression
Azathioprine	Bone marrow suppression, hepatitis and pneumonitis
Prednisone	Hypertension, hyperlipidaemia, diabetes, peptic ulcer disease, skin bruising, Cushing's syndrome and osteoporosis

Top tip: All live vaccines should be avoided while on immunosuppression therapy. All the above immunosuppression medications increase risk of infections and malignancy.

COMPLICATIONS OF RENAL TRANSPLANT

- Rejection.
- Infections.
- Cardiovascular disease: Leading cause of death after renal transplant.
- Diabetes.
- Osteoporosis.
- Malignancy: SCC, BCC, post-transplant lymphoproliferative disorder, Kaposi's sarcoma.
- Persistent hyperparathyroidism.
- Hyperuricemia and gout.
- Surgery-specific complications: Vessel/ureter anastomosis leakage, ureteric obstruction, renal vein/artery thrombosis, haematuria, haematoma, lymphocele, haemorrhage.

NB: Frequent follow-up is required to monitor and manage any potential complications.

Table 10.14   Types of Transplant Rejection

Hyperacute (immediate to days)	Hyperacute antibody mediated response.
Acute (weeks to months)	Acute T-cell-mediated rejection and antibody mediated response.
Chronic (months to years)	T-cell-mediated process. Interstitial fibrosis and tubular atrophy.

SIGNS OF ACUTE REJECTION

- Increase in creatinine ≥25% from baseline
- Worsening hypertension

- Proteinuria >1 g/day
- Plasma donor-derived cell-free DNA (dd-cfDNA) >1%.

NB: Renal biopsy is used to grade the severity of rejection.

MCQs FOR SELF-ASSESSMENT

Chapter 11

CARDIOTHORACIC SURGERY

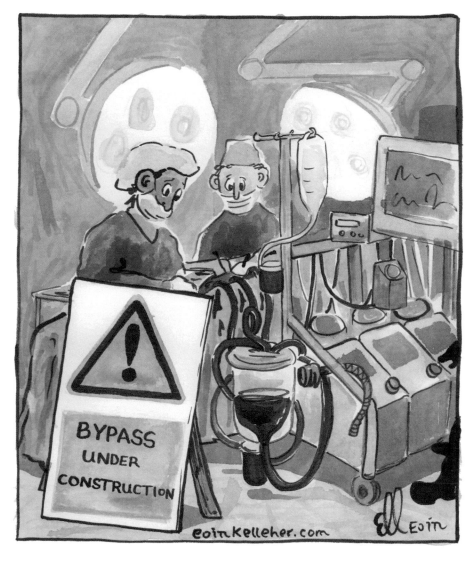

eoinkelleher.com

DOI: 10.1201/9781003207184-11

CONTENTS

Pre-Operative Investigations for Cardiothoracic Surgery	235
Coronary Artery Bypass Grafting (CABG)	235
Valvular Heart Disease	237
Aortic Stenosis (AS)	238
Mitral Regurgitation (MR)	239
Mitral Stenosis (MS)	240
Aortic Regurgitation (AR)	240
Pneumothorax	241
Primary Spontaneous Pneumothorax	241
Secondary Spontaneous Pneumothorax	243
Chest Tube Insertion	243

PRE-OPERATIVE INVESTIGATIONS FOR CARDIOTHORACIC SURGERY

1. **Full history and exam:**
   - Including full neurological exam
   - NYHA and GOLD scoring systems
2. **Full bloods:**
   - Including FBC, U&E, coagulation screen, type and screen
3. **ECG**
4. **CXR:** AP + lateral views
5. **Pulmonary function tests** (PFTs):
   - FEV1 is important to assess patient's ability to undergo lung reducing surgery
   - Include a diffusion capacity of the lung for carbon monoxide (affected with fibrosis and emphysema)
6. **Cardiopulmonary exercise stress test**
7. **CT thorax +/- contrast**
8. **Carotid Doppler ultrasound:** To assess for carotid atherosclerotic disease
9. **Transthoracic/Transoesophageal echocardiogram** (TTE/TOE):
   - Assessment of valves including degree of prolapse/stenosis
   - Assessment for regional wall motion abnormalities
10. **Coronary angiography:**
    - A planned CABG or those undergoing valvular surgery who would benefit from surgical revascularisation in the same operation
    - May consider revascularisation before surgery in stable angina
11. **Pulmonary wedge capillary pressures:**
    - Via right heart catheterisation
    - Before complex valvular surgery
12. **Cardiac MRI:**
    - If specified by surgeon
13. **Dental review:**
    - If surgery on valves

CORONARY ARTERY BYPASS GRAFTING (CABG)

INDICATIONS FOR SURGERY

- >70% left main stem (LMS) stenosis.
- Symptomatic patients with >70% proximal left anterior descending (LAD) stenosis.
- Symptomatic patients with >70% disease in all three vessels.
- Concomitant valvular disease which requires replacement.
- Vessel disease (as above) in a diabetic.

PROCEDURE

- Performed via median sternotomy Figure 11.1.
- A piece of conduit (saphenous vein, left internal mammary artery [LIMA], radial artery) is anastomosed to the coronary artery beyond the lesion and then to the ascending aorta.

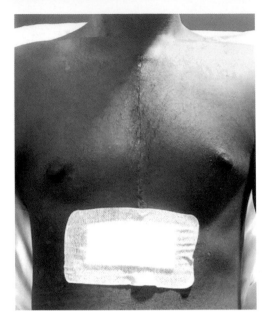

Figure 11.1 Midline sternotomy scar. Courtesy of Dr Jaclyn Croyle

SELECTION OF CONDUITS

- **Venous grafts**
  - The great saphenous vein (GSV) is the most common vein used as a conduit. The 10-year patency rate is 50–60%.
- **Arterial grafts**
  - The LIMA/internal thoracic artery is the conduit of choice for the LAD artery. The 10-year patency rate is 90%.
  - Radial artery can also be used as a second choice but it is prone to vasospasm.

COMPLICATIONS

- Death: 0–1% in low-risk patients.
- Stroke: 1–2% in low-risk patients.
- Re-sternotomy for bleeding or tamponade: 5%.
- Chest infection, atrial fibrillation, wound infection, renal failure.

PROGNOSIS

- In untreated patients with symptoms severe enough to warrant coronary angiography, 10% have an acute MI within 1 year and 30% have an acute MI within 5 years. Hospital mortality of MI is 7–10%.
- In three-vessel disease, the 5-year survival is 50%, lower if LV function is impaired.
- LMS disease has a 2-year survival of 50%.

> **Top tip:** Standard 'triple bypass' includes:
>
> - LIMA to LAD
> - Portion of harvested GSV from aorta to circumflex artery
> - Portion of harvested GSV from aorta to distal right coronary artery (RCA) Figure 11.2

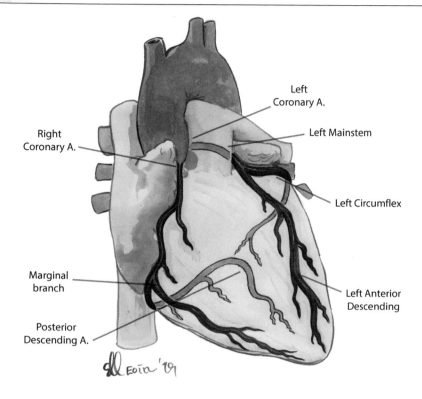

Figure 11.2 Anatomy of the coronary vessels.

VALVULAR HEART DISEASE

CHOICE OF VALVE TYPE

Table 11.1 Types of Valves

Mechanical Valve	Bio-prosthetic (Bovine/Porcine) Valve
Lifelong (>20 years)	Shorter life (10–15 years)
Requires warfarin	No need for warfarin
Noisy (metallic click)	Silent

AORTIC STENOSIS (AS)

AETIOLOGY
- Calcific degeneration.
- Bicuspid valve.
- Rheumatic disease.

CLINICAL PRESENTATION
- **Triad of symptoms**
  - Syncope, Angina, Dyspnoea.
- **Signs**
  - Ejection systolic murmur loudest in aortic region and radiates to carotids.
  - Heaving apex beat.

INVESTIGATIONS
- ECG may show left ventricular hypertrophy.
- TTE needed to assess the degree of stenosis.

INDICATIONS FOR SURGERY
- Mean gradient across valve >40 mmHg.
- Symptomatic aortic stenosis.

SURGICAL APPROACH
- Open surgical aortic valve replacement (SAVR) via thoracotomy Figure 11.3.
- Transcatheter aortic valve implantation (TAVI).

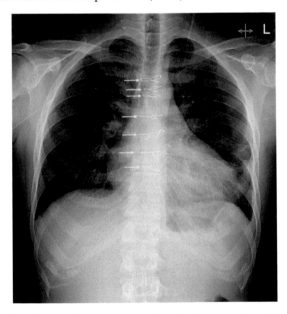

Figure 11.3 CXR showing midline sternotomy wires (yellow arrows) post-aortic valve replacement. Courtesy of Dr Jaclyn Croyle

PROGNOSIS

- When combined with coronary artery disease, aortic stenosis is associated with a high risk of sudden death.
- Post-operative prognosis is good.
- Type of valve used is of importance to length of patency.

MITRAL REGURGITATION (MR)

AETIOLOGY

- Second most common valvular lesion.
- Mitral valve prolapse due to ischaemia (papillary muscle dysfunction/chordae tendinae rupture).
- Rheumatic disease.
- Infective endocarditis.
- Connective tissue disorders.

CLINICAL PRESENTATION

- Holosystolic murmur loudest at apex +/- third heart sound that can radiate to axilla.
- **Acute MR**
  - Signs of CCF.
- **Chronic MR**
  - Exertional dyspnoea.
  - Orthopnoea.
  - Displaced apex beat.
  - Atrial fibrillation in 80%.

INVESTIGATIONS

- TTE/TOE.

INDICATIONS FOR SURGERY

- Acute MR.
- Severe chronic MR.

SURGICAL APPROACH

- Open valve replacement.
- Endovascular MitraClip if open surgery contraindicated.

PROGNOSIS

- Mortality of untreated severe MR is 5% per year.
- Operative mortality is 2–3% for low-risk cases.

MITRAL STENOSIS (MS)

KEY FACTS

- Prevalence <1%.
- Rheumatic heart disease is the most common cause.

CLINICAL PRESENTATION

- Rumbling mid-diastolic murmur at apex.
- Signs of right heart failure (due to increased pulmonary vascular resistance).
- Atrial fibrillation.
- Left parasternal heave.
- Tapping apex beat.

NB: Many patients may be asymptomatic.

INVESTIGATIONS

- CXR shows splaying of carina (enlarged left atrium).
- TTE/TOE.

SURGICAL APPROACH

- Percutaneous valvotomy.
- Open mitral valve replacement.

PROGNOSIS

- Poor once symptoms of heart failure are present.

AORTIC REGURGITATION (AR)

KEY FACTS

- Prevalence <1%.

AETIOLOGY

- Rheumatic disease.
- Marfan's syndrome and other connective tissue disorders.
- Large vessel vasculitis.
- Infective endocarditis.
- Aortic dissection.

CLINICAL PRESENTATION

- Early diastolic murmur.
- **Acute AR**
    - Two most common causes of acute AR are endocarditis and aortic dissection.
    - Signs of left ventricular failure.
    - Usually a medical emergency.

- **Chronic AR**
  - Often asymptomatic.
- Wide pulse pressure (Corrigan's/water hammer pulse).

INVESTIGATIONS

- CXR: Shows cardiomegaly.
- TTE.

INDICATIONS FOR SURGERY

- Acute AR is a surgical emergency.
- Chronic AR.
- Left ventricular dilatation >5.5 cm.

PROGNOSIS

- Acute AR has a poor prognosis.
- Chronic AR has a good outcome until failure occurs (50% 2-year mortality).
- Operative mortality is 3–5%.

PNEUMOTHORAX

DEFINITION

- Presence of air in the pleural space with varying degrees of secondary lung collapse.

CLASSIFICATION

- **Primary spontaneous pneumothorax:** Occurs without obvious reason or apparent lung disease.
- **Secondary spontaneous pneumothorax:** Due to a known underlying lung or systemic disease.
- **Traumatic pneumothorax:** The result of iatrogenic or non-iatrogenic blunt and/or penetrating chest interventions and injuries.

PRIMARY SPONTANEOUS PNEUMOTHORAX

KEY FACTS

- More common in tall, young men.
- More common on the right side.
- Caused by rupture of small subpleural blebs.
- Usually found in the apex.

CLINICAL FEATURES

- Dyspnoea.
- Chest pain.
- Tachypnoea.
- Hyperresonant hemithorax.
- Absent breath sounds.

INVESTIGATIONS

- CXR Figure 11.4.
- CT thorax provides a more accurate estimate of the size of pneumothorax.

COMPLICATIONS

- Tension pneumothorax.
- Pneumomediastinum.
- Haemopneumothorax.
- Recurrent pneumothorax.

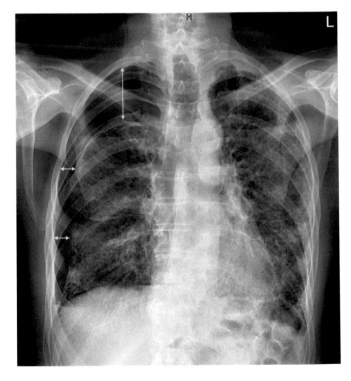

Figure 11.4   CXR showing pneumothorax (yellow arrows). Courtesy of Dr Jaclyn Croyle

MANAGEMENT

- Conservative if small (<20%) pneumothorax and asymptomatic
  - Supplemental oxygen, repeat CXR.
- Needle aspiration if >2 cm rim of air seen.
- Chest tube insertion (fourth to fifth intercostal space [ICS] in the mid-axillary line) indicated if aspiration fails.

SURGERY

- Video-assisted thoracoscopic surgery (VATS) is being increasingly used for **bullectomy and pleurodesis**.
- Recurrence rate is <2% following surgery.

SECONDARY SPONTANEOUS PNEUMOTHORAX

AETIOLOGY

- **Underlying lung or systemic disease**
  - **Chronic airway and alveolar diseases:** E.g. severe asthma, cystic fibrosis, emphysema, bullae and cysts.
  - **Systemic connective tissue diseases:** E.g. rheumatoid arthritis, ankylosing spondylitis, scleroderma, Marfan and Ehlers–Danlos syndromes.
  - **Malignant lung and chest diseases:** E.g. bronchial cancer, sarcoma.

NOTES ON THORACIC SURGERY

- **Pleurodesis**
  - Kaolin talc insufflation ('snowstorm') promotes inflammation and pleural adherence.
  - Pleurectomy (pleural stripping) creates raw surface for inflammatory adhesive reaction.
  - Post-operative pyrexia is common and is seen as a sign of success associated with inflammation.
  - Pleurodesis must be avoided if the patient may be considered for a lung transplant.
- **Empyema**
  - May be associated with infection post thoracic surgery or spontaneous following a pneumonia.
  - Approximately 40% associated with streptococcal species.
  - **Symptoms and signs include** persistent pyrexia, dyspnoea and pleuritic chest pain.
  - Decortication of the empyema may be necessary if medical management has failed.

CHEST TUBE INSERTION

DEFINITION

- The insertion of a chest tube into the pleural cavity to drain air, blood, pus or other fluids.

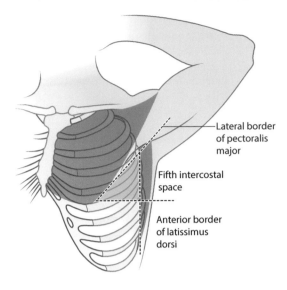

Figure 11.5   Borders of the 'safe triangle' in the axilla. Illustrated by Dr Jaclyn Croyle

KEY FACTS

- Allows for continuous, large-volume drainage until the underlying pathology can be more formally addressed.
- A **'safe triangle'** has been described as the preferred site of insertion Figure 11.5.

CHEST TUBE INSERTION TECHNIQUE

- Inserted in the **fourth to fifth ICS just anterior to the mid-axillary line, just above the rib to avoid the neurovascular bundle.**
- Blunt dissection of the subcutaneous tissues is used to access the pleural space. Keep dissection tools on the upper edge of the rib to avoid the neurovascular bundle on the underside of the rib above.
- Chest tube is inserted under direct vision and attached to an underwater seal.
- To avoid water entering the pleural space, never lift the underwater seal above the level of the bed.

CONFIRMATION OF TUBE PLACEMENT

1. Bubbling of air in the underwater chamber.
2. Oscillation of fluid in the tube connecting the chest tube to the underwater seal with patient's respiration.
3. Post-insertion CXR.

Top tip:

Safe triangle: Preferred insertion site for chest tube which lies between:

The lateral border of pectoralis major
The anterior border of latissimus dorsi
The fifth ICS (usually at level of the nipple line)

Top tip: Chest drains are inserted at the level of the fourth to fifth ICS, just anterior to the mid-axillary line and at the upper border of the inferior rib, so as to avoid damaging the neurovascular bundle.

MCQs FOR SELF-ASSESSMENT

Chapter 12

MAJOR TRAUMA

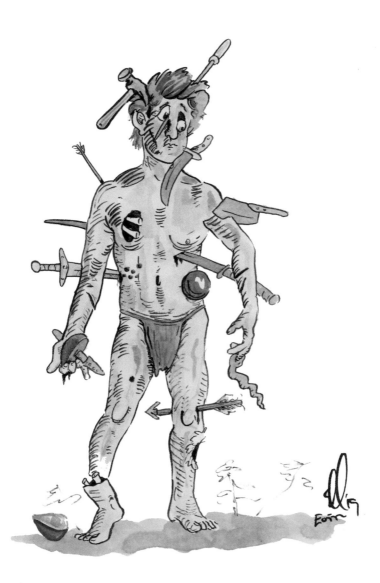

DOI: 10.1201/9781003207184-12

CONTENTS

Major Trauma	249
Advanced Trauma Life Support (ATLS®) System (Tenth Edition)	250
Thoracic Trauma	254
Abdominal Trauma	258

MAJOR TRAUMA

DEFINITION

- An injury or combination of injuries that are life or limb-threatening and potentially life-changing as they may result in long-term disability.

COMMON AETIOLOGY

- Road traffic accident (RTA)
- Violent assaults
- Stabbing
- Gunshot
- Fall-from-height (e.g. fall from roof)
- Suicide attempt

GLOBAL BURDEN OF FATAL INJURY

- Injuries account for 5.8 million deaths each year worldwide, representing 10% of total deaths.

GLOBAL INJURY MORTALITY BY CAUSE

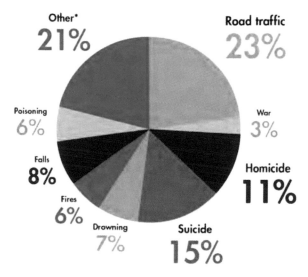

* Other includes smothering, asphyxiation, choking, animal and venomous bites, hypothermia and hyperthermia, as well as natural disasters.

Figure 12.1 Global injury mortality graph. From the World Health Organisation, Injuries & Violence: The Facts, 2010

ADVANCED TRAUMA LIFE SUPPORT (ATLS®) SYSTEM (Tenth Edition)

GENERAL INFORMATION

- The international standard for care during the 'golden hour' following trauma Figure 12.2.
- Emphasises that injury kills in certain reproducible time frames in a common sequence:
  - Loss of airway
  - Inability to breathe
  - Loss of circulating blood volume
  - Expanding intracranial mass.
- Primary survey (ABCDEs) is performed **simultaneously** with resuscitation.

Top tip:

Primary Survey: The goal of primary survey is to identify and treat life-threatening conditions according to priority (**ABCDE**).

KEY POINTS

1. Always consider the cohort of person you are treating:
   - Children, athletes, elderly and the multi-morbid all respond in different ways to shock.
2. Always **remember to reassess** after any intervention by monitoring vitals and clinical response.
- **Airway maintenance with cervical spine protection**
- **Assess airway patency**
  - If the patient can speak, airway is not immediately threatened (Exception: Burn victims due to rapid laryngeal oedema).

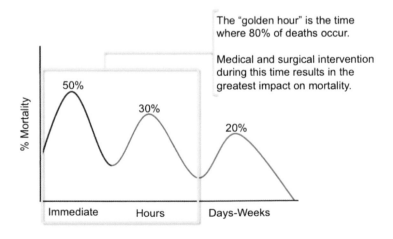

The "golden hour" is the time where 80% of deaths occur.

Medical and surgical intervention during this time results in the greatest impact on mortality.

Figure 12.2   Trimodial pattern of mortality following trauma. Illustrated by Dr Jaclyn Croyle

- **If there is airway impairment**, consider the following causes and the need to establish a definitive airway:
  - Reduced level of consciousness.
  - Secretions (can be suctioned).
  - Foreign body (if visible, can be removed with a finger sweep).
  - Mandibulofacial fractures (e.g. Le Fort fractures).
  - Tracheal/laryngeal fractures.
- **Assume C-spine injury**, and manage with manual in-line immobilisation or immobilisation devices in the following situations:
  - Substantial mechanism of injury.
  - Unconscious patient.
  - Significant facial/head injury.
  - Neurological deficit.
- **Action sequence in airway impairment**
  1. Perform jaw thrust +/– chin lift with in-line C-spine immobilisation.
  2. Consider nasopharyngeal/oropharyngeal airway.
     - If tolerated, the patient likely requires a definitive airway.
     - Often used in the intermediate phase until possible to establish definitive airway (e.g. equipment assembly).
  3. If patient is unable to maintain airway integrity, secure a **definitive airway** (orotracheal/nasotracheal intubation, cricothyroidotomy).
- **Breathing and ventilation**
- Administer 100% O_2 using a non-rebreathing mask/reservoir.
- Full cardiorespiratory exam with appropriate chest and neck exposure.
  1. **Inspecting specifically for**
     - Tracheal deviation.
     - Neck vein distention.
     - Chest wall expansion and any asymmetry.
     - Respiratory rate.
     - Thoracic wounds.
  2. **Percussion and auscultation specifically for**
     - Hyper-resonance or dullness.
     - Reduced air entry.
- Identify and treat life-threatening conditions (see "Thoracic Trauma" section)
  - Tension pneumothorax.
  - Open pneumothorax.
  - Flail chest with pulmonary contusion.
  - Massive haemothorax.
- **Circulation with haemorrhage control**
- **Assess for signs of shock** Table 12.1.
  - Altered level of consciousness.
  - Cold, clammy skin.
  - Reduced capillary refill.
  - Hypotension.
  - Tachycardia.
- Control external bleeding with **pressure**.
- Obtain IV access using two 14G cannula.

- Send blood for cross-match, FBC, coagulation profile and U&E.
- Commence bolus of **warmed** Hartmann's solution.
- If ongoing, immediately life-threatening blood loss, activate the massive transfusion protocol (accessible in Emergency Department, **always** contact Blood Transfusion Laboratory to alert possible need for further products).
  - 4 units RBC (O-negative until cross-matched).
  - 2 units plasma (e.g. Octaplex).
  - 1 adult therapeutic dose platelets.
- Consider surgical control of haemorrhage.
  - Laparotomy or thoracotomy.

 Top tip: Hypotension in trauma is due to blood loss until proven otherwise.

Table 12.1   Signs and Symptoms of Haemorrhage by Class

Parameter	Class 1	Class 2 (Mild)	Class 3 (Moderate)	Class 4 (Severe)
Approximate blood loss	<15% Up to 750 ml	15–30% 750–1500 ml	31–40% 1500–2000 ml	>40% >2000 ml
Heart rate	<100	100–120	120–140	>140
Blood pressure	Normal	Normal	Decreased	Decreased
Pulse pressure	Normal/Increased	Decreased	Decreased	Decreased
Respiratory rate	14–20	20–30	30–40	>35
Urine output (ml/hr)	>30	20–30	5–15	Negligible
Glasgow Coma Scale	Normal	Normal	Reduced	Reduced
CNS mental state	Slightly anxious	Slightly anxious	Anxious, Confused	Confused, lethargic
Base deficit (mEq/L)	0 to −2	−2 to −6	−6 to −10	−10 or less
Need for blood products	Monitor	Possible	Yes	Massive transfusion protocol

- **Disability**
  - Rapid neurological evaluation using the Glasgow Coma Scale (GCS)
- **Exposure/Environment control**
  - Completely expose patient for thorough examination.
  - **Prevent hypothermia** by covering with blankets/warming device.
  - Use warm IV fluids.

Table 12.2   Glasgow Coma Scale

The Glasgow Coma Scale (GCS):

- Used for rapid neurological evaluation
- The GCS runs from 3-15, i.e. 3 is the lowest possible score
- A GCS of 8 or less indicates a need to intubate the patient

Assessment Area	Score
Eye-Opening (E):	
• Spontaneous	4
• To sound	3
• To pressure	2
• None	1
• Non-testable	NT
Verbal Response (V):	
• Orientated	5
• Confused	4
• Words	3
• Sounds	2
• None	1
• Non-testable	NT
Motor Response (M):	
• Obeys commands	6
• Localising	5
• Normal flexion	4
• Abnormal flexion	3
• Extension	2
• None	1
• Non-testable	NT

Note: GCS Score = (E[4] + V[5] + M[6]) = Best possible score 15; worst possible score 3. *If an area cannot be assessed, no numerical score is given for that region, and it is considered "non-testable." Source: www.glasgowcomascale.org

THE TRAUMA TRIAD OF DEATH

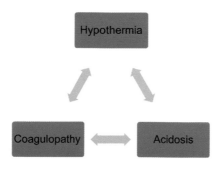

Figure 12.3   The trauma triad of death.

ADJUNCTS TO PRIMARY SURVEY

- **Monitoring of vital signs**
  - Pulse
  - Non-invasive BP
  - ECG
  - Pulse oximetry
- **Bladder catheterisation**
  - Urine output is a sensitive measure of end organ perfusion
  - Always exclude urethral injury first
  - If concerned, contact urology
  - Urethral injury can be indicated by blood at urethral meatus, perineal bruising, or non-palpable prostate on DRE
- **Diagnostic studies**
  - X-rays of lateral cervical spine, AP chest, and AP pelvis
  - US scan
  - CT scan
  - Diagnostic peritoneal lavage (rarely performed in ED, however, forms part of field trauma protocols)

SECONDARY SURVEY

- Begin only after the primary survey is complete and while adequate resuscitation is taking place.
- Use the **AMPLE** method to take a history
  - Allergy
  - Medication
  - Past medical history
  - Last meal
  - Events of the incident
- Perform a head-to-toe physical examination and **continue to reassess all vital signs**
- Perform any specialised diagnostic tests that may be required

THORACIC TRAUMA

KEY FEATURES

- Thoracic injuries account for 25% of deaths from trauma.
- 50% of patients who die from multiple injuries also have a significant thoracic injury.
- **Open injuries** are caused by penetrating trauma from knives or gunshots.
- **Closed injuries** occur after blasts, blunt trauma and deceleration.
  - Most commonly post-RTA.

MANAGEMENT–ATLS PROTOCOL

- Identify and treat major thoracic life-threatening injuries.
- **Tension pneumothorax** Figure 12.4
- Clinical diagnosis–**You should not delay management for imaging.**

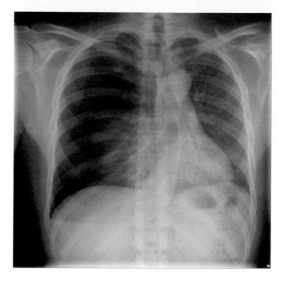

Figure 12.4 Tension pneumothorax. Courtesy by Dr Niamh Adams

NB: Tension pneumothorax is a clinical diagnosis. You should never see an X-ray like this!

- Air enters the pleural space via injury to the lung or the chest wall.
- Expanding pneumothorax
  - Impedes venous return to the heart
  - Leading to respiratory distress, tachycardia and hypotension
- Examination reveals
  - Decreased expansion, hyper-resonant percussion note
  - Absent breath sounds over the affected hemithorax
- Tracheal deviation <u>away</u> from affected side is a late sign associated with massive pneumothorax.
- Management:
  - Requires immediate needle decompression followed by chest drain insertion.
  - Insert a 14G cannula into the second intercostal space in the mid-clavicular line[1] (expect a hissing noise as the pressure is released!).
  - Place a surgical chest drain into the triangle of safety attached to an underwater seal drain.

Top tip:

Triangle of Safety: Chest drains can be safely inserted in the space bordered by the anterior edge of latissimus dorsi, the lateral edge of pectoralis major and the fifth intercostal space. The space ends at the base of the axilla. See chest tube insertion in Chapter 11.

---

[1] According to the Tenth Edition, ATLS now recommends that needle decompression is performed at the fourth or fifth intercostal space mid-axillary line for adults.

UNDERWATER SEAL DRAIN

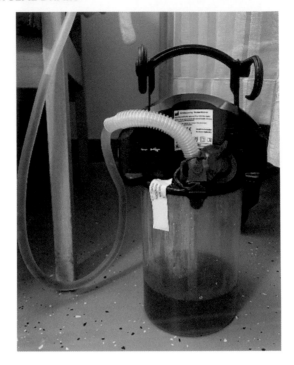

Figure 12.5   Underwater seal with portable suction. Courtesy of Dr Jaclyn Croyle

- **Open pneumothorax**
- Associated with a chest wall defect >3 cm.
- Air flows through path of least resistance, i.e. if thoracic opening >2/3 diameter of trachea.
- Radiographic appearance as of tension pneumothorax.
- **Management**
  - Cover with a three-sided occlusive dressing to create a valve that allows air out of the pleural cavity but not into it.
  - Follow by immediate insertion of an intercostal drain through a separate incision.
- **Flail chest**
- **Definition:** Two or more ribs fractured in two or more locations.
- Causes paradoxical motion of the chest wall.
- Restricted chest wall movement and underlying lung contusion result in hypoxia.
- **Management**
  - If the segment is small and respiration is not compromised, transfer patient to the HDU with adequate analgesia.
  - Encourage early ambulation and vigorous physiotherapy. Perform regular blood gas analysis.
  - In more severe cases, endotracheal intubation with positive pressure ventilation is required.
- **Massive haemothorax**

- Accumulation of >1500 mL of blood in pleural cavity.
- Suspect when circulatory shock is associated with dull percussion note and absent breath sounds on one side of chest.
- CXR may show a 'white out' in the hemi-thorax.
- **Management**
  - Restore blood volume.
  - Decompress by inserting a wide bore (>32 Ch) chest drain.
  - Consider need for urgent thoracotomy to control bleeding if there is continued brisk bleeding and need for persistent blood transfusion.
  - Consult with a regional thoracic centre immediately.
- **Cardiac tamponade**
- Most commonly results from penetrating injuries, but blood can also accumulate in pericardial sac after blunt trauma.
- Recognised by haemodynamic instability–tachycardia, pulsus paradoxus.
- **Remember Beck's Triad:** Hypotension, raised JVP and faint heart sounds.
- **Management**
  - If critically ill with suspected tamponade, perform 'blind' pericardiocentesis.
  - Call cardiothoracic or general surgeons to consider emergency thoracotomy.
  - If responding to treatment, arrange urgent TTE and eFAST scan in the ED.

MANAGEMENT–SECONDARY SURVEY

- Perform a complete examination.
- In stab injuries, expose the patient fully and position them so that you can assess the entire chest.
- Obtain erect CXR looking for pneumothorax/haemothorax.
- Treat with a chest drain if large or symptomatic or in any patient likely to require mechanical ventilation.

FURTHER READING

Radiopaedia playlist
https://radiopaedia.org/playlists/34761?lang=gb
This playlist contains radiological images and associated cases for your further understanding of the following entities.

Table 12.3 Other Thoracic Injuries

Pulmonary Contusion:
Most common potentially lethal chest injury
Associated consolidation and pulmonary oedema cause increasing respiratory distress and may lead to cardiac arrest
Treatment:
Analgesia, physiotherapy, oxygenation
Consider supplemental respiratory support for a patient with significant hypoxia

(continued)

Table 12.3 Other Thoracic Injuries (*continued*)

Tracheobronchial Rupture: Suspect when there is a persistent large air leak after chest drain insertion. Air leak is seen as rapid bubbling of the underwater seal drain Seek immediate surgical (cardiothoracic) consultation CT thorax is usually diagnostic
Blunt Cardiac Injury: Myocardial contusion or traumatic infarction Suspect when there are significant abnormalities on ECG or TTE Seek cardiology or cardiothoracic surgical advice
Thoracic Aortic Injury: *Transection/partial transection* Most common area affected is the proximal descending aorta, where the mobile aortic arch is fixed at the ligamentum arteriosum Patients survive immediate death if the haematoma is contained **Suspect when:** History of decelerating force, and where there is widened mediastinum on CXR CT thorax is usually diagnostic Consider cardiothoracic and/or vascular surgical referral as appropriate
Diaphragmatic Rupture: Usually secondary to blunt trauma in restrained car passengers (seat belt compression causes 'burst' injury commonly on the left side) **Suspect in:** A patient with a suitable history and a raised left hemidiaphragm on CXR Penetrating trauma below the fifth intercostal space can produce a perforation Commonly missed on CT scans **Laparoscopy** is diagnostic in cases where diaphragmatic injury is highly suspected

ABDOMINAL TRAUMA

KEY FEATURES

- Abdominal injuries are present in 7–10% of trauma patients.
- If intra-abdominal haemorrhage is uncontrolled or unrecognised, it can lead to preventable death.

CATEGORIES OF ABDOMINAL TRAUMA

- **Blunt trauma:**
  - Blunt trauma may cause:
    - Compression or crushing, causing rupture of solid or hollow organs.
    - Deceleration injury due to differential movement of fixed and non-fixed parts of organs, causing tearing or avulsion from their vascular supply, e.g. liver tear and vena caval rupture.
    - Most frequent injuries are spleen (45%), liver (40%) and retroperitoneal haematoma (15%).

- Blunt abdominal trauma is very common in RTAs where:
  - There have been fatalities.
  - Any casualty has been ejected from the vehicle.
- The closing speed is >50 km/hr.
- **Penetrating trauma:**
  - Stab wounds and low velocity gunshot wounds.
    - Cause damage by laceration or cutting.
    - Stab wounds commonly involve the liver (40%), small bowel (30%), diaphragm (20%) and colon (15%).
  - High velocity gunshot wounds transfer more kinetic energy and cause further injury by cavitation effect, tumble and fragmentation of ammunition.
    - Commonly involve the small bowel (50%), colon (40%), liver (30%) and vessels (25%).
- **Blast trauma:**
  - Occurs as a combination of blunt and penetrating injuries.
  - Thorough inspection for penetrating fragments is required, as they may be multiple.
  - Patients close to explosion may incur blast overpressure injuries, specifically to the bowel, lungs and tympanic membranes.
    - These can present later and must not distract from identifying and treating penetrating/blunt trauma.

INITIAL EXAMINATION

- **Primary survey of the abdomen.**
  - In the setting of trauma, persistent hypotension in the absence of obvious blood loss should be assumed to be due to intra-abdominal haemorrhage.
  - Focused abdominal sonography in trauma (FAST) scanning is used as part of primary survey.
  - If the patient is stable, an emergency CT abdomen and pelvis is indicated.
  - If the patient remains critically unstable, an emergency laparotomy is usually indicated.
- **Secondary survey of the abdomen.**
  - AMPLE history structure.
  - Consider need for collateral history to obtain a true picture of the event.
    - Emergency response team, staff, witnesses.
  - Important to establish mechanism of injury:
    - RTA: Seat belt usage, steering wheel deformation, speed, damage to vehicle, ejection of victim, etc.
    - Gunshot injury: Velocity, calibre, presumed path of bullet, distance from weapon, etc.
    - Penetrating injury: Weapon used (if known), number of injuries, etc.
  - Prehospital condition and treatment of patient.
- **Physical examination**
  - Inspect anterior abdomen which includes lower thorax, perineum and log roll to inspect posterior abdomen, specifically for:
    - Abrasions
    - Contusions

- Lacerations
- Penetrating wounds
- Distension
- Evisceration of viscera
- Exit wounds
- Palpate abdomen for tenderness, involuntary muscle guarding, rebound tenderness, gravid uterus.
- Percuss to elicit subtle rebound tenderness.
- Assess pelvic stability.
- Penile, perineum, rectal, vaginal examinations and examination of gluteal regions as indicated.

FURTHER READING

Radiopaedia playlist
https://radiopaedia.org/playlists/34776?lang=gb
This numbered playlist contains radiological images and associated cases for your further understanding of the following entities.

Table 12.4   Investigations for Abdominal Trauma

Bloods	• ABG, FBC, U&E, LFTs • Coagulation screen, group and crossmatch • Ethanol level, toxicology screen, β-HCG
Urinalysis	• Urine dipstick, urine toxicology, pregnancy test
Plain radiography	• Supine CXR is unreliable in the diagnosis of free intra-abdominal air
Focused abdominal sonography for trauma (FAST)	• **Imaging of the 4 P's:** Morrison's Pouch, Pouch of Douglas (or Pelvic), Perisplenic, and Pericardium • Used to identify the peritoneal cavity as a source of significant haemorrhage
	• Sensitive, but user dependent and not specific enough to identify the site of intra-abdominal haemorrhage • Cannot adequately assess for retroperitoneal haematoma
Diagnostic peritoneal lavage (DPL)	• Superseded by FAST and CT scanning • Aspiration of blood, GI contents, bile or faeces through the lavage catheter indicates laparotomy • *Rarely performed in ED setting, mentioned here as reference only, used in mass casualty settings or field trauma when there is reduced access to imaging*
CT-AP	• The investigation of choice in haemodynamically stable patients in whom there is no apparent indication for an emergency laparotomy • It provides detailed information of specific organ injury and may guide/inform conservative vs. operative management

INDICATIONS FOR RESUSCITATIVE LAPAROTOMY

- Blunt abdominal trauma.
- Unresponsive hypotension despite adequate resuscitation and no other cause for bleeding found.

INDICATIONS FOR URGENT LAPAROTOMY

- Blunt trauma with positive DPL or free blood on ultrasound and an unstable circulatory status.
- Blunt trauma with CT features of solid organ injury not suitable for conservative management.
- Clinical features of peritonitis.
- Any knife injury associated with visible viscera, clinical features of peritonitis, haemodynamic instability or developing fever/signs of sepsis.
- Any gunshot wound.

MCQs FOR SELF-ASSESSMENT

Chapter 13

PLASTIC SURGERY

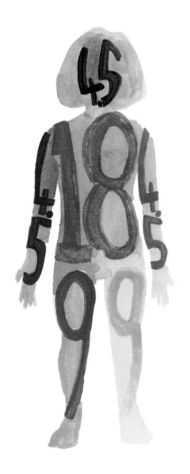
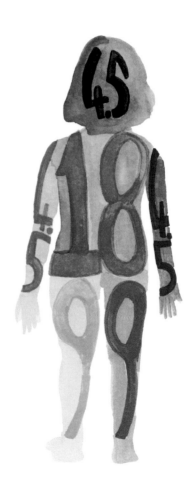

DOI: 10.1201/9781003207184-13

CONTENTS

Malignant Melanoma	265
Basal Cell Carcinoma versus Squamous Cell Carcinoma	268
Burns	270
Wound Healing	273
Dupuytren's Disease	278
Hand Trauma	280
Upper Limb Compression Neuropathy	281
Compartment Syndrome	283
Infectious Flexor Tenosynovitis	285
Trigger Finger (Stenosing Flexor Tenosynovitis)	286

MALIGNANT MELANOMA

DEFINITION

- A malignant neoplasm of melanocytes.

INCIDENCE

- Fifth most common cancer in the UK; 4% of all new cancers
- Global incidence doubled in last 20 years
- 80% of skin cancer deaths

RISK FACTORS: ENVIRONMENTAL AND GENETIC

- Fitzpatrick skin type 1 and 2: Pale skin, freckles, fair hair.
- Multiple benign naevi.
- Atypical naevi.
- UV exposure: UVB more strongly related to melanoma development compared to UVA. Intermittent, intense episodes of sun exposure increase the likelihood of melanoma development.
- Family history: Atypical melanoma syndrome, familial atypical multiple mole melanoma (FAMMM) syndrome.
- Personal history of melanoma.
- Immunosuppression.

CLINICAL PRESENTATION

- The **American System: 'ABCDE' system** Figure 13.1
  - Asymmetry, Border, Colour, Diameter, Evolution.

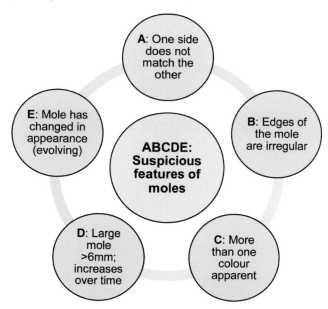

Figure 13.1 Clinical presentation of melanoma (American system).

- Metastatic melanoma may present with palpable lymph nodes. It may be the only clinical finding as the primary site of the melanoma may not be clinically evident.
- The **Glasgow system (7-point checklist)** Table 13.1
  - A score of 3 or more needs specialist referral.

Table 13.1 Clinical Presentation of Melanoma (Glasgow System)

Major (2 points)	Minor (1 point)
Change in size	Diameter ≥7 mm malignant melanoma
Irregular pigment	Inflammation
Irregular border	Oozing/Bleeding/Crusting
	Itching/Altered sensation

DIFFERENTIAL DIAGNOSIS

- Junctional or compound naevi.
- Campbell de Morgan spot (cherry angioma).
- Pigmented BCC.
- Seborrheic keratosis.
- Kaposi sarcoma.

PATHOLOGICAL SUBTYPES

STAGING

- **Breslow thickness:**
  - Depth of the tumour: The distance measured in mm from the epidermis to the maximum depth of the tumour Table 13.2.

Table 13.2 Breslow Thickness

Depth	5-Year Survival (%)
In situ	95–100
<1 mm	95–100
1–2 mm	80–95
2–4 mm	60–75
>4 mm	50

KEY POINT

Breslow thickness is the single most important prognostic variable. Other prognostic indicators include the presence of ulceration and number of mitoses.

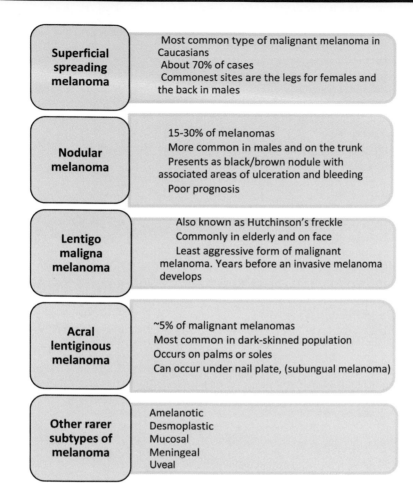

Superficial spreading melanoma	Most common type of malignant melanoma in Caucasians About 70% of cases Commonest sites are the legs for females and the back in males
Nodular melanoma	15-30% of melanomas More common in males and on the trunk Presents as black/brown nodule with associated areas of ulceration and bleeding Poor prognosis
Lentigo maligna melanoma	Also known as Hutchinson's freckle Commonly in elderly and on face Least aggressive form of malignant melanoma. Years before an invasive melanoma develops
Acral lentiginous melanoma	~5% of malignant melanomas Most common in dark-skinned population Occurs on palms or soles Can occur under nail plate, (subungual melanoma)
Other rarer subtypes of melanoma	Amelanotic Desmoplastic Mucosal Meningeal Uveal

Figure 13.2   Pathological subtypes.

- Sentinel lymph node biopsy is generally indicated if Breslow thickness is ≥0.8 mm. Any decisions made in relation to the management of melanoma are done through the MDT.

MANAGEMENT

- **Specific investigations**
  - Excision biopsy with a 2 mm margin (not a punch biopsy) for histopathology diagnosis.
  - A staging CT scan to rule out metastatic disease for tumours ≥1 mm thickness.
    - For all Stage 3 and considered in Stage 2.
  - Baseline blood tests.

- **Surgery**
  - Wide local excision is performed with a margin of 1–3 cm, depending on the Breslow thickness of the tumour.
  - Sentinel lymph node biopsy for tumours with ≥0.8 mm Breslow thickness, in the absence of regional lymphadenopathy and recommended by melanoma MDT.
  - The presence of metastatic disease in the sentinel node mandates completion lymphadenectomy.
- **Adjuvant therapy**
  - Immunotherapy (interferon)–for metastatic or recurrent disease, however trials of its efficacy are still ongoing
  - Ipilimumab (monoclonal antibody)–for metastatic disease
- **Local recurrence**
  - Surgical excision if lesions are solitary.
  - CO_2 laser useful for smaller dermal lesions.
  - Isolated chemotherapeutic limb perfusion has been demonstrated to aid in patients with multiple recurrences isolated to one limb.
- **Radiotherapy**
  - For metastatic disease and palliative symptom control, i.e. bone or brain metastases.

BASAL CELL CARCINOMA VERSUS SQUAMOUS CELL CARCINOMA

Table 13.3   Features of Basal Cell Carcinoma and Squamous Cell Carcinoma

	BCC	SCC
Definition/ Epidemiology	• Malignant neoplasm of the basal cells of the epidermis; also known as 'rodent ulcer' • Most common non-melanoma skin cancer (NMSC) • More common age >40 & Caucasians • Slow growing; **metastases are rare** • Cause extensive local damage if left untreated	• Malignant neoplasm of keratinising cells of the epidermis • Second most common NMSC • Higher mortality than BCC • More common age >50 & Caucasians • Metastases in SCC are more common than BCC; spread via lymphatics • Lesions on the lip, ears and perineum metastasise early; poorer prognosis
Risk factors	• Exposure to sunlight (i.e. working outdoors) • Fair skin, light hair, blue or green eyes • Male preponderance • Family history • Immunosuppression • Smoking • Previous BCC	

Table 13.3   Features of Basal Cell Carcinoma and Squamous Cell Carcinoma *(Continued)*

	BCC	SCC
Prevention	• **Primary:** Minimising sun exposure, protective clothing and sunscreen • **Secondary:** Early detection and appropriate management (regularly examining patients with previous BCC and biopsy of any suspicious skin lesions to confirm diagnosis)	
Presentation	• Shiny, translucent or pearly pink or skin coloured papule or nodule • The lesion may also be tan, black or brown and may be confused with a mole • Open sore that bleeds, oozes or crusts and remains open for 3 or more weeks. May ulcerate • A reddish patch or irritated area, which may crust or itch • Telangiectasia • A white, yellow or waxy scar-like area with poorly defined borders and shiny, taut skin may represent a more aggressive tumour	• Hyperkeratotic indurated crusted nodule • Reddish, scaly patch or plaque • Ulcerated • May bleed
Management	• Depends on the size, depth and location of the tumour • Surgical excision: simple excision (3 mm margins) or Mohs micrographic surgery • Cryotherapy/curettage • Radiotherapy: For medically unfit • Topical creams (Imiquimod 5% or Fluorouracil 5% [5-FU])–for smaller superficial lesions	• Excision of primary tumour with a 5–10 mm clearance margin • Block dissection of affected lymph nodes if lymphatic involvement • Radiotherapy: For unresectable tumours, unfit for surgery or local control of distant metastases • Cryotherapy/curettage • Topical creams (Fluorouracil 5% [5-FU])– for smaller superficial lesions
Prognosis	• Previous BCC diagnosis increases risk of having recurrent BCC's within 3 years by ~40%	• Good, with ~95% of patients remaining disease free at 5 years in those with clear margins

BURNS

AETIOLOGY

- Most **thermal burns** are caused by a flame, boiling water or contact with hot objects, e.g. hot stove.
- **Chemical burns** are much less common and most often occur with:
  - Industrial chemicals, e.g. splashes or inhalation of fumes.
  - Household chemicals, e.g. caustic soda.
- **Electrical burns** act like thermal burns: Heat is produced. Injury is proportional to the voltage of the source.
- **Cold thermal** injury occurs in frostbite.

EMERGENCY BURN CARE

- Manage as per ATLS guidelines.
- Stop the burning process.
- Flames: Stop, drop and roll, remove from burning source.
- Scalds: Remove wet clothing.
- Cool the burn:
  - Cool running water for at least 20 minutes.
  - Do not use ice.
  - Wet towels work less efficiently and should be changed regularly to ensure they are cold.

SEVERITY OF BURN INJURY DEPENDS ON MULTIPLE FACTORS

- Depth.
- Size: Calculated as a percentage of the total body surface area (TBSA).
- Location.
- Patient risk factors.

ASSESSING DEPTH OF THE BURN

- **Epidermal**
  - Erythematous/bright red, shiny.
  - Brisk capillary refill, painful to touch.
  - Heals within a few days with simple dressings.
- **Partial thickness (superficial or deep, can be mixed)**
  - Dark red, blotchy, may have blisters.
  - Slow capillary refill, may not have any sensation.
  - May heal with dressings, but if there is mixed depth, some require surgery.
- **Full thickness**
  - Leathery appearance, usually white.
  - No capillary refill or sensation.
  - Most require excision and reconstruction.

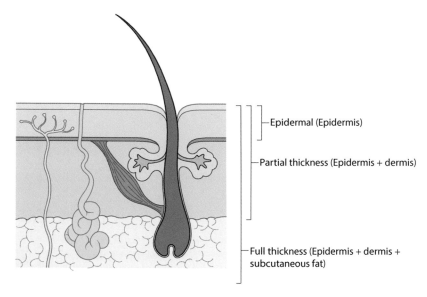

Epidermal (Epidermis)

Partial thickness (Epidermis + dermis)

Full thickness (Epidermis + dermis + subcutaneous fat)

Figure 13.3 Depth of burns.

- TBSA
- **Lund-Browder chart**
  - The most accurate method.
  - Note: There are different percentages for small children, as the head is proportionately larger.
  - For small burns, the 'palm rule' can be useful, the patient's palm (not the assessor) is worth ~1%.
- **Wallace rule of Nines** (less accurate)
  - Each entire arm (posterior and anterior surface) is worth 9%, each leg is 18%, anterior and posterior trunk is 18% each, etc. The head is 9% and the perineum is 1%.

BURN RESUSCITATION

- Burns cause vasodilation and increase vascular permeability.
- This causes oedema and loss of circulating fluid.
- May lead to organ failure.
- The burn area itself also has a direct loss of fluid due to evaporation.
- **Fluid resuscitation in the first 24 hours is paramount** to improve mortality and morbidity. Indicated in adults with >15% and children with >10% TBSA burns.

Top tip: The Parkland formula is the gold standard for guiding fluid replacement:

(4mls Hartmann's solusion) × (Bodyweight in kg) × (%TBSA)

Half of the fluid is given in the first 8 hours and the other half in the next 16 hours. Response should be monitored by urine output.

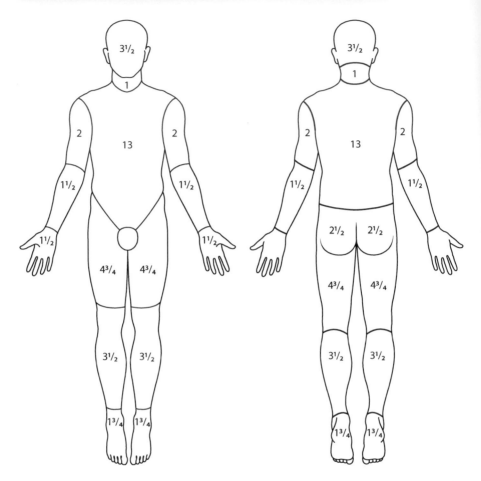

Figure 13.4 Lund-Browder chart for assessing burn size. Arun Murari, Kaushal Neelam Singh. Lund and Browder chart–modified versus original: a comparative study. Acute Crit. Care 2019;34(4):276–281. Published online November 29, 2019 https://doi.org/10.4266/acc.2019.00647

MANAGEMENT

- **General**
  - Early aggressive fluid resuscitation is key.
  - Early enteral feeding in more severe burns.
  - Drug therapy in burns includes IV analgesics and sedatives for the patient's comfort.
  - Tetanus immunisation is routinely given and antibiotics are usually administered topically due to no blood supply to the burn eschar.

- Proton pump inhibitors: To reduce the incidence of associated stress ulceration.
- Consider DVT prophylaxis.
- **Conservative treatment**
  - For small superficial or mixed partial thickness burns.
  - Simple dressings changed infrequently to allow healing.
- **Surgery**
  - For deeper burns or full thickness burns.
  - The burn is excised down to healthy viable tissue.
  - Usually the wounds are reconstructed using a split thickness skin graft.
  - For specialised areas such as the hand and face, full thickness skin graft may be indicated.

COMPLICATIONS

- **Circumferential burns can act like a tourniquet** and reduce blood supply to the affected limb resulting in ischaemia.
  - Treatment is by escharotomy (incision through the eschar/burn) to release the stricture and restore circulation to the compromised extremity.
- **Respiratory compromise**
  - Upper airway burns that cause oedema and obstruction of the airway.
  - Inhalation injury causing decreased gas exchange.
- **Renal compromise occurs secondary to acute tubular necrosis**
  - Because of the hypovolaemic state, blood flow decreases to the kidneys causing ischaemia.
  - If this persists, renal failure may ensue with severe metabolic acidosis and myoglobinuria.
- **Infection**
  - The most serious threat to further tissue injury and possible sepsis.
  - Survival may be dependent on the prevention of wound contamination.
  - Burns may be protected from contamination by application of topical antibiotics with or without dressings.
  - Excision of the burn and adequate skin coverage is the primary goal for these wounds.

WOUND HEALING

CLASSIFICATION

- **Primary intention:** May be further subdivided into the following categories:
  - Immediate closure of incised wound through apposition of wound edges.
  - Delayed primary closure in cases where time is allowed for oedema or infection to resolve before definitive wound closure.
- **Secondary intention:** Wound healing occurs by concomitant wound contraction and migration of fibroblasts and keratinocytes from the wound edges.

Table 13.4   Abnormal Scarring

Hypertrophic	Keloid
Abnormal proliferation of scar tissue limited to original wound margins.	Abnormal proliferation of scar tissue **extending beyond original wound margins.**
Hypertrophic more common than keloid.	More common in dark-skinned populations and often have family history.
Occur within 8 weeks of injury, grows rapidly and regresses over time.	Persist for many years and often do not regress spontaneously.
Typical locations are areas where there is scar tension such as pre-sternal region, shoulders and crossing joint surfaces.	May develop after minor trauma such as acne scars or ear piercing.
Type III collagen.	Type I and II collagen.
May lead to pruritus due to increased numbers of mast cells.	Treatment modalities may be combined and include pressure garments, silicone sheeting, topical silicone gel, intra-lesional corticosteroid injection, excision, and radiation (each of which carry high risk of keloid recurrence).

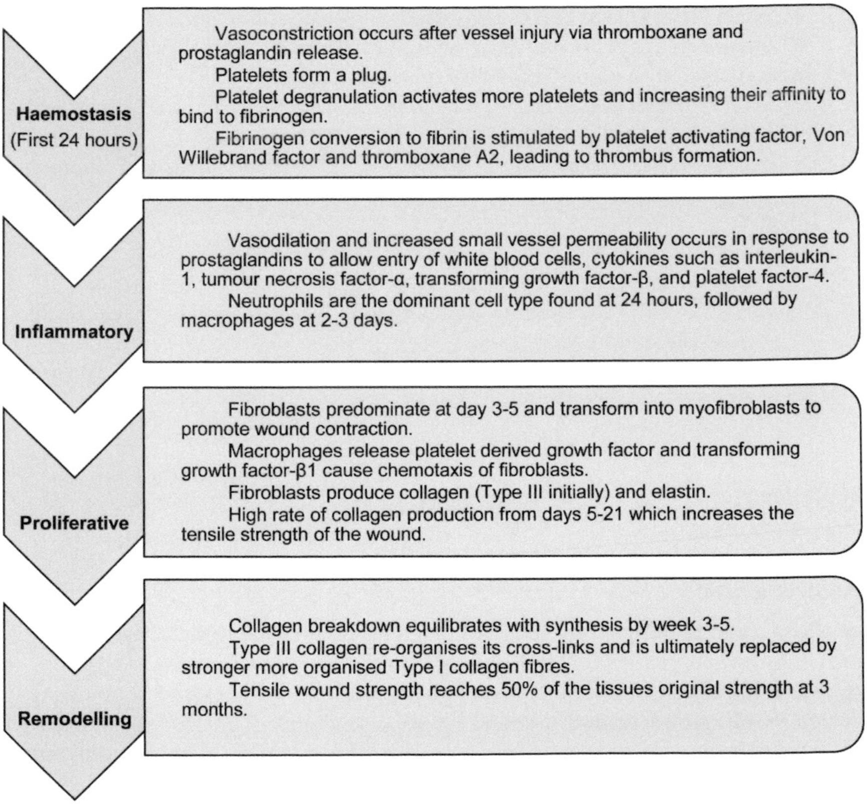

Haemostasis (First 24 hours)

Vasoconstriction occurs after vessel injury via thromboxane and prostaglandin release.

Platelets form a plug.

Platelet degranulation activates more platelets and increasing their affinity to bind to fibrinogen.

Fibrinogen conversion to fibrin is stimulated by platelet activating factor, Von Willebrand factor and thromboxane A2, leading to thrombus formation.

Inflammatory

Vasodilation and increased small vessel permeability occurs in response to prostaglandins to allow entry of white blood cells, cytokines such as interleukin-1, tumour necrosis factor-α, transforming growth factor-β, and platelet factor-4.

Neutrophils are the dominant cell type found at 24 hours, followed by macrophages at 2-3 days.

Proliferative

Fibroblasts predominate at day 3-5 and transform into myofibroblasts to promote wound contraction.

Macrophages release platelet derived growth factor and transforming growth factor-β1 cause chemotaxis of fibroblasts.

Fibroblasts produce collagen (Type III initially) and elastin.

High rate of collagen production from days 5-21 which increases the tensile strength of the wound.

Remodelling

Collagen breakdown equilibrates with synthesis by week 3-5.

Type III collagen re-organises its cross-links and is ultimately replaced by stronger more organised Type I collagen fibres.

Tensile wound strength reaches 50% of the tissues original strength at 3 months.

Figure 13.5   Phases of wound healing.

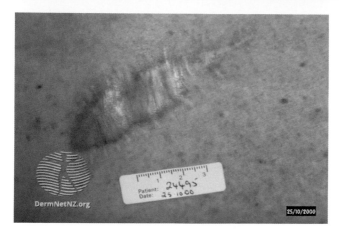

Figure 13.6   Hypertrophic scar. Image from DermNet NZ. https://creativecommons.org/licenses/by-nc-nd/3.0/nz/legalcode

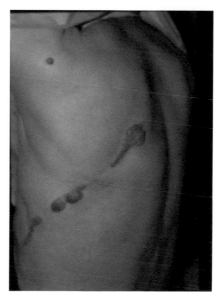

Figure 13.7   Keloid scar. Courtesy of Prof Tom Walsh

DISORDERED WOUND HEALING

- **Factors affecting wound healing**
  - Local factors
    - Infection, vascularity, trauma, radiation therapy, denervation.
  - Systemic factors
    - Congenital: Ehlers-Danlos syndrome, Werner syndrome, epidermolysis bullosa.
    - Acquired: Nutritional deficiency, steroid use, immunosuppression, diabetes mellitus (DM), hypothyroidism, smoking.

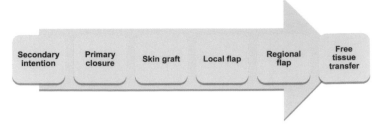

Figure 13.8   Reconstructive ladder.

- **Pathologic wound healing**
  - Acute failure of wound healing
    - Post-operative separation of a surgical incision
    - Local causes: Haematoma, seroma, infection, oedema, excess tension
  - Chronic failure of wound healing
    - Failure to achieve anatomical or functional integrity over 3 months.
    - Common causes: DM, venous stasis, ischaemic tissue, pressure necrosis, osteo-myelitis, hidradenitis suppuritiva, pyoderma gangrenosum, occult malignancy, e.g. SCC/Marjolin's ulcer.

WOUND MANAGEMENT

- **Reconstructive ladder:** Algorithm or spectrum of reconstructive options applied to manage wounds or defects that advocates the use of the least complicated techniques necessary for optimum functional and aesthetic outcome.
- **Skin grafts**
  - A graft is a subunit of tissue transferred from one part of the body to another without its own blood supply, e.g. skin, bone, cartilage.

Table 13.5   Types of Skin Grafts

Split-Thickness Skin Graft	Full-Thickness Skin Graft
Epidermis with a variable amount of dermis.	Epidermis with the entire dermis.
Harvested from thigh or buttock.	Harvested from eyelids, postauricular area, supraclavicular area, and less commonly flexor creases of the elbow, buttock or groin.
Deep dermis is preserved at donor site to allow healing by secondary intention.	Donor sites are areas with thin skin and allows direct closure of the donor defect.
Recipient site must have reasonable blood supply for skin graft to 'take'. The graft is usually tacked to the recipient site around the edges and covered for a week without any dressing change.	Requires good blood supply for survival and graft take.
If there is insufficient graft to cover the recipient site the graft may be meshed to allow it to spread out over a wider area.	Used to cover more sensitive areas, e.g. nose or eyelids, when pigment matching.

A dermatome is a surgical instrument used to produce thin slices of skin from a donor area, to use them for making skin grafts. A skin graft mesher is used to perforate skin sections. See the QR Code below for videos of both instruments.

AIR-POWERED DERMATOME AND SKIN GRAFT MESHER VIDEOS:

- **Flaps:**
  - A flap is a subunit of tissue that is transferred from one part of the body to another **with its own blood supply.**
  - Differs from skin graft in that it does not rely on revascularisation from the recipient bed.

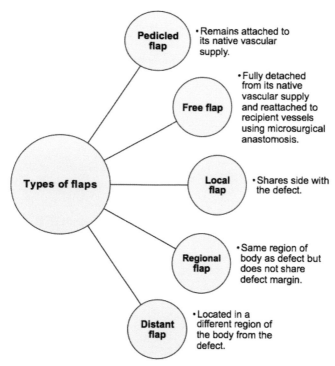

Figure 13.9 Types of flaps.

DUPUYTREN'S DISEASE

DEFINITION
- An abnormal, benign and progressive fibroproliferative disorder affecting the fascial layers of the digits and palm.

EPIDEMIOLOGY
- Caucasians, most commonly northern Europeans.
- Strong genetic predisposition. Autosomal dominant inheritance with variable penetrance.
- Male predominance, with approximately 7 to 10 times greater incidence.
- Peaks between 40 and 60 years of age.

AETIOLOGY
- Cause unknown.
- More common in diabetics (type 1 > type 2).
- Increased risk with smoking and heavy alcohol consumption according to population studies.
- Trauma can hasten the onset of Dupuytren's disease in those predisposed.

PRESENTATION
- **Discrete nodules, longitudinal cords**
- Skin thickening and pitting
- Progressive flexion contractures
- Affects the palm and most commonly the ring and small fingers

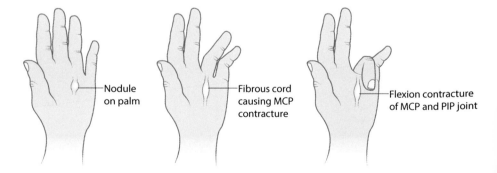

Figure 13.10   Progression of Dupuytren's disease.

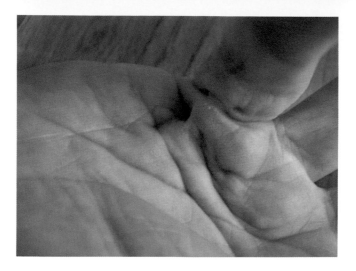

Figure 13.11   Dupuytren's contracture. Courtesy of Prof Tom Walsh

DUPUYTREN'S DIATHESIS (DD)

- An aggressive cohort which has an earlier onset of disease and an early recurrence.
- Features in patients with increased disease severity and recurrence risk:
  - Bilateral palmar lesions.
  - Family history of DD.
  - Ectopic lesions.
  - Ethnicity (northern European).
  - Male.
  - Age of onset (<50 years old).
- Ectopic disease
  - Knuckle pads: **Garrod pads.**
  - Foot involvement: **Ledderhose disease.**
  - Penis involvement: **Peyronie's disease.**

SURGICAL INDICATIONS

- MCPJ contracture is usually correctable.
  - Interference with daily activities.
  - If contracture 30°–45°.
- PIPJ contracture is difficult to fully correct.
  - Early intervention.
- Contracture causing maceration or hygiene difficulties.
- Rapid rate of progression.
- If patient is not able to have both the digit and palm simultaneously on the table surface (**Hueston's tabletop test**).

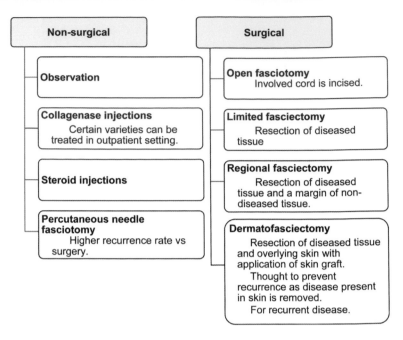

Figure 13.12 Management of Dupuytren's disease.

COMPLICATIONS (SURGERY)
- Wound healing issues, infection
- Pain
- Recurrence
- Neurovascular injury
- Finger stiffness
- Complex regional pain syndrome

HAND TRAUMA

TENDON INJURIES
- **Flexor tendon injuries**
  - Commonly result from volar lacerations and may be associated with neurovascular injury.
  - Surgical repair.
  - Early hand therapy and ROM exercises is extremely important.
- **Extensor tendon injuries**
  - Commonly from dorsal lacerations.
  - If injury proximal to juncturae tendinum, may be a normal range of motion as disruption to extensor mechanism is masked.
  - Surgical repair.

FRACTURES
- Rigid fixation allows for early movement.
- Aim to move hand early to reduce stiffness.

AMPUTATIONS
- **Indications for replantation**
  - Thumb, multiple digit, or whole hand amputations.
  - Transmetacarpal and partial hand amputations.
  - Any amputated part in a child.
  - Sharp injuries at elbow, proximal forearm, or humeral-level amputations.
  - Single-digit amputations distal to flexor digitorum superficialis (FDS) insertion.
  - Single-digit amputations in athletes/musicians/persons needing full complement of fingers and cosmesis.
- **Management of the amputated part**
  - Amputated part is wrapped in moist saline gauze.
  - Placed in a waterproof ziplock plastic bag/container and placed in icy water.
  - Get X-ray to rule out fracture.
- **Management of patient**
  - Stabilise.
  - Optimise.
  - Surgical repair.
- **Post-operative**
  - Keep patient and digit warm and well perfused.
  - Urine output >0.5 ml/kg/hr.
  - Look for changes in the colour of digit.
  - Post-operative use of therapeutic heparin/LWMH.
  - Examine finger every hour, and if any change from baseline, notify the surgeon as may need to go back to theatre.

UPPER LIMB COMPRESSION NEUROPATHY

MEDIAN NERVE
- **Carpal tunnel syndrome**
  - Most common mononeuropathy of upper limb.
  - Compression of the median nerve in the fixed rigid space of the carpal tunnel.
- **Aetiology**
  - Reduction in size of the tunnel.
    - Acromegaly, trauma (e.g. dislocation), osteophytes due to osteoarthritis.
  - Increase in the volume of contents.
    - Ganglia, lipomas, inflammation (gout, rheumatoid), metabolic changes (DM, pregnancy).
  - Congenital (rare)
    - Persistent median artery, abnormally long FDS muscle belly.

- ● **Risk factors of carpal tunnel syndrome**
  - ● Female sex, DM, pregnancy, rheumatoid arthritis, hypothyroidism, connective tissue disorders, wrist fracture or dislocation, or arthritis that deforms the small bones in the wrist.
- ● **Carpal tunnel anatomy**
  - ● Boundaries:
    - – Scaphoid and trapezium radially.
    - – Pisiform and hook of hamate ulnarly.
    - – Transverse carpal ligament forms the roof.
    - – Carpal bones form the floor.
  - ● Contents:
    - – Median nerve.
    - – Flexor pollicis longus (FPL).
    - – Flexor digitorum superficialis (FDS) × 4.
    - – Flexor digitorum profundus (FDP) × 4.
- ● **Presentation**
  - ● Pain and paraesthesia of thumb, index, middle, and radial border ring finger, worse at night and relieved by shaking hands.
- ● **Clinical exam**
  - ● Thenar muscle wasting and weakness of abduction.
  - ● Thenar sensory disturbance spared due to innervation by palmar cutaneous branch.
  - ● Special tests: Phalen's, Tinel's, and Durkan's tests. Pen touch test can be used to isolate abduction.
- ● **Electromyography studies**
  - ● Aid in diagnosis and localisation of nerve compression site.
  - ● Prolonged motor and sensory latencies and reduced conduction velocities are diagnostic for carpal tunnel syndrome.
- ● **Management**
  - ● Conservative treatment
    - – Analgesia, NSAIDs, corticosteroid injection.
    - – Splint in neutral position continuously at night time.
  - ● Surgery
    - – Open carpal tunnel release.
- ● **Post-operative complications**
  - ● Infection, haematoma, scar, tenderness.
  - ● Complex regional pain syndrome.
  - ● Pillar pain, incomplete resolution of symptoms due to 'double-crush' phenomenon.
  - ● Injury to palmar cutaneous branch, and recurrent motor branches of median nerve.

ULNAR NERVE

- ● **Cubital tunnel syndrome**
  - ● Compression at multiple sites at or adjacent to cubital tunnel.
- ● **Ulnar tunnel syndrome**
  - ● Compression in Guyon's canal.
- ● **Presentation**
  - ● Hypoesthesia/paraesthesia of little and ulnar half ring fingers and dorsoulnar hand.

- Sensory disturbance at dorsoulnar hand is spared in ulnar tunnel syndrome innervated by dorsal sensory branch of ulnar nerve.
- Weakness of grip strength and intrinsic wasting in advanced cases causing functional issues with fine motor control.
- **Tinel's test**–positive over site of compression.
- **'Ulnar paradox'**–more likely to get clawing with distal compared to proximal ulnar nerve compression due to sparing of the FDP.
- **Management**
  - Conservative treatment
    - Analgesia/NSAIDs.
    - Splint wrist in neutral position.
  - Surgery
    - Decompression of cubital tunnel or ulnar tunnel as per site of compression.

RADIAL NERVE

- **Posterior interosseous syndrome**
  - Compression at or adjacent to radiocapitellar joint.
- **Radial tunnel syndrome**
  - Compression at radial tunnel running from radiocapetellar joint to the distal edge of the supinator.
- **Wartenberg syndrome**
  - Compression of superficial sensory branch of radial nerve
- **Diagnosis**
  - Gradual weakness of finger and wrist extensors
  - Posterior interosseous syndrome: Motor symptoms predominates.
  - Radial tunnel syndrome: Pain predominates.
  - Wartenberg syndrome: Pain and paraesthesia is exacerbated by pinch grip.
- **Management**
  - Conservative treatment
    - Analgesia/NSAIDs.
    - Splint/Steroid injection.
  - Surgery
    - Nerve exploration/decompression.

COMPARTMENT SYNDROME

DESCRIPTION

- Surgical emergency.
- Raised pressure within a closed anatomical space, which as it continues to rise, will eventually compromise tissue perfusion resulting in **necrosis** as a result of microvascular compromise.
- Can occur in the lower limb (below knee, most common), thigh, forearm, foot and hand.

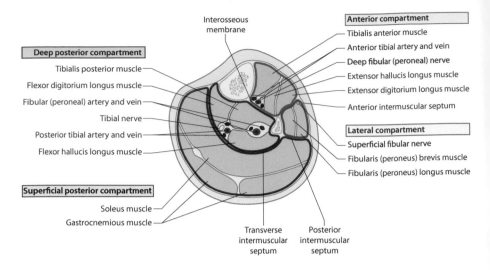

Figure 13.13   Left leg axial view from below showing compartments of the lower leg.

PRESENTATION

- Pain out of proportion to the injury (most significant) and worse on passive stretch of the compartment muscles Figure 13.13.
- Paraesthesia.
- Pallor (may be present).
- Arterial pulsation may still be felt but pulselessness tends to be a sign of irreversible damage.
- Paralysis of the muscle group may occur.

CAUSES

- Blunt trauma.
- Crush injury.
- Fractures–tight cast.
- Burns.
- Penetrating trauma–vascular injury.
- Malignancy.

DIAGNOSIS

- Clinical suspicion.
- Measurement of intracompartmental pressures:
  - Compartment pressure of >40 mmHg or >30 mmHg with clinical suspicion (can be measured using Stryker needle and is especially useful in unconscious patients).
  - Difference between diastolic pressure and compartment pressure of <30 mmHg.
  - Follow the trend of pressures.

MANAGEMENT

- Prompt and extensive **fasciotomies** within 4–6 hours of symptom onset.
- If the extremity is being compressed by dressings, reduce them.

COMPLICATIONS

- Muscle fibrosis and death–Volkmann ischaemic contracture.
- Nerve injury and dysfunction.
- Myoglobinuria and renal failure–aggressive IV fluid resuscitation.
- Amputation–consider if muscle groups necrotic at fasciotomy.

INFECTIOUS FLEXOR TENOSYNOVITIS

DEFINITION

- Infection of the tendon and synovial sheath leading to inflammatory products in the potential space between the visceral and parietal paratenon.

KEY POINTS

- Infectious source may be from local trauma, spread from surrounding soft tissues, or haematogenous spread.
- Progresses from exudative (Stage 1) to suppurative (Stage 2) to septic necrosis of the tissue (Stage 3) if not treated promptly.

COMPLICATIONS

- Rupture of tendon sheath.
- Compartment syndrome.
- Ischaemia and necrosis.

KANAVEL'S CARDINAL SIGNS

- Tenderness on percussion or palpation over the flexor sheath.
- Finger held in slight flexion.
- Pain on passive extension.
- Fusiform swelling.

MANAGEMENT

- Surgical emergency: Early antibiotics plus surgical intervention.
  - Initially empiric antibiotics guided by mechanism of injury then tailored if possible.
- Surgery is almost always required to decompress the flexor space:
  - **Brunner's incision:** 'Z' shape incision allows surgical access to tendon sheath and avoids contracture and functional complication of a linear incision.
  - **Stage 1:** Tendon sheath irrigation and drainage +/– debridement.
  - **Stage 2/3:** Debridement of tendon sheath and necrotic tissue.

TRIGGER FINGER (STENOSING FLEXOR TENOSYNOVITIS)

KEY POINTS

- This occurs due to difficulty in the tendon to pass through a relatively stenosed fibro-osseous canal due to thickening of the first annular (A1) pulley overlying MCP joint.
- This leads to an inability to smoothly flex or extend the affected digit with associated painless locking of the finger in flexion or extension which may only be overcome with passive manipulation.
- The cause is unknown but may be due to overuse or repetitive use.

MANAGEMENT

- **Conservative/medical**
  - Limit exacerbating activities and use splinting.
  - May involve a trial of NSAIDs.
  - Local glucocorticoid injection if above fails.
- **Surgical:** Reserved for those that fail conservative treatment and glucocorticoid injections.
  - Surgical release of the A1 pulley ligament.
  - Open approach most common.

COMPLICATIONS FROM SURGERY

- Infection.
- Digital nerve damage.
- Bowstringing of the flexor tendon.
- Scarring of the tendon.

MCQs FOR SELF-ASSESSMENT

Chapter 14

ORTHOPAEDIC SURGERY

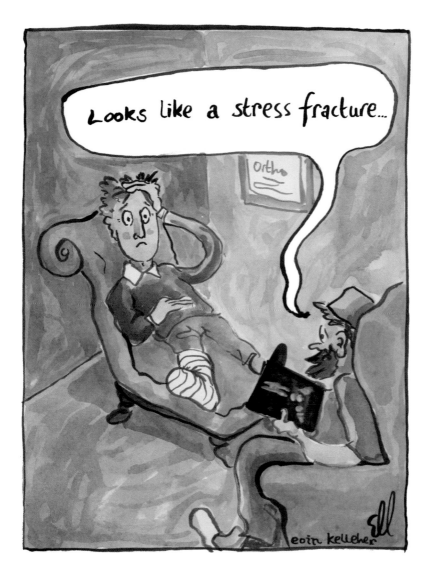

DOI: 10.1201/9781003207184-14

CONTENTS

Principles of Orthopaedics	289
Upper Limb Injuries	292
Distal Radial Fracture	292
Humeral Fracture	295
Clavicle Fracture	297
Anterior Shoulder Dislocation	298
Posterior Shoulder Dislocation	299
Scaphoid Fracture	300
Lower Limb Injuries	301
Hip Fracture	301
Slipped Upper Femoral Epiphysis (SUFE)	303
Ankle Fractures	304
Tibial Fracture	307
Open Fractures	307
Compartment Syndrome in Orthopeadics	308
Pelvic Fractures	309
Septic Arthritis	311
Back Pain	312
Cauda Equina Syndrome	312
Sciatica	313
Osteoarthritis	313

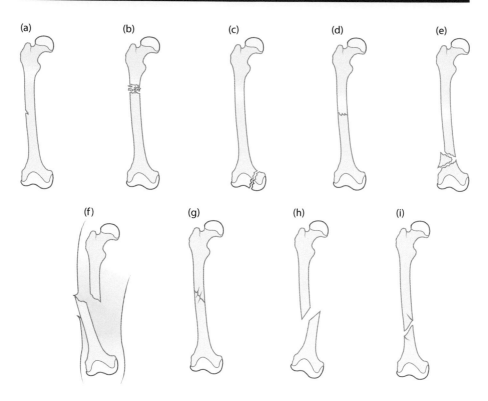

Figure 14.1 (a)–(i): Types of fractures.

PRINCIPLES OF ORTHOPAEDICS

DEFINITIONS

- A fracture is a break in the continuity of bone cortex, whether it's complete or incomplete Figure 14.1.
- **A closed fracture** is a fracture with intact skin, and there is no communication with the external environment.
- **An open fracture** is a type of fracture where there is fracture site communication with the external environment, due to a breach in the skin.
- **Reduction** is the manipulation of a fracture to restore normal alignment at the fracture site.
- In medical notes, the '#' symbol is used instead of the word 'fracture.'
- Fracture-dislocation occurs when the fracture is associated with joint dislocation (complete loss of contact of the joint surfaces).

GENERAL FRACTURE MANAGEMENT

- Follow the ATLS guidelines: Treat life-threatening injuries first.
- Provide adequate analgesia.
- Always check neurovascular status before and after interventions.
- Fracture dislocations need to be reduced ASAP.
- Wounds require antibiotics ideally within one hour of injury, and tetanus cover.
- Irrigation of wounds needs to be done in the operating theatre, e.g. open fractures.
- Reduction promotes healing and reduces pain.
- A back-slab, rather than a full cast, is applied initially to allow room for swelling.
- Obtain X-rays:
  - Two views
  - Two joints (above and below)
  - Two eyes (confer with a colleague/senior)
- Unstable fractures, intraarticular fractures, displaced fractures and poorly reduced fractures are the ones most likely to require operative intervention.

PRINCIPLES IN FRACTURE TREATMENT

- **Reduction** of the fracture (closed or open surgical reduction).
- **Immobilisation:** Cast/splint/internal or external surgical device.
- **Rehabilitation:** Mobilisation and exercise.

WHY DO WE REDUCE FRACTURES?

- Stabilise the fracture
- Reduce pain
- Preserve the blood supply
- Restore anatomical relationships
- Aid bone healing and remodelling
- Avoid deformity and mal-union
- Reduce the chance of non-union
- Reduce the risk of osteoarthritis

FRACTURE REDUCTION

- **Open or closed reduction**
  - **Closed reduction**
    - The fracture is reduced manually without surgically exposing the fracture site.
    - This may be done with the patient awake or under general anaesthetic.
    - Immobilisation could be achieved with a cast, brace or surgical devices (e.g. percutaneous wires, or intramedullary nailing).
  - **Open reduction**
    - The fracture site is exposed surgically.
    - The fracture is then usually immobilised by internal fixation with plates and screws.
    - This is generally referred to as open reduction and internal fixation (**ORIF**).

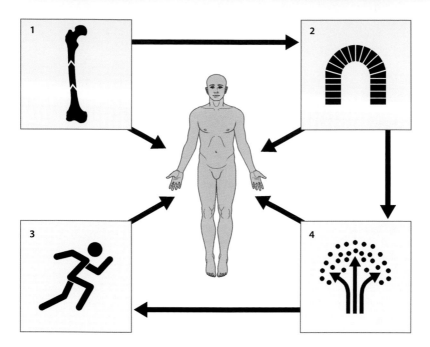

Figure 14.2. The principles of fracture fixation.

THE PRINCIPLES OF FRACTURE FIXATION

KEY POINT

- **Fracture reduction** to restore anatomical relationship.
- **Fracture fixation** to provide absolute or relative stability.
- Preservation of blood supply.
- Early and safe mobilisation.

STAGES IN FRACTURE HEALING

1. Tissue destruction and haematoma formation (immediate)
2. Inflammation and cellular proliferation (acute)
3. Callus formation (days to weeks)
4. Consolidation (weeks to months)
5. Remodelling (months up to more than one year)

Top tip:

Factors Adversely Affecting the Healing of Fractures:

Age, poor nutrition, smoking, drugs, local trauma, mal-reduction and immobilisation, infection and fracture location.

UPPER LIMB INJURIES

DISTAL RADIAL FRACTURE

KEY FACTS

- Distal radius fracture is the most common orthopaedic injury with a bimodal distribution.
  - Younger patients: High-energy mechanisms, fall from a height, RTA, sports injuries.
  - Older patients: Low-energy mechanisms, e.g. fall from standing position.
- 50% intra-articular.
- Distal radio-ulnar joint (DRUJ) injuries must be evaluated.
- Radial styloid fracture indicates higher energy.

RISK FACTORS

- Decreased bone mineral density
- Female sex
- Caucasian
- Early menopause

Top tip:

Mechanism of Injury: The most common mechanism is a fall onto an outstretched hand (FOOSH) with wrist in dorsiflexion.

PRESENTATION

- Wrist deformity, swelling, pain, bruising and loss of function.
- The neurovascular examination is essential; median nerve symptoms are common, carpal tunnel compression (13–23%).

EPONYMS

- **Colles' Fracture**
  - Extra-articular distal radius fracture with dorsal angulation (apex volar), dorsal displacement, radial shift and radial shortening.
  - Classical 'dinner fork' deformity.
- **Smith's fracture** (reverse Colles)
  - Extra-articular fracture with volar angulation (apex dorsal). With a 'garden spade' deformity or volar displacement of the hand and distal radius.
  - Fall onto a flexed wrist with forearm fixed in supination.
  - This unstable distal radius almost always needs surgical fixation with a volar buttress plate.

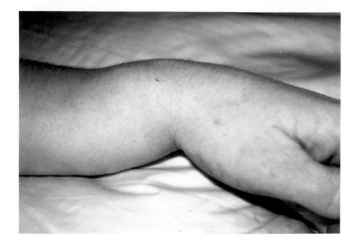

Figure 14.3 Dinner fork deformity. Courtesy of Prof Joe O'Beirne

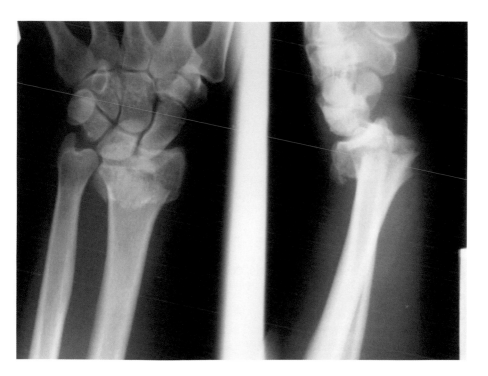

Figure 14.4 Colles' fracture. Courtesy of Prof Joe O'Beirne

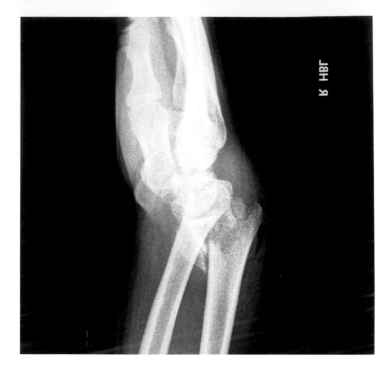

Figure 14.5 Smith's fracture. Courtesy of Prof Joe O'Beirne

TREATMENT

- **Non-operative**
  - Cast immobilisation for non-displaced or minimally displaced fractures.
  - Closed reduction and cast immobilisation for displaced fractures.
  - Low demand patients, e.g. significant surgical risk patient or severe dementia.
- **Operative**
  - Indications include:
    - Intra-articular fracture with 2 mm displacement
    - Failed closed reduction
    - Significant radial tilt or loss of radial height
    - Metaphyseal comminution or bone loss, loss of volar buttress with displacement (e.g. Smith's fracture)
    - DRUJ instability
    - Open fractures
  - Techniques include:
    - Percutaneous wiring
    - Open reduction internal fixation (ORIF)–dorsal or volar plating
    - External fixation–some of the open fractures when adequate soft tissue coverage can't be achieved)

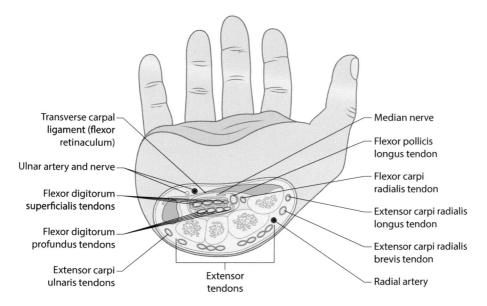

Transverse carpal ligament (flexor retinaculum)

Ulnar artery and nerve

Flexor digitorum superficialis tendons

Flexor digitorum profundus tendons

Extensor carpi ulnaris tendons

Extensor tendons

Median nerve

Flexor pollicis longus tendon

Flexor carpi radialis tendon

Extensor carpi radialis longus tendon

Extensor carpi radialis brevis tendon

Radial artery

Figure 14.6   The right carpal tunnel.

COMPLICATIONS

- Carpal tunnel syndrome and median nerve dysfunction
- Mal-union and non-union
- Posttraumatic osteoarthritis
- Tendon rupture (extensor pollicis longus EPL tendon)
- Complex regional pain syndrome CRPS

HUMERAL FRACTURE

KEY FACTS

- Increased incidence in older population is related to osteoporosis.
- 300,000 per year (more common than hip fractures)
- 85% are undisplaced
- Female:male = 2:1, likely related to issues of bone density

MECHANISMS OF INJURY

- Fall onto outstretched hand from standing height typically in old, osteoporotic women.
- Younger patients present following high-energy trauma e.g. RTA.

- Other mechanisms:
  - Electrical shock, seizure, direct trauma (greater tuberosity fracture), malignancy.

PRESENTATION

- Pain in shoulder or proximal arm, with arm held close to chest.
- Swelling, tenderness, reduced range of motion and crepitus.
- Possible paraesthesia or numbness of lateral arm over deltoid (regimental patch), secondary to *axillary nerve injury*.

NEER CLASSIFICATION

- Based on the number of fragments displaced: Ranges from 1 to 4 parts. Also may have articular subtypes.
- The four described fragments include:
  - Greater tuberosity (GT)
  - Lesser tuberosity (LT)
  - Surgical neck (SN).
- The classification then describes the number of fragments displacement:
  - One-part fractures are minimally displaced (<45° angulation or <1 cm displacement).
  - A way of remembering this is, in minimally displaced fractures, the humerus can still be thought of as 'one complete part' → 1-part).
- For each number of parts that is displaced (e.g. GT, LT, SN) the classification goes up by 1-part. Thus a 2-part has one fragment displaced, a 3-part has 2 fragments displaced.

TREATMENT

- **Non-operative treatment:**
  - Minimally or non-displaced fractures
  - Immobilisation with broad arm sling, shoulder immobiliser, humeral brace, U-slab or hanging cast
- **Operative treatment:**
  - Any significant displacement of 2-part or more fractures
  - ORIF or intramedullary nail as option
  - 3-part or more fractures are unstable and are almost always surgically treated
  - Primary shoulder arthroplasty is an option for elderly patients

COMPLICATIONS

- Vascular injury (5–6%); axillary artery most common site
- Neural injury (brachial plexus, axillary nerve injuries)
- Myositis ossificans
- Joint stiffness
- Avascular necrosis
- Non-union or Malunion

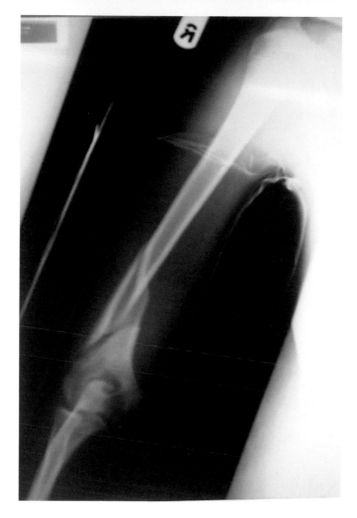

Figure 14.7   Humeral shaft fracture. Courtesy of Prof Joe O'Beirne

CLAVICLE FRACTURE

KEY FACTS

- Fall or direct blow to lateral shoulder
- 75% occur in middle of clavicle, 20% lateral/distal clavicle

TREATMENT

- **Middle third:**
  - Most treated conservatively with broad arm sling
  - ORIF is for: Open fractures, significant displacement or shortening, skin tenting by fracture, neurovascular injury
- **Lateral/medial third:**
  - Non-displaced–sling, displaced–ORIF

COMPLICATIONS

- Neurovascular injury: Brachial plexus
- Pneumothorax
- Non-union
- Operative complications:
  - Infection, vascular injury, pneumothorax
  - Paraesthesia secondary to supraclavicular nerve injury

ANTERIOR SHOULDER DISLOCATION

KEY FACTS

- Anterior dislocation is most common
- **Trauma:** Forced abduction and external rotation, or a direct all on the shoulder.
- Shoulder looks 'square,' loss of normal contour
- Patients support affected arm with their other arm

TREATMENT

- Reduction of dislocation with various methods
- **Assess neurovascular status before and after reduction**–axillary nerve sensation
- **External rotation technique:**
  - The patient's arm is adducted with the elbow flexed
  - The forearm is then gently and very slowly externally rotated
- **Stimson technique:**
  - The patient lays prone on a trolley with their arm hanging off the side with a weight and allowed to drop towards the ground
- **Cunningham:**
  - The clinician sits in front of the patient who is in a comfortable sitting position
  - The patient places the hand of the dislocated shoulder on the clinician's shoulder who then rests one arm on the patient's elbow crease while gently massaging the patient's biceps, deltoid and trapezius to encourage relaxation.
  - The patient is then encouraged to pull the shoulder blades together while straightening the back.

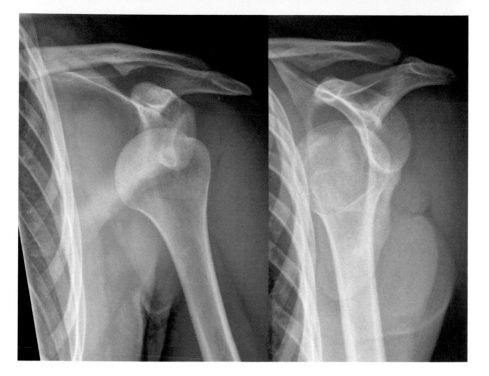

Figure 14.8   Left and Right: Anterior shoulder dislocation. Courtesy of Prof Joe O'Beirne

POSTERIOR SHOULDER DISLOCATION

KEY FACTS

- Epileptic seizure or electrocution.
- A fall on outstretched arm, while arm is in an internally rotated, flexed, adducted position.
- Arm is held in internal rotation, unable to externally rotate. Can palpate humeral head posteriorly.

 Top tip: Do not miss a posterior dislocation. Look for the 'lightbulb sign' and always get three X-ray views of the shoulder.

MANAGEMENT

- A humeral head defect <25% of articular surface + a duration of injury <3 weeks means **closed reduction can be tried**
- **Otherwise:** Surgical intervention may be best

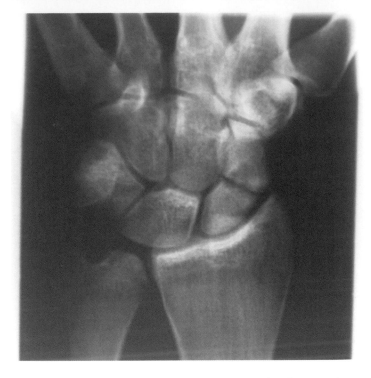

Figure 14.9 Scaphoid non-union following fracture. Courtesy of Prof Joe O'Beirne

SCAPHOID FRACTURE

KEY FACTS

- FOOSH (Fallen onto an outstretched hand)
- Tender at anatomical snuffbox
- Treat on clinical suspicion:
  - Repeat X-ray at 2 weeks. If still no fracture, perform CT/MRI
- Risk of avascular necrosis (AVN)
  - More proximal fractures = higher risk AVN

 Top tip: Scaphoid fractures may not be visible on initial X-ray.

Treat based on clinical suspicion and repeat X-rays at 2 weeks.

LOWER LIMB INJURIES

HIP FRACTURE

KEY FACTS

- Most common fracture site in the elderly
- 80% occur in women
- Bimodal distribution: Majority in elderly, minority in young patients (road traffic accident/high energy trauma)
- Other risk factors:
  - Caucasian
  - Osteoporosis or osteopenia
  - Diabetes mellitus
  - Recurrent falls
  - Tobacco and alcohol use

PRESENTATION

- Pain and unable to weight bear on the affected limb
- Shortened and externally rotated limb
- If high clinical suspicion but X-ray unequivocal perform CT or MRI (gold standard)

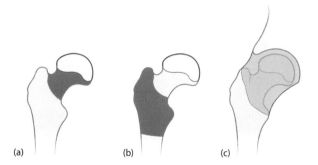

(a)   (b)   (c)

Figure 14.10   (a)–(c). Classification of hip fractures.

Intracapsular Fractures	Extracapsular Fractures	The Joint Capsule Demarcates the Area for Intra-Capsular Fractures
• Any fracture in the yellow shaded area shown above • These must be classified according to **Garden classification** to determine whether to:	• Any fractures in the green shaded area shown above • Includes intertrochanteric and sub-trochanteric fractures	• The femoral head can also be fractured and these fractures should not be confused with intracapsular neck of femur fractures

(continued)

• **Fix** the fracture, with cannulated screws or dynamic hip screw (DHS) OR • **Replace** it (hemi-arthroplasty or total hip arthroplasty)	• These **must be fixed**; they cannot be replaced • Fix using DHS or intramedullary (IM) nail	• These fractures are classified differently altogether

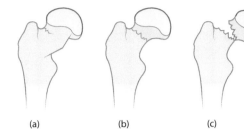
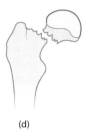

(a)   (b)   (c)   (d)

Figure 14.11 (a)–(d). Classification of intracapsular neck of femur fractures. Garden classification.

Garden I	• Incomplete fracture • Not displaced but impacted • Called 'valgus impacted'–due to valgus deformity at the neck
Garden II	• Complete fracture • Non-displaced fracture
Garden III	• Complete fracture • Partially displaced
	• Risk of AVN of the femoral head after fixation, so replacement by hemi-arthroplasty or total hip arthroplasty is recommended • In very young patients fixation rather than replacement may still be attempted
Garden IV	• Complete fracture • Fully displaced • High risk AVN • Should be treated with hemiarthroplasty or total hip arthroplasty • In very young patients fixation rather than replacement may still be attempted

COMPLICATIONS

- AVN of femoral head
- Osteoarthritis
- Non-union
- Mortality (**pre-injury mobility** is the most significant determinant of post-operative survival)
- Wound infection
- Haematoma
- DVT/PE

Top tip: Hip fractures should be operated on the day of, or day after admission to improve patient outcomes.

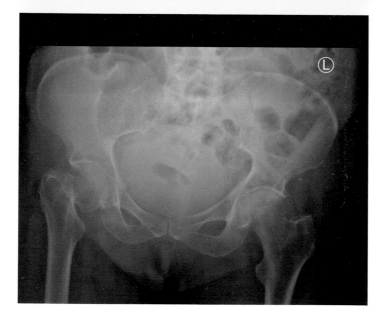

Figure 14.12　Right displaced intracapsular fracture (Garden III). Courtesy of Prof Joe O'Beirne

SLIPPED UPPER FEMORAL EPIPHYSIS (SUFE)

KEY FACTS

- Paediatric/adolescent presentation
- Not usually associated with trauma
- Instability of the proximal femoral growth plate

CLINICAL PRESENTATION

- Can include hip pain, thigh pain, knee pain
- Limp (acute or chronic)
- Decreased ROM of the hip
- Shortening of the affected limb is possible

X-RAY FEATURES

- **Displaced femoral head:** Posterior and inferior to femoral neck, within the limits of the acetabulum

---

Top tip:

Do not miss: Often presents as knee pain. Always examine the joint above and below the site of pain.

MANAGEMENT

- Non-weight bearing with crutches, and typically includes surgical fixation
- Fixation of the unaffected side may be a necessary preventative measure

ANKLE FRACTURES

KEY FACTS

- The ankle is complex hinge joint composed of articulations among the fibula, tibia and talus held by ligaments.
- Usual mechanism of injury include torsional (foot inversion) or axial loading (fall from height).

CLINICAL PRESENTATION

- Pain, swelling of ankle, clinical deformity, non-weight bearing on ankle.
- Fractures can involve just one malleolus, both medial and lateral malleoli (bimalleolar), or all three 'malleoli' i.e. medial, lateral and posterior (trimalleolar).

CLASSIFICATIONS

- **Denis–Weber classification**
  - Based on level of fibular fracture; the more proximal the injury, greater risk of syndesmosis disruption and instability.

Denis–Weber Classification	
Normal ankle joint	• The syndesmosis (shown in grey below) consists of the ligament complex at the distal tibiofibular joint and the lower thickened portion of the intraosseous membrane • As it is ligamentous it is not visible on X-ray
Weber A	• Fracture line (red) below the level of the syndesmosis • Usually treated in below knee walking cast
Weber B	• Fracture at the level of the syndesmosis • Some possibility of syndesmosis disruption and instability • Needs surgical fixation if significant displacement, or non-weight bearing in below knee cast if non-displaced
Weber C	• Fracture above the level of the syndesmosis • High likelihood of syndesmosis disruption and instability • Needs surgical fixation

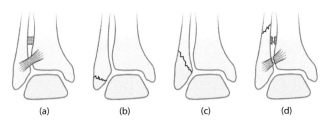

Figure 14.13   (a)–(d). Denis–Weber classification.

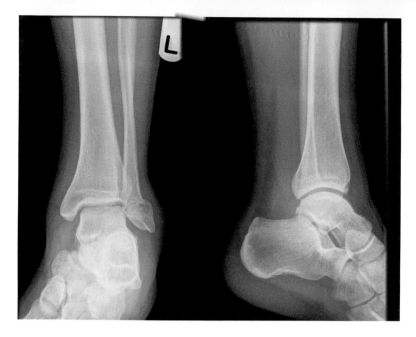

Figure 14.14   Weber A ankle fracture. Courtesy of Prof Joe O'Beirne

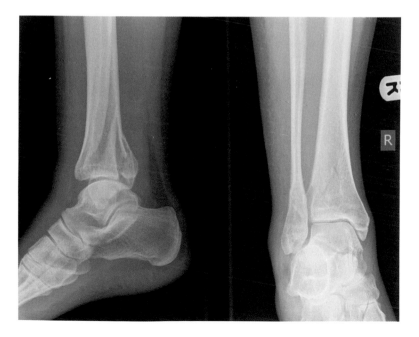

Figure 14.15   Weber B ankle fracture. Courtesy of Prof Joe O'Beirne

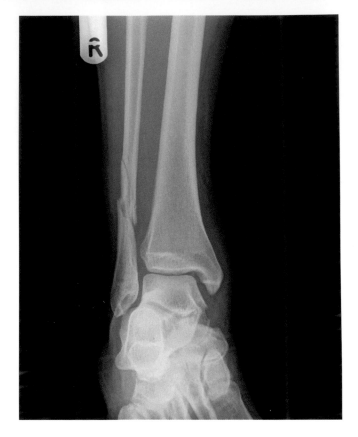

Figure 14.16   Weber C ankle fracture. Courtesy of Prof Joe O'Beirne

MAISONNEUVE FRACTURE

- Medial malleolar fracture OR a deltoid ligament rupture

WITH

- A fracture at proximal third of fibula.
- It may be associated with a syndesmosis injury.
- Always remember to examine the knee as well as the ankle.

COMPLICATIONS OF ANKLE FRACTURES

- Malunion, non-union
- Osteoarthritis
- Infection
- Prosthesis failure
- DVT

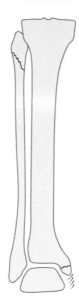

Figure 14.17 Maisonneuve fracture.

TIBIAL FRACTURE

KEY FACTS

- **Mechanism:** High-energy, young people with sporting injuries or a fall from a height
- **Common site for open fractures** as the tibia lies just below the skin. (Also poor blood supply which affects healing)
- Susceptible to compartment syndrome

TREATMENT

- **Conservative:** If undisplaced and closed
- **Surgical:** In unstable fractures or open fractures
  - Locking plate
  - Intramedullary nail–most common
  - External fixation

OPEN FRACTURES

DEFINITION

- A fracture where there is a skin breach allowing exposure of the fracture to the external environment.

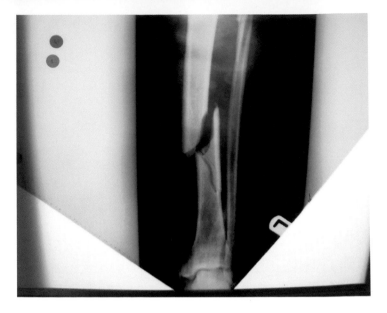

Figure 14.18   Open tibial fracture. Courtesy of Prof Joe O'Beirne

KEY POINTS

- The skin breach may even be a small puncture near the fracture.
- Examine for associated neurovascular injury.
- Large skin defects need immediate plastic surgery involvement.

MANAGEMENT

- Check and document neurovascular status
- Reduce fracture, **recheck** neurovascular status
- Remove only gross contamination
- Photograph
- Place dressing over wound
- Place in backslab
- Give IV antibiotics and tetanus prophylaxis
- Arrange for early surgical management (immediate/within 12 hr/within 24 hr)
- In open **tibial** fractures, also monitor for compartment syndrome

COMPARTMENT SYNDROME IN ORTHOPEADICS

KEY FACTS

- An orthopaedic emergency.
- Increased pressure in an osseofascial compartment above the capillary pressure, which may lead to irreversible neural and muscular damage.

- **Permanent damage occurs if not treated within 4–6 hours.**
- The diagnosis is clinical. In patients who cannot report pain e.g. ICU patients, or if there is clinical uncertainty a compartment pressure monitor may be used.

> **Top tip:** Compartment syndrome is a clinical diagnosis.
>
> Pain is the hallmark symptom as well as increased pain with passive stretch of the affected muscles.
>
> Neurovascular symptoms are NOT part of the initial diagnosis as these are late signs. Surgery should be performed **within 1 hour** of diagnosis.

CLINICAL FEATURES
SYMPTOMS

- PAIN
- Pain out of proportion to the injury
- Do not simply try to manage pain with increasing opioid use. Look for signs of compartment syndrome and plan to operate immediately if signs are present and other short-term measures (below) fail

SIGNS

- Swollen 'tense' limb/muscle compartment
- Pain worsens with **passive stretch** of the affected muscle compartment, e.g. passive plantarflexion of the ankle increases pain in the anterior leg

TREATMENT

- **Remove all circumferential dressings:** Split and remove casts, backslabs, splints and even bandage dressings
- **Maintain a normal blood pressure:** Avoid hypotension, this improves circulation to the affected compartment
- If symptoms do not resolve within 30 minutes, **surgical decompression by fasciotomy** must be performed. This must be done within 1 hour of diagnosis

PELVIC FRACTURES

KEY FACTS

- Apart from pubic rami and insufficiency fractures, pelvic fractures indicate a major trauma to the patient.
- In young patients this may be from high energy trauma e.g. RTA.
- In the elderly major trauma is most often caused by a fall from standing height.
- An X-ray of the pelvis is part of the **'trauma series'** of X-rays (Chest, C-spine, AP pelvis) required in the initial assessment of polytrauma cases. Some centres with adequate facilities have replaced trauma series X-rays with trauma CTs.

- Mortality 15–25% for closed fractures, as much as 50% for open fractures.
- **Haemorrhage from venous plexus is leading cause of death, especially in open book pelvic fracture.**
- Associated injuries include thoracic and intra-abdominal injuries with genitourinary or gastrointestinal injuries and other fractures.
- Multidisciplinary approach with early general surgeon/vascular surgeon or urologist involvement when suspect other injuries.

 Top tip: Reduce haemorrhage into the pelvis by applying a pelvic binder for unstable pelvic fractures 'close the tap.'

TYPES

- **Isolated pelvic fractures are usually stable:**
  - If the fracture doesn't extend to acetabulum, early mobilisation, bed rest and analgesia usually suffice.
  - If the fracture extends into acetabulum, patient may require operative management.
- **Multiple ring fractures are usually unstable:**
  - They also have a significant probability of massive haemorrhage.
  - Early stabilisation with pelvic binder essential. Definitive treatment with an external fixator or ORIF within 72 hours.
- Lateral compression, anteroposterior compression, vertical shear or a combination of forces are involved.
- So-called **open book fractures** can be especially serious.

INITIAL MANAGEMENT

- ATLS guidelines
- Apply pelvic binder or bedsheet around the pelvis at the level of the GREATER TROCHANTERS
- Some vertical shear type fractures may require traction–get specialist help
- Two Large IV Cannulae and Warm Crystalloid + O negative blood
- Crossmatch 4–6 units

 Top tip: Avoid 'springing' the pelvis as this may disrupt any pre-formed clot.

COMPLICATIONS

- Death from haemorrhage
- Osteoarthritis
- Urogenital Injury
- DVT/PE

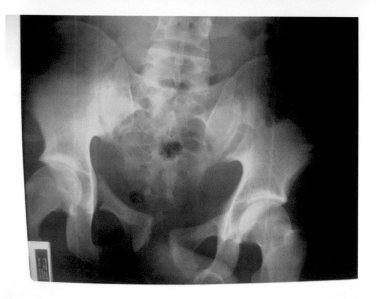

Figure 14.19   Pelvic fracture. Courtesy of Prof Joe O'Beirne

SEPTIC ARTHRITIS

KEY FACTS

- An orthopaedic emergency–chondral damage and risk of sepsis and death
- Adult/paediatric
- Native/prosthetic joint
- 'Spontaneous' or post procedure
- Usually spreads haematologically but may develop from contiguous osteomyelitis/ skin puncture
- Usually *Staph aureus*/gonococcus/strep
- Red, hot, swollen, painful joint
- Painful to move
- Fever and rigors

INVESTIGATIONS

- FBC, CRP, blood cultures, joint aspirate and X-ray
- Kocher's criteria in children

TREATMENT

- IV flucloxacillin and benzylpenicillin (or according to local hospital guidelines)
- Refer to orthopaedics ASAP for surgical washout of joint

BACK PAIN

KEY FACTS

- Lower back pain is very common
- Need to rule out AAA, cauda equina, spinal cord compression, metastatic disease
- Perform an ASIA (American Spinal Injury Association) assessment

CAUDA EQUINA SYNDROME

DEFINITION

- Acute compression of the cauda equine, usually by herniated intervertebral disc, fracture or other lesion resulting in typical symptoms.
- If not urgently treated surgically, cauda equina syndrome (CES) may result in permanent urinary and faecal incontinence.

CLINICAL PRESENTATION

- Pain: Lower back, buttocks, posterior thighs, legs
- Paraesthesia:
  - Saddle/perineal/perianal
  - Weakness in legs or feet
  - **Sphincter disturbance:** Urinary or faecal incontinence or retention

DIAGNOSIS

- Urgent MRI of Lumbar spine

TREATMENT

- Urgent surgical decompression

 Top tip: Time from clinical suspicion of cauda equina syndrome to MRI is paramount: Delays may have huge clinical and medicolegal consequences. Order and discuss the MRI promptly and document the timeline.

KEY POINTS

Back Pain Red Flags

Back Pain Symptoms
  Night pain
  Progressive unrelenting pain

Associated Symptoms–Legs/ Perineum

Altered perineal/perianal sensation
Sphincter disturbance; retention or incontinence of urine/faeces
Lower limb weakness
Bilateral lower limb symptoms

Systemic Symptoms

Trauma
Systemic symptoms, e.g. weight loss

Patient Factors

Previous Ca history
<20 years of age or >55 years of age

SCIATICA

DEFINTION

- Pain and/or parasthaesia caused by irritation or compression of the sciatic nerve
- Disc protrusion or herniation is the most common cause of the pain

CLINICAL PRESENTATION

- Pain usually radiates from the lower back through the buttock and lower limb on the affected side
- Pain can become very severe and easily exacerbated by activities of daily living, such as prolonged sitting, coughing or sneezing

INVESTIGATIONS

- Rule out more sinister manifestations including spinal stenosis, space occupying lesion, spinal infection, trauma, cauda equina, spondylolisthesis

MANAGEMENT

- Sciatica can be self-limiting, or may be treated with anti-inflammatories, physiotherapy and surgery in rare cases

OSTEOARTHRITIS

KEY FACTS

- Osteoarthritis (OA) is a form of non-inflammatory arthritis
- May represent a failed attempt of chondrocytes to repair damaged cartilage

- **OA is the most common form of arthritis**
  - Knee is the most commonly affected joint
  - Other affected joints include hips, ankles, facet joints of vertebrae, etc.
- **Osteoarthritis can either be**
  - Primary: Intrinsic defect, genetic predisposition
  - Secondary: Trauma, infection or congenital

CLINICAL PRESENTATION

- **Pain and stiffness**
  - Especially in the morning, on movement and increasing with age or chronicity of condition
- Swelling
- Reduced range of movement

INVESTIGATIONS
CHARACTERISTICS OF OSTEOARTHRITIS ON RADIOGRAPHS

1. Joint space narrowing
2. Osteophyte formation
3. Subchondral sclerosis
4. Subchondral cysts

MANAGEMENT

- The primary goal of treatment is to manage pain
- **Non-operative:**
  - Analgaesia
  - Lifestyle modifications
  - Physiotherapy
  - Weight loss
  - Corticosteroid joint injections
- **Operative:**
  - Arthroscopic debridement is not routinely indicated in osteoarthritis
- **Total joint arthroplasty** for advanced disease with disabling pain refractory to conservative measures
- Total hip and total knee replacement/arthroplasty are among the most commonly performed elective procedures

TOTAL HIP ARTHROPLASTY (THA)

- Involves replacing the femoral head (ball) and acetabulum (socket) with artificial prostheses
- These may be cemented or non-cemented or a combination
  - e.g. non cemented acetabulum and cemented femur
- **THA risks:**
  - Infection
  - Nerve injury (e.g. Sciatic)
  - Intra-operative fracture
  - Dislocation
  - Leg length discrepancy

TOTAL KNEE ARTHROPLASTY (TKA)

- Involves replacing the surface of the distal femur and proximal tibia with artificial prosthesis +/– patellar resurfacing
- **TKA risks:**
  - Infection
  - Nerve injury (Peroneal)
  - Intra-operative fracture
  - Chronic pain
  - Instability

MCQs FOR SELF-ASSESSMENT

Chapter 15

NEUROSURGERY

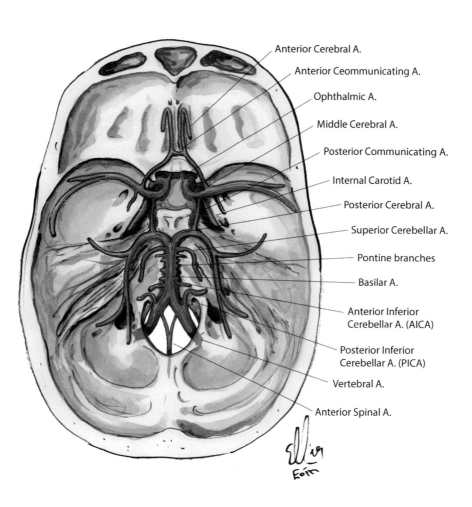

Anterior Cerebral A.

Anterior Ceommunicating A.

Ophthalmic A.

Middle Cerebral A.

Posterior Communicating A.

Internal Carotid A.

Posterior Cerebral A.

Superior Cerebellar A.

Pontine branches

Basilar A.

Anterior Inferior
Cerebellar A. (AICA)

Posterior Inferior
Cerebellar A. (PICA)

Vertebral A.

Anterior Spinal A.

DOI: 10.1201/9781003207184-15

CONTENTS

Cranial Trauma	319
Extradural Haemorrhage	325
Subdural Haemorrhage	326
Subarachnoid Haemorrhage (SAH)	328
Spinal Injury	329
Spinal Cord Injury	332
Brain Tumours	334

CRANIAL TRAUMA

KEY POINTS
- Must be promptly and systematically assessed
- Intracranial injuries are surgical emergencies
- Scalp lacerations can result in large volume blood loss

SCALP LAYERS
- **S:** Skin
- **C:** Connective tissue (contains blood vessels)
- **A:** Galea aponeurotica
- **L:** Loose areolar tissue (LAT) (allows scalp free movement)
- **P:** Periosteum or pericranium

 Top tip: The blood vessels in the connective tissue layer cannot shrink back and therefore bleed heavily when scalp is lacerated.

- If the galea (aponeurosis) layer is lacerated, the wound edges will need suturing (or closure with skin clips) as aponeurosis will pull back and separate the wound edges.
- Loose areolar tissue layer is referred to as the danger zone, infection can be spread within this layer and intracranially via emissary veins.

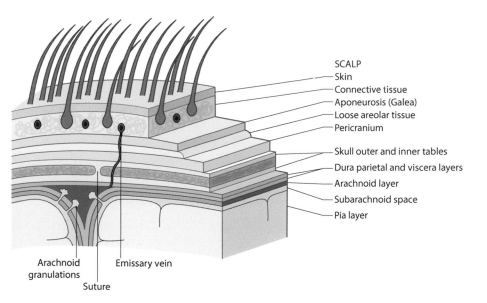

SCALP
Skin
Connective tissue
Aponeurosis (Galea)
Loose areolar tissue
Pericranium

Skull outer and inner tables
Dura parietal and viscera layers
Arachnoid layer
Subarachnoid space
Pia layer

Arachnoid granulations
Emissary vein
Suture

Figure 15.1 The scalp.

CONCUSSION

- Minor head injury
- Common symptoms include confusion, amnesia, headache, visual problems
- Usually carries good prognosis and full recovery
- Important to avoid a second hit especially in contact sports

SKULL FRACTURES: CLASSIFICATION

- <u>Simple</u>: Linear closed fracture
- <u>Open</u>: Continuity with external environment
  - E.g., skin breach, sinus mucosa
  - Risk of infection
  - Wash and close overlying laceration
  - Pneumovax for sinus breach but no antibiotics needed
- <u>Depressed</u> fractures
- <u>Base of skull</u> fractures
  - Racoon eye or Battle sign (images included further on)
  - CSF rhinorrhoea (nose leak), usually resolves spontaneously
  - CSF otorrhea (ear leak), conductive hearing loss

 Top tip: Occipital bone is thick and a fracture suggests high energy injury. Caution when inserting NG tube if anterior cranial fossa BOS fracture is suspected.

AETIOLOGY OF HEAD INJURIES

- **Direct trauma**
  - Coup injury: Brain injury under the area of impact
  - Contrecoup injury: Brain injury on the area opposite the impact
- **Contusions**
  - Bruising of the brain
  - Risk of swelling and mass effect over the next 5–7 days
- **Traumatic haemorrhage**
  - Extradural
  - Subdural
  - Traumatic subarachnoid haemorrhage (SAH)
  - Traumatic parenchymal haemorrhage
- **Diffuse axonal injury (DAI)**
  - Shearing of axons with rapid acceleration deceleration
  - Worse neurological function than what is expected on imaging

CEREBRAL BLOOD FLOW

- Cerebral blood flow (CBF) depends on:
  - Systemic blood pressure
  - Intracranial pressure (ICP)
  - Cerebral vascular resistance
- **Autoregulation** is the ability to regulate and maintain constant blood flow to vital organs, such as brain, kidneys and heart across a range of systemic blood pressure

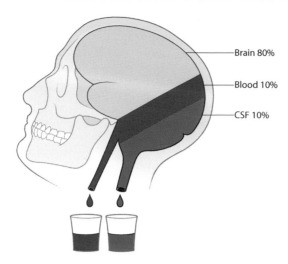

Figure 15.2   The Munro-Kellie doctrine.

- **Cerebral autoregulation** is lost in head injury and therefore CBF depends on the:
  - ICP and MAP (mean arterial pressure)

MUNRO-KELLIE DOCTRINE

- The skull is a rigid box
- It contains three things: Brain, blood, CSF
- **If the volume of one of the contents increases, the others must reduce to accommodate the change, or the ICP rises quickly**

APPLICATION IN HEAD INJURY

- ICP is usually maintained at **10–15 mmHg**, and is measured at the level of foramen of Monro
- As ICP rises, **CSF acts as a buffer** and will be sacrificed first
- Blood is the next component to be lost
- ICP then rises very quickly and leads to hypoxic brain injury

CEREBRAL HERNIATION

- Subfalcine
- Uncal
- Central
- Tonsillar/coning

Top tip:

Uncal herniation: Compresses third cranial nerve and causes a dilated pupil.
Tonsillar herniation: Causes compression of cardiorespiratory centres, coma and death.

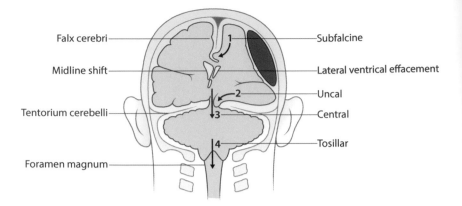

Figure 15.3   Cerebral herniation.

Top tip:

Cushing's Triad:

Hypertension, bradycardia and irregular respiration.
Occurs in raised ICP due to brainstem compression.

ASSESSMENT OF HEAD INJURY

- **Airway, Breathing, Circulation, Disability, Exposure** as per ATLS guidelines
- **History:**
  - May need to obtain collateral from ambulance personnel, police or witnesses
  - Establish mechanism of injury:
    - In falls, establish height
    - In road traffic accidents, establish speed, seat belt use, position of patient before and after accident
- **Examination:**
  - Glasgow Coma Scale (GCS) Table 15.1
  - Trauma survey as per ATLS guidelines
  - Neurological observations should be monitored and recorded:
    - GCS
    - Pupil size and reaction
    - Focal neurological deficits
  - Bruising: Racoon eye and Battle sign suggest the presence of base of skull fracture.

Top tip: The aim of assessment and observation is to prevent secondary brain injury as a result of hypoxia. **Investigations should not be delayed.**

Early communication with senior staff, including anaesthetics, and liaising with specialist centres is an important component of management.

Table 15.1   Glasgow Coma Scale

The Glasgow Coma Scale (GCS):	
• Used for rapid neurological evaluation • The GCS runs from 3-15, i.e. 3 is the lowest possible score • A GCS of 8 or less indicates a need to intubate the patient	
Assessment Area	**Score**
Eye-opening (E):	
• Spontaneous	4
• To sound	3
• To pressure	2
• None	1
• Non-testable	NT
Verbal response (V):	
• Orientated	5
• Confused	4
• Words	3
• Sounds	2
• None	1
• Non-testable	NT
Motor Response (M):	
• Obeys commands	6
• Localising	5
• Normal flexion	4
• Abnormal flexion	3
• Extension	2
• None	1
• Non-testable	NT

Note: GCS Score = (E[4] + V[5] + M[6]) = Best possible score 15; worst possible score 3. *If an area cannot be assessed, no numerical score is given for that region, and it is considered "non-testable." Source: www.glasgowcomascale.org

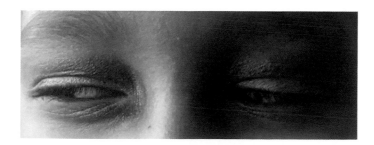

Figure 15.4   Raccoon eye. Courtesy of Dr Wail Mohammed

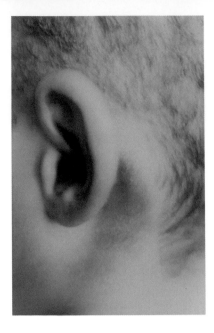

Figure 15.5   Battle sign. Courtesy of by Dr Wail Mohammed

INVESTIGATIONS

- **Imaging**
  - CT brain shows fractures, contusions and haematomas.
  - CT angiogram may be used to assess intracranial vasculature.
  - CT head and neck/CT TAP if injury suspected on clinical examination or mechanism of injury.
  - MRI is not usually used in acute phase as slower to organise in unwell patients.

MANAGEMENT

- **ABCDE** as per ATLS guidelines.
- Maintain spinal precautions until injury is excluded.
- Position the patient with their head end up and ensure nothing compresses neck veins and impairs venous return (ties, collar, etc.). **This reduces ICP.**
- If there is a suspicion of raised ICP, invasive monitoring may be necessary.
- **Airway management is essential** and patients with head injuries often require ventilation.
- Sedation may be needed for imaging or for intubation to protect airway.
- Hypertonic saline or mannitol may be administered to reduce ICP.
- **Obtain early neurosurgical advice** and consider transfer to specialist centre.
- **Surgery:** Patients may require surgical decompression or haematoma evacuation.

EXTRADURAL HAEMORRHAGE

MECHANISM OF INJURY

- Impact injury.
- Blow injury (pterion most common)

CLINICAL PRESENTATION

- Classic but rare lucid interval.
- May be conscious or unconscious.
- Bleeding occurs between the skull and dura mater.
- Space occupying.
- Middle meningeal artery (MMA) affected in 80% of cases.
- Signs include fixed, dilated pupil on the affected side (CN III damage).
- Can lead to uncal/transtentorial herniation, which leads to respiratory arrest.
- **CT brain features:**
  - Biconvex/Lentiform.
  - Midline shift.
  - Ventricular compression.
  - Usually does not cross sutures.

MANAGEMENT

- Craniotomy and evacuation of hematoma.
- Haemostasis and diathermy of the bleeding vessel.

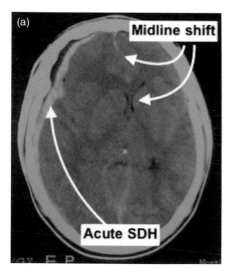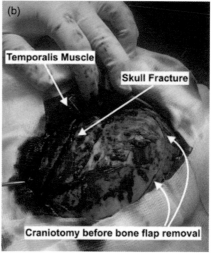

Figure 15.6 (a–c). *Axial CT* shows EDH with lateral ventricle effacement and midline shift, and *intraoperative images* show skull fracture and underlying extradural haematoma. Courtesy of Dr Hamzah Soleiman

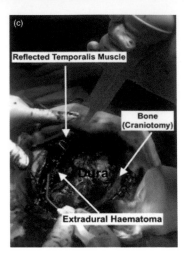

Figure 15.6 (a)–(c) (*continued*)

SUBDURAL HAEMORRHAGE

KEY FACTS
- Between dura and arachnoid (ruptured bridging veins).
- Can be acute, subacute or chronic, the latter having a better prognosis.

MECHANISM OF INJURY
- Acceleration/deceleration/shearing injuries
- In 50% of chronic cases, no discrete cause is found
- Usually associated with brain injury and has a worse prognosis

CLINICAL PRESENTATION
- Confusion
- Worsening headache
- Symptoms from raised ICP
- Focal neurological deficit such as hemiparesis or dysphasia
- **CT brain features:**
  - Will cross suture lines, but not the falx cerebri or tentorium cerebelli
  - Crescent shaped
  - Chronic bleeds may be isodense to the brain

RISK FACTORS
- Elderly (cerebral atrophy increases tension on bridging subdural veins)
- Alcoholics (cerebral atrophy)
- Anticoagulated patients

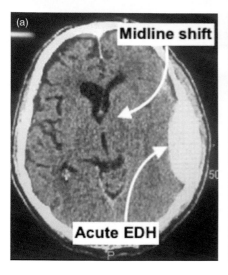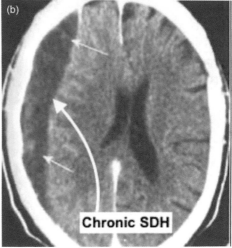

Figure 15.7   Axial CT brain scans show acute (a) and chronic (b) subdural haematomas. Courtesy of Dr Hamzah Soleiman

TREATMENT

- Depends on size, onset and patient factors.
- Small SDHs may be treated conservatively.
- Larger ones may require evacuation of the clot by burrhole for chronic haematoma or craniotomy and washout for acute haematoma.

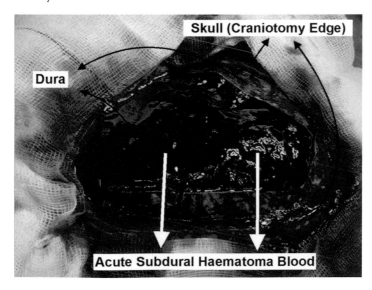

Figure 15.8   Acute subdural haematoma before evacuation. Courtesy of Dr Hamzah Soleiman

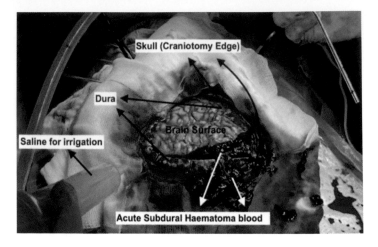

Figure 15.9 Acute subdural haematoma during washout and evacuation. Courtesy of Dr Hamzah Soleiman

SUBARACHNOID HAEMORRHAGE (SAH)

DEFINITION

- Bleed between pia and arachnoid matter due to arterial or venous origin.

Table 15.2 Clinical Features of Subarachnoid Haemorrhage

Causes	• Rupture of cerebral **berry aneurysms** • Rupture of vascular malformation (AVM, AV fistula) • Vasculitis • Drugs • Cerebral venous sinus thrombosis • Tumours • **Trauma:** The most common cause

Presentation: Non-traumatic	• Sudden onset headache
	  • Pain at its worst on onset
	• May have had earlier sentinel bleeds
	• **Other features: (Not always present)**
	  • Confusion
	  • Poor conscious level
	  • Signs of raised ICP
	  • May develop hydrocephalus

INVESTIGATIONS (NON-TRAUMATIC)

- **Non-contrast CT:**
  - Blood within the cisterns (CSF spaces) Figure 15.10
  - Can be associated with hydrocephalus

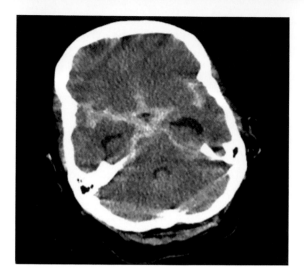

Figure 15.10   Subarachnoid haemorrhage. Courtesy of Dr Wail Mohammed

- LP (if CT is negative): Xanthochromia
- CT angiogram
- Cerebral catheter angiography

MANAGEMENT OF ANEURYSMAL SAH

- **Prevention of vasospasm:** (Non-traumatic SAH)
    - Hydration
    - Oral Nimodipine
- **Prevention of rebleed:**
    - Endovascular coiling
    - Surgical clipping
- **Treatment of hydrocephalus:**
    - LP
    - External ventricular drainage
    - VP shunt

SPINAL INJURY

GENERAL PRINCIPLES

- Chief concerns relate to:
    - Underlying primary neurological injury to the spinal cord, nerve roots or cauda equine
    - Preventing secondary injury by systemic (hypotension, hypoxia, etc.) or local factors (compression)

- Assess and protect:
  - Assess level of current injury, while taking precautionary measures to prevent further injury occurring (ATLS principles)

GENERAL ANATOMY POINTERS

- Spinal cord ends at L1/2

Any injury distal to this involves the cauda equina not the spinal cord.

- All the lumbar and sacral segments of the cord lie between T10 and L1.
- Phrenic nerve arises from C3,4,5.

Cord section proximal to C3 leads to respiratory arrest.

- C2 and C3 supply the vertex and occiput.
- C5-T1 supply the brachial plexus.

ASSESSMENT OF INJURIES TO VERTEBRAL COLUMN

- **Clinical history and examination:**
  - High yield information of injury mechanism and structures involved
- **X-ray and CT:**
  - Define bony anatomy clearly
- **MRI:**
  - Used for soft tissues (ligaments, intervertebral discs, nerve roots, spinal cord).

Top tip:

'Stability' is the ability of spine to bear physiological loads.
'Instability' implies further damage may occur leading to deformity and/or pain and/or neurological deficit.

CLINICAL EXAMINATION

- Full neurological examination with additional reflexes needed.
- Ascertain whether 'complete' or 'incomplete' neurological injury.
  - **Complete:**
    - 'No motor or sensory function more than 3 segments below the level of the injury'.
    - Alternatively, 'no motor or sensory function in lowest sacral segments'.
  - **Incomplete:**
    - Preservation of sacral function, toe flexion, sphincter contraction.
- Always document perianal sensation (sensory) AND anal tone (motor) AND presence of anal reflex separately.
- **Motor (myotomes)**
  - Find the spinal cord level supplying the lowest functioning motor nerve to ascertain the level of injury Table 15.3.

Top tip: Myotome = muscles supplied by a particular spinal nerve root.

- **Sensory (dermatomes)**
  - Nipple line–T4
  - Middle finger–C7
  - Lower limbs–'You stand on S1, sit on S3 and the first three lumbars run down to the knee'

Table 15.3   Muscle Myotomes

Key Muscle Myotomes	
Upper Limb	
Myotome	Muscles
C5	Elbow flexors
C6	Wrist extensors
C7	Elbow extensors
C8	Finger flexors
T1	Finger abductors (little finger)
Lower Limb	
L2	Hip flexors
L3	Knee extensors
L4	Ankle dorsiflexors
L5	Long toe extensors
S1	Ankle plantar flexors

Table 15.4   MRC Grading for Strength Examination

Grade	Strength
0	No active contraction
1	Flicker of contraction
2	Contraction producing movement if gravity eliminated
3	Weak contraction and movement against gravity
4	Active movement against some resistance
5	Full resistance, full strength
NT	

Top tip: Dermatome = area of skin mainly supplied by a single spinal nerve.

- **Reflexes:**
  - Deep tendon reflexes–rated 'Absent' to 4+
  - Anal reflex ('wink')–stimulation of perineum = anal contraction

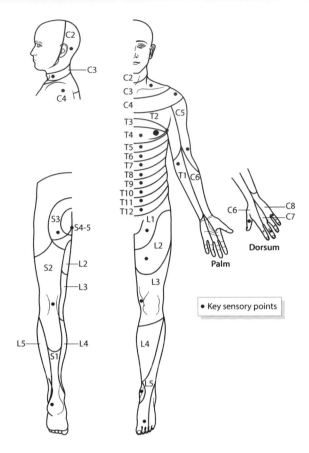

Figure 15.11 Sensory dermatomes.

SPINAL CORD INJURY

SPINAL CORD SYNDROMES

- **Anterior cord syndrome**
  - Anterior ⅔ of cord affected
  - Burst fracture with extrusion of fragments into canal/trauma to anterior spinal artery
  - Dorsal columns preserved
    - Proprioception
    - Vibration sense
    - Deep touch
  - Motor: Complete paralysis
  - Sensory: Light touch and pain loss
  - Worst prognosis

- **Brown-Sequard**
  - Unilateral facet joint trauma causing hemitransection of cord.
  - Motor: Ipsilateral loss of motor and proprioceptive function.
  - Sensory: Contralateral loss of pain and temperature sensation as spinothalamic tracts cross over in the lower cord.
  - Best prognosis.
- **Cauda equina syndrome**
  - Surgical emergency.
  - Compression of the cauda equina.
  - Essentially a nerve root compression.
  - Causes:
    - Large central/paracentral disc herniation
    - Neoplasms
    - Infection
    - Trauma
  - Bladder dysfunction most consistent finding
    - Overflow urinary incontinence with large residual volumes.
  - Areflexic, asymmetrical lower limb flaccid paralysis.

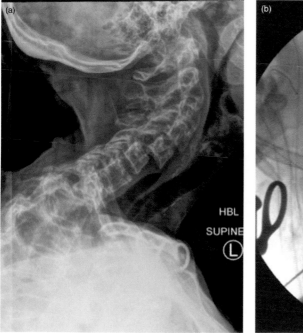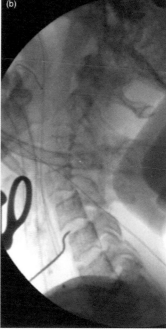

Figure 15.12 (a)–(d). Pre- and post-operative images of a patient admitted with C5/6 dislocation, underwent cervical traction which reduced the dislocation in image b before anterior fixation, anterior fusion and posterior fixation and fusion with cement augmentation seen on intraoperative X-ray in image c, and post-operative CT in image d. Courtesy of Dr Hamzah Soleiman

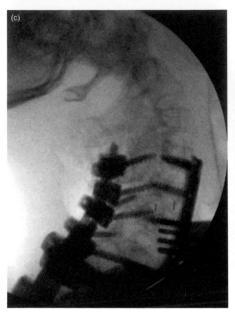

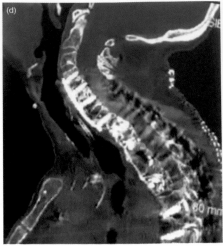

Figure 15.12   (a)–(d) (continued)

- Asymmetrical lower limb sensory changes.
- 'Saddle anaesthesia' (loss of perianal sensation) due to affected sacral nerve roots.

INITIAL MANAGEMENT OF SPINAL INJURIES
- Utmost caution in turning and lifting the patient
- Spine should be stabilized with collar/brace/spinal board
- Hypotension and hypoventilation must be treated
- Careful attention to body temperature
- Nasogastric tube and urinary bladder catheter should be passed
- Instability and neurological compression may need surgical decompression and fixation/fusion

BRAIN TUMOURS

KEY FACTS
- 2% of cancer-related deaths.
- **Cerebral metastasis** is the most common brain tumour.
- Primary brain tumours may arise from cells of the brain parenchyma or from its intracranial linings.
- Brain tumours are the second most common solid cancer in children, comprising 15–25% of all paediatric malignancies.

- Location:
  - **Adults**–supratentorial is more common
  - **Children**–infratentorial is more common

CLINICAL PRESENTATION

- Symptoms and signs of brain tumours depend on the location, size, degree of brain invasion and infiltration and surrounding brain oedema.
- **The most common presentations of brain tumours are:**
  - Headache with or without vomiting (symptoms of raised ICP), progressive neurological deficit and seizures.

CLINICAL PRESENTATION OF SUPRATENTORIAL TUMOURS

- *Symptoms due to increased ICP*
  - Headache (especially early morning)
  - Nausea/vomiting
  - Diplopia
  - Reduced visual acuity
  - Papilloedema
- *Progressive focal deficit*
  - Weakness (posterior frontal primary motor cortex or pyramidal tracts)
  - Dysphasia (dominant lobe Broca's and Wernicke's speech areas or connecting fibre tracts)
  - Visual disturbance (occipital lobe or optic pathway)
- Apathy and behaviour change (anterior frontal lobe)
- Headache (may occur with or without raised ICP)
- Seizures
- Change in cognitive function, memory, confusion and drowsiness

CLINICAL PRESENTATION OF INFRATENTORIAL TUMOURS (POSTERIOR FOSSA TUMOURS)

- Does not cause seizures
- Symptoms secondary to increased ICP due to hydrocephalus
  - Headache (especially early morning)
  - Nausea/vomiting
  - Diplopia
  - Reduced visual acuity
  - Papilloedema
- Cerebellar signs
  - Truncal ataxia (vermian tumour)
  - Intention tremor
  - Dysmetria
  - Slurred speech
  - Nystagmus
- Brain stem involvement
  - Cranial nerve palsies
  - Weakness of extremities
  - Drowsiness, and cardiorespiratory dysfunction (Cushing's triad)

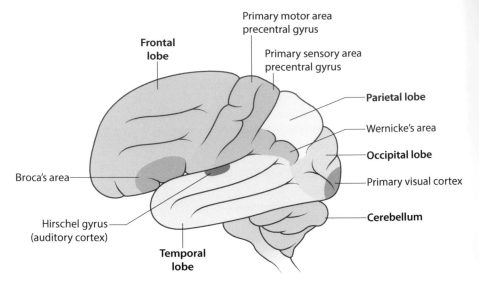

Figure 15.13 Anatomy of the brain.

KEY POINTS

Eloquent Functions Localisation
- Speech:
  - In the dominant hemisphere which is usually the left in right-handed and most left-handed individuals
  - Broca's (expressive dysphasia) inferior frontal gyrus Figure 15.13
  - Wernicke's (receptive dysphasia). Parietal lobe Figure 15.13
  - Fibre tracts connecting Broca's, Wernicke's and other involved areas.
- Motor:
  - Primary motor area is in precentral gyrus in posterior frontal lobe.
  - Pyramidal tracts cross over or 'decussate' at the medulla.
- Sensory:
  - Primary sensory cortex is in postcentral gyrus in anterior parietal lobe. Also crossed sensation, so right hemisphere signal is from left.
- Vision:
  - Visual cortex is on occipital lobe, also crossed so left lobe dysfunction causes right visual field defect.
  - Optic chiasm compression causes bitemporal field defects or tunnel vision.
  - Optic nerve compression causes field defects in the eye supplied.

- Hearing:
  - Primary auditory area is in Herschel gyrus in superior temporal gyrus but bilateral representation.
- Coordination:
  - Cerebellar vermis lesion causes truncal ataxia and mutism while hemispheres lesions cause ipsilateral limbs coordination difficulties.

PATHOGENESIS

- Unknown
- Radiation
- Immunosuppression–lymphoma
- Genetic–neurofibromatosis, Von Hippel-Lindau syndrome

INVESTIGATIONS

- **History:** Symptoms, past history of cancer, rate of progression of symptoms
- **Physical examination:** (neurological findings)
  - Detailed neurological examination can aid in lesion localisation
  - Body systems examination is essential for identification of a primary tumour in metastasis, e.g. breast, lung, melanoma
- **Radiological investigations:**
  - CT brain is usually the initial imaging test
  - MRI is the best imaging modality
    - T1 pre- and post-gadolinium MRI shows tumour enhancement
    - T2 shows extent of oedema

PATHOPHYSIOLOGY

- **Gliomas (neuroepithelial tumours)**
  - **Astrocytomas** (WHO grade 1–4)
  - **Oligodendroglioma** (WHO grade 1–3)
  - Ependymoma
- **Meningeal tumours**
  - Meningioma: 20%
  - Usually benign
- **Nerve sheet tumours**
  - Vestibular schwannoma
- **Pituitary adenoma**
  - Functioning
    - Acromegaly: Growth hormone adenomas
    - Cushing disease: ACTH
    - Galactorrhoea: Prolactinomas
      - Prolactinomas can be treated medically with dopamine agonists
    - Acromegaly and Cushing disease impact on life expectancy and are usually treated with surgery when comorbidities allow

- Non-functioning
  - Mass effect
  - Visual disturbance such as bitemporal hemianopia (tunnel vision) due to their proximity to the optic chiasm
- Apoplexy is bleeding into pituitary adenoma, and can cause an Addisonian crisis.
  - It is a medical emergency and must be managed in liaison with the endocrinology team, with urgent pituitary function tests, hydration, hydrocortisone and hormone supplements.
  - Emergency surgery may be indicated when stable for acute visual disturbance.
- **Tumour of the sellar region**
  - Craniopharyngioma
- **Embryonal tumours**
  - Medulloblastoma
- **Tumour-like malformations**
  - Colloid cyst
- **Metastatic tumours**
  - Most common brain tumour
  - Common primary sites are:
    - Lungs–50%
    - Breast
    - GIT
    - Renal
    - Melanoma
  - Management is mostly palliative

MANAGEMENT

- **Surgery**
  - The goals of surgery are as follows:
    - Relief of mass effect
    - Histological diagnosis
    - Resection or debulking when possible
    - CSF diversion in hydrocephalus
  - Adjuncts to surgery:
    - Surgical navigation systems (for tumour localisation)
    - Awake craniotomy and debulking (in eloquent areas such as speech)
    - Intraoperative mapping (in tumours close to the motor or sensory cortex)
    - Intraoperative MRI (to confirm gross or total resection)
  - Curative resection is mostly for benign tumours
  - Debulking of tumour is usually followed by adjuvant radiotherapy and chemotherapy in higher grade gliomas
  - Stereotactic tissue biopsy performed when surgery is not possible
- **Radiotherapy**
  - External beam radiotherapy.
  - Goal of radiation treatment is to cause cell death or to stop cell replication.

- In certain tumours it can be curative and in the majority of cases it will prolong survival.
- Stereotactic radiosurgery delivers a large dose of radiation to the tumour in one dose, based on imaging that has accurately outlined the lesion (useful in well-defined tumours <3 cm).
- **Chemotherapy**
  - Temozolomide for HGG
    - Alkylating agent
    - Good penetration of the BBB

MCQs FOR SELF-ASSESSMENT

Chapter 16

OTORHINOLARYNGOLOGY (ENT)

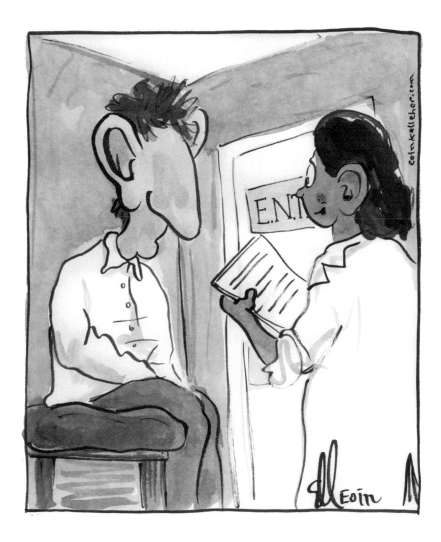

DOI: 10.1201/9781003207184-16

CONTENTS

General ENT	344
Acute Tonsillitis	345
Head and Neck Masses	347
Otology	348
Pinna (Auricular) Hematoma	348
Prominent Ears	349
Otitis Externa	349
Acute Otitis Media (AOM)	350
Otitis Media with Effusion (OME)	351
Chronic Suppurative Otitis Media	352
Cholesteatoma	353
Acoustic Neuroma	355
Rhinology	356
Epistaxis	356
Allergic Rhinitis	357
Nasal Polyps	358
Sinusitis	359
Acute Rhinosinusitis	359
Chronic Rhinosinusitis	360
Head and Neck Anatomy	361
Human Papilloma Virus	363
Laryngeal Cancer	365
Oral Cancer	366
Oropharyngeal Cancer	367
Nasopharyngeal Carcinoma (NPC)	368
Surgical Procedures	368
Tonsillectomy	368
Ventilation (Tympanostomy) Tubes	369
Mastoidectomy	370
Parotidectomy	371
Neck Dissection	372

Common Symptoms: Ear		
Symptom	Description	Notes
Otalgia	Pain in the ear	• Referred pain: Pathology affecting anatomy with shared sensory pathways • Mainly oropharynx/larynx
Otorrhea	Discharge from the ear	• Often associated with infection • Clear/blood stained/purulent?
Hearing loss		• Timeline important • Sudden onset: Urgent attention
Tinnitus	Perception of sound in the ear: No external stimuli	• Character: Ringing/pulsatile?
Vertigo	Hallucination of movement	• True vertigo: Rotary • Central/peripheral cause? • Establish triggers + duration • Triggers: Sudden movement, spontaneous, ongoing infection
Facial nerve	Palsy/anaesthesia/paraesthesia	• Pathology may originate from the ear • Facial nerve: Intrinsically related to middle/inner ear anatomy • Terminal branches: Possible parotid gland pathology
Common Symptoms: Nose		
Symptom	Description	Notes
Epistaxis	Nose bleeding	• Document risk factors: Anticoagulants/HTN/bleeding disorders/trauma • Site/volume/duration • Anterior bleed: From anterior nasal septum • Posterior nasal cavity bleed: Clots often swallowed/coughed up • First aid measures undertaken?
Nasal Blockage		• May be unilateral/bilateral • Can interfere with sleep/exercise • Acute nasal obstruction post trauma: Rule out septal haematoma
Rhinorrhea	Nasal discharge	• Clear/mucopurulent/blood-stained? • Seasonal/perennial? • Clear rhinorrhea with recent head trauma/nasal surgery: Possible CSF leak • Anterior/postnasal drip? • Associated respiratory symptoms?

Intermittent unilateral epistaxis, nasal blockage and atypical facial pain: Concerning for a sino-nasal or postnasal space malignancy.

(continued)

Common Ontological Symptoms: Head and Neck		
Symptom	Description	Notes
Pain		• Anatomical location • Referred pain most often to the ear
Odynodysphagia	Painful/difficulty swallowing	• Timeline, liquids-solids?
Dysphonia	Impaired inability to vocalise	
Stridor	High pitched sound: Partial airway obstruction at or below level of larynx	• <u>Inspiratory</u>: Laryngeal obstruction • <u>Expiratory</u>: Tracheobronchial obstruction • <u>Biphasic</u>: Subglottic/glottic obstruction
Dyspnoea		• Associated breathlessness?
Neck mass/ non-healing ulcer		• Several causes: Malignant/benign conditions
Trismus	'Lockjaw' spasm of jaw muscles (tetanus) causing mouth to remain tightly closed	• Quinsy (peritonsillar abscess)

GENERAL ENT

FOREIGN BODY IN THE EAR

- Common in the paediatric population, attempts to remove the foreign body by an adult may compound the problem
- Patient may present with otitis externa or perichondritis
- Removal can be attempted if child is compliant: Prevent iatrogenic tympanic membrane perforation
- If child is not compliant, removal can be done under general anaesthetic
- Treatment commonly involves syringing
- Insects in the ear should be first killed with an oil-based solution and then removed

FOREIGN BODY IN THE NOSE

- May present with unilateral rhinorrhoea
- Unwitnessed foreign body insertion should be investigated with lateral nasal, inspiratory and expiratory CXR
- All nasal foreign bodies should be removed on an **urgent basis** to prevent aspiration with anterior rhinoscopy and atraumatic extraction
- Removal under general anaesthetic is indicated if initial attempts fail
- Bronchoscopy is indicated if nasal foreign body is aspirated during removal or not visible under anaesthesia
- Button batteries may cause burns and septal perforation
- Complications may include epistaxis, inhalation or ingestion

FOREIGN BODY IN THE UPPER OESOPHAGUS

- Fish bone, dentures, coins and many others may lodge in the hypopharynx or oesophagus
- Often obstructing oesophagus at four constricted sites:
  1. Level of the cricoid cartilage
  2. Arch of aorta
  3. Left main bronchus
  4. Diaphragm

> **If the foreign body is a battery**, this is an ENT emergency requiring immediate removal to prevent chemical burn.

ACUTE TONSILLITIS

DEFINITION

- Tonsils are paired lymphatic organs that form part of Waldeyer's ring and are thought to have a protective/immunological role Figure 16.1

KEY FACTS

- Each tonsil has a fibrous capsule and is separated from the pharyngobasilar covering of the superior constrictor muscle by a layer of areolar tissue
- **Blood supply to the tonsils is through the external carotid artery branches**
  - Superior pole
    - Ascending pharyngeal artery
    - Lesser palatine artery

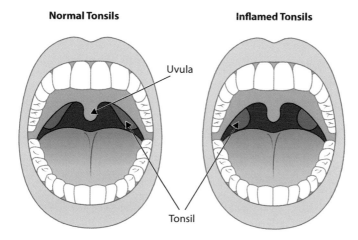

Normal Tonsils   **Inflamed Tonsils**

Uvula

Tonsil

Figure 16.1   Normal/inflamed tonsils.

- Inferior pole
    - Facial artery branches
    - Dorsal lingual artery
    - Ascending palatine artery
- Venous drainage is a diffuse peritonsillar plexus that drains into the **lingual and pharyngeal veins** that anastomose with the internal jugular vein

PATHOGENS

- Predominantly viral (influenza, parainfluenza, adenovirus, enterovirus)
- *Streptococcus pneumoniae*
- *Haemophilus influenzae*
- Anaerobes

CLINICAL PRESENTATION

- **Symptoms**
    - Sore throat
    - Odynodysphagia
    - Otalgia (referred pain)
    - Dysphonia
    - Trismus
    - Painful cervical lymphadenopathy
    - Pyrexia
    - Malaise
- **Signs**
    - Hyperaemic tonsils
    - Peritonsillar erythema

INVESTIGATIONS

- Clinical diagnosis
- **Centor Score** indicates likelihood of bacterial infection as cause
- Referred to hospital in cases of no oral intake, severe dehydration, sepsis or airway concerns
- Hospital-referred cases are investigated with FBC, CRP, LFTs and Monospot test (glandular fever)

Centor Score:	Score
Presence of tonsillar exudate	1
Tender anterior cervical lymphadenopathy	1
History of fever	1
Absence of cough	1

- **Score 0–2:** Do not treat with antibiotics
- **Score 3–4:** Treat with antibiotics

COMPLICATIONS OF ACUTE TONSILLITIS

- Local and spread of infection; quinsy, parapharyngeal abscess, retropharyngeal abscess, chronic tonsillitis, acute otitis media
- **Rheumatic fever, post-streptococcal glomerulonephritis (PSGN), scarlet fever**

MANAGEMENT

- Most cases are managed in the community with analgesia, bed rest and continued oral intake
- Oral antibiotics are often prescribed if symptoms are persistent
- If hospital referred, intravenous antibiotics, fluids and analgesia
- **First-line antibiotic:** Penicillin (clarithromycin if penicillin allergic)
- **Tonsillectomy indicated if:** ≥7 episodes in 1 year

HEAD AND NECK MASSES

PERITONSILLAR ABSCESS (QUINSY)

- A **clinical diagnosis:**
  - Peritonsillar swelling
  - Dysphagia
  - Trismus
  - A deviated uvula
- This is a complication of tonsillitis
- Urgent incision and drainage under local anaesthetic is indicated plus intravenous antibiotics
- Incision is made midway between the uvula and site of upper wisdom tooth

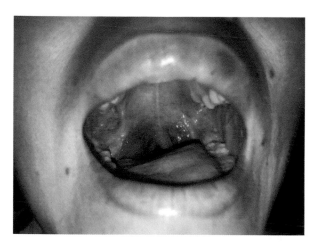

Figure 16.2 Trismus and right peritonsillar abscess. Image by Niwadee Laophaibulkul; reproduced under licence from Shutterstock

PARAPHARYNGEAL ABSCESS

- A deep neck space infection
- **Symptoms:**
  - Sore throat
  - Odynodysphagia
  - Lateral neck mass
- **Diagnosis:** CT neck
- **Management:** Incision and drainage under general anaesthetic and intravenous antibiotics

RETROPHARYNGEAL ABSCESS

- The retropharyngeal space is from the skull base to the T3 vertebral level in the mediastinum
- **Clinical presentation:**
  - Sore throat
  - Neck stiffness
  - Odynodysphagia
  - Stridor
- A large abscess in a child can compromise the airway
- **Investigations:**
  - A lateral neck X-ray will show soft tissue widening at level of C2 and C6
  - +/− CT scan to confirm diagnosis
- **Management:**
  - Abscess should be drained urgently under general anaesthetic to prevent spread to the mediastinum causing mediastinitis
  - IV antibiotics are indicated
  - Intubation or an emergency tracheostomy should be considered in cases of airway compromise

---

OTOLOGY

PINNA (AURICULAR) HEMATOMA

KEY FACTS

- Complication of direct trauma to the anterior pinna
- Shearing of blood vessels from the perichondrium to the cartilage leads to hematoma formation
- Persistent hematoma between the perichondrium and cartilage could lead to **avascular necrosis** of the cartilage
- Immediate management is indicated to prevent long-standing deformity (cauliflower ear)

CLINICAL PRESENTATION

- Pain
- Pinna laceration
- Bleeding
- Hematoma

MANAGEMENT

- Urgent incision and drainage under local anaesthetic
- Splinting to prevent reformation of hematoma at incision site

PROMINENT EARS

DEFINITION

- Pinna malformation during intrauterine development

KEY FACTS

- Can be bilateral or unilateral
- Associated with psychological sequelae due to bullying in school or teen years

CLINICAL PRESENTATION

- Cosmetic appearance
- Psychological

MANAGEMENT

- Operative intervention is to prevent bullying
- Done prior to child commencing school
- **Pinnaplasty or otoplasty** are cosmetic procedures aimed to augment the over projection of the cartilage

OTITIS EXTERNA

DEFINITION

- Infective inflammation of the external auditory canal

KEY FACTS

- Bacterial overgrowth is due to skin maceration from moisture exposure, canal trauma or obstruction
- Loss of protective lipid layer lining the canal

RISK FACTORS

- Water exposure (swimmers)
- Immunosuppression
- Retained foreign body
- Auditory canal stenosis
- Dermatological conditions (eczema, psoriasis, dermatitis)
- Canal trauma (cotton bud)

PATHOGENS

- *Pseudomonas aeruginosa*
- *Staphylococcus aureus*
- Fungal (aspergillus, candida)

CLINICAL PRESENTATION
SYMPTOMS

- Otalgia
- Otorrhea (muco-purulent, green)
- Hearing loss in the affected ear
- Fullness

SIGNS

- Canal oedema and erythema
- Muco-purulent discharge filling the canal
- Tympanic membrane may not be visible due to canal oedema

MANAGEMENT

- Aural toilet under microscope visualisation
- Extensive canal oedema may prevent topical treatment from infiltrating the canal
- If tympanic membrane is not visible due to canal oedema, a topical antibiotic laced wick is inserted
- If a wick is placed, a follow-up review after 2 days is indicated
- Once canal oedema is reduced, topical antibiotic drops can be commenced
- Routine analgesia is required
- **IV antibiotic therapy for immunocompromised patients** due to risk of infective spread to the pinna or skull base (malignant otitis externa)

ACUTE OTITIS MEDIA (AOM)

DEFINITION

- Acute infective inflammation of the middle ear

KEY FACTS

- High incidence in children aged 3–7 years
- Can occur **following an URTI**

PATHOGENS

- Viral
- *Streptococcus pneumoniae*
- *Haemophilus influenza*
- *Moraxella catarrhalis*

CLINICAL PRESENTATION
SYMPTOMS

- Otalgia and hearing loss
- Otorrhoea following tympanic perforation
- Coexisting nasal symptoms

SIGNS

- Middle ear effusion
- Bulging inflamed tympanic membrane
- Tympanic membrane perforation and otorrhoea
- Nasal endoscopy is indicated in adults

MANAGEMENT

- Analgesia
- Oral antibiotics
- Nasal decongestants
- Failure to resolve may require intravenous antibiotics and myringotomy

COMPLICATIONS OF AOM

- **Extracranial/intratemporal:**
  - Tympanic membrane (TM) perforation
  - Acute mastoiditis and subperiosteal abscess
  - Facial nerve palsy
  - Labyrinthitis
  - Petrositis
  - Tympanosclerosis (conductive hearing loss)
- **Intracranial:**
  - Meningitis
  - Extradural abscess
  - Subdural abscess
  - Brain abscess
  - Lateral sinus thrombosis (may lead to internal jugular vein thrombosis and cavernous sinus thrombosis)

OTITIS MEDIA WITH EFFUSION (OME)

DEFINITION

- Chronic accumulation of non-purulent effusion within the middle ear and mastoid air cell system

KEY FACT

- The most common cause of conductive hearing loss in children

RISK FACTORS

- Eustachian tube dysfunction
- Craniofacial abnormalities
- Cleft palate
- Adenoid hypertrophy
- Allergic rhinitis
- Recurrent acute otitis media
- Passive smoking
- Bottle feeding

CLINICAL PRESENTATION

SYMPTOMS

- Asymptomatic
- Hearing loss
- Tinnitus
- Aural fullness

SIGNS

- Air bubbles or fluid level behind the drum
- Amber yellow drum
- Retracted drum

INVESTIGATIONS

- Hearing assessment
- Tympanogram

MANAGEMENT

- Watchful waiting for at least 3 months
- Ventilation tube insertion if the effusion is persistent

COMPLICATIONS OF OME

- Hearing loss
- Retraction pockets
- Cholesteatoma
- Tympanosclerosis

CHRONIC SUPPURATIVE OTITIS MEDIA

DEFINITION

- Persistent inflammation of the middle ear or mastoid cavity

KEY FACTS

- Characterised by recurrent or persistent ear discharge (otorrhoea) through a perforation of the tympanic membrane
- The most commonly isolated microorganisms are *Pseudomonas aeruginosa* and *Staphylococcus aureus*

MANAGEMENT

- To improve symptoms of otorrhoea: Heal perforations, improve hearing and reduce complications, with minimum adverse effects of treatment

CHOLESTEATOMA

DEFINITION

- An expanding keratinizing squamous epithelium within the middle ear

KEY FACTS

- Locally destructive
- Has a tendency to recur after surgical management

CLASSIFICATION

- **Congenital**
  - Due to a persistent epidermoid ectoderm
  - Presents as a white anterior attic mass/pearl behind an intact tympanic membrane in the 1st year of life
  - Disease can be extensive if diagnosed later in childhood
- **Acquired**

AETIOLOGY

- It is normal for squamous epithelium to migrate from the surface of the tympanic membrane outwards along the external auditory canal
- Keratin builds up within the retraction pocket and may get infected or expand further into the middle ear

CLINICAL PRESENTATION
SYMPTOMS

- Painless foul-smelling discharge
- Hearing loss secondary to ossicular erosion
- Vertigo (erosion of the vestibular organ)
- Tinnitus
- Facial nerve palsy
- Meningitis–intracranial extension

SIGNS

- Attic retraction with keratin build up observed on otoscopy or micro-otoscopy

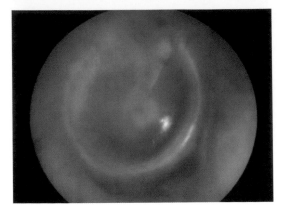

Figure 16.3 Normal tympanic membrane. Image courtesy of Mr Michael Saunders

INVESTIGATIONS

- Audiogram
- High-resolution CT temporal bone (inadequate views of the temporal bone with CT brain alone)

MANAGEMENT

- Aural toilet and topical antibiotic treatment
- Mainstay of treatment is operative

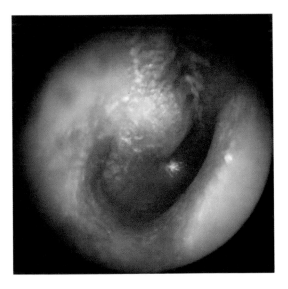

Figure 16.4 Showing right acute otitis media. Image by Mikhail V Komarov; reproduced under licence from Shutterstock

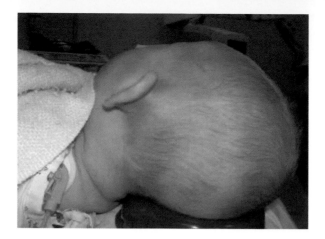

Figure 16.5   Acute otitis media. Image courtesy of Mr Rogan J Corbridge

- **Mastoidectomy** to remove disease
- If disease (cholesteatoma) is causing intracranial complications (meningitis, cerebral abscess), urgent mastoid exploration is indicated

ACOUSTIC NEUROMA

DEFINITION
- Common benign tumour of the cerebellopontine angle

KEY FACTS
- Benign tumour arising from the **schwann cells**
- Often unilateral; bilateral is seen in neurofibromatosis type 2 (NF2)

CLINICAL PRESENTATION
- Unilateral sensorineural hearing loss (SNHL)
- Tinnitus
- Vertigo
- Facial nerve palsy
- Headaches
- Ataxia
- Raised CSF (papilloedema, altered consciousness)

INVESTIGATIONS
- Audiology (unilateral SNHL)
- MRI of the internal auditory meatus

MANAGEMENT

- Guided by tumour size, growth rate, hearing level and patient preference
- Conservative
  - Stereotactic radiosurgery
  - Surgery

RHINOLOGY

EPISTAXIS

LOCAL CAUSES

- Idiopathic
- Traumatic (nasal bone or septum fracture, foreign body, digit trauma)
- Inflammatory (rhinitis)
- Neoplastic
- Iatrogenic

SYSTEMIC CAUSES

- Anticoagulation drugs
- Inherited bleeding disorders
- Acquired coagulopathy (liver failure, vitamin K deficiency, platelet dysfunction)
- Hypertension

CLINICAL PRESENTATION
SYMPTOMS

- Anterior bleeding (via nostrils)
- Posterior bleeding (ingestion of blood)

SIGNS

- Circulatory shock
- Bleeding on anterior nasal inspection
- Posterior bleeding visible on nasal endoscopy
- Haematoma noted on posterior pharyngeal wall on oral examination

BLOOD VESSELS INVOLVED

- 90% of bleeds originate from **Little's area (Kiesselbach's plexus):**
  - An anterior-inferior naso-septal anastomosis
- Internal and external carotid artery branches
- Ophthalmic artery (internal carotid artery)
- Anterior and posterior ethmoid arteries
- Greater palatine and superior labial artery (internal maxillary artery)
- Posterior bleeds involve posterolateral branches of sphenopalatine artery

INVESTIGATIONS

- FBC (haemoglobin and platelets)
- Coagulation screen
- Renal function
- Group and hold or crossmatch
- CXR and ECG (*pre-operative assessment*)
- Examination of nose with nasal speculum to identify source

MANAGEMENT

- Most cases are managed in the community
- **Head flexed forward and nasal alar compression for 15 minutes**
- Profuse bleeding or failure of conservative measures indicate hospital assessment
- Gain intravenous access
- Correct coagulopathy if medically indicated or contributing factor such as hypertension
- Anterior bleeding can be visualised and cauterised (silver nitrate or electrocautery)
- Anterior nasal packing
- Posterior nasal packing
- Oral antibiotics are indicated with nasal packing to prevent sinusitis, otitis media (Eustachian tube obstruction) and cavernous sinus thrombosis
- Persistent bleeding may require operative intervention
- Functional endoscopic sinus surgery (FESS) with sphenopalatine artery ligation
- Anterior ethmoid artery ligation
- External carotid artery ligation
- Radiological embolisation

ALLERGIC RHINITIS

DEFINITION

- IgE mediated type 1 hypersensitivity reaction in the nasal mucous membranes

KEY FACTS

- Can be seasonal or perennial
- Allergen–IgE interaction triggers release of prostaglandins, leukotriene and other factors that cause **nasal mucosal oedema, increased capillary permeability and rhinorrhoea**

TYPICAL ALLERGENS

- Pollens
- Mould
- House dust mite
- Animals (cats, dogs, birds)

CLINICAL PRESENTATION
SYMPTOMS

- Rhinorrhoea
- Sneezing
- Nasal itch
- Epiphora (watery eyes)
- Nasal obstruction
- Postnasal drip

SIGNS

- Mucosal oedema
- Turbinate hypertrophy
- Nasal polyps (variable)

INVESTIGATIONS

- Skin prick test
- Total plasma IgE and radioallergosorbent test (RAST)

MANAGEMENT

- Managed in the primary care setting once diagnosis established
- Avoid allergen
- Oral antihistamines
- Topical steroid nasal sprays
- Oral steroids if symptoms severe
- Desensitisation (oral or injection depot) to proven pollen allergy
- Surgical intervention to reduce nasal obstruction (septoplasty, turbinate reduction) for better aeration or access for topical therapy
- Coexisting sinusitis should be treated

NASAL POLYPS

KEY FACTS

- Polyp formation secondary to inflammatory nasal mucosal oedema
- Often at middle meatus
- Inflammatory process may be due to allergy, chronic infection or idiopathic

CLINICAL PRESENTATION
SYMPTOMS

- Nasal blockage
- Rhinorrhoea
- Post nasal drip
- Large polyps can be visible at nasal nares or cause intercanthal widening

SIGNS

- Visible polyps on nasal endoscopy

INVESTIGATIONS

- Allergic rhinitis investigations (skin prick, IgE and RAST)
- CT of paranasal sinuses
- **Biopsy if suspicious of malignancy**

MANAGEMENT

- Medical management is first-line if not suspicious of malignancy
- Intranasal steroid spray +/− tapering oral steroids
- Surgical management if failed medical therapy causing persistent nasal blockage
- FESS and polypectomy
- Continue medical management post-operative
- Long-term recurrence is inevitable

SINUSITIS

KEY FACTS

- Paranasal sinuses are maxillary, **frontal, ethmoidal and sphenoidal**.
- Obstruction of paranasal sinus openings either in the middle meatus or superior meatus can lead to secretion retention within the sinuses and reduced aeration

LOCAL CAUSES

- Infective rhinitis or upper respiratory tract infection
- Allergic or nonallergic rhinitis
- Nasal polyposis
- Retained foreign body
- Anatomical variations (deviated nasal septum, abnormal uncinate process and turbinate hypertrophy)
- Tumour
- Fractures involving the paranasal sinuses

ACUTE RHINOSINUSITIS

DEFINITION

- Acute inflammation of the sinuses, most often the maxillary sinuses
- Often during upper respiratory tract infection

KEY FACTS

- Infective inflammation leads to mucosal oedema, increased mucous production and sinus cilia dysfunction
- Subsequent obstruction of sinus openings leads to mucus stasis and secondary bacterial infection
- Fungal sinusitis is rare but may affect immunocompromised patients

CLINICAL PRESENTATION
SYMPTOMS

- Nasal blockage
- Malaise
- Pyrexia
- Atypical facial pain
- Upper molar pain

SIGNS

- Nasal mucosal oedema and erythema
- Mucopurulent pus in the middle meatus
- Tenderness over the cheek

INVESTIGATIONS

- Flexible nasal endoscopy under local anaesthetic vasoconstrictor spray (co-phenylcaine)
- Raised inflammatory markers (WCC, CRP/ESR)
- CT of paranasal sinuses (gold standard)

MANAGEMENT

- Antibiotics
- Analgesia
- Nasal decongestant to aid aeration of sinuses and prevent secretion stasis
- Failure of medical therapy may indicate FESS

CHRONIC RHINOSINUSITIS

DEFINITION

- Inflammatory condition of the paranasal sinuses and nasal passage lasting three months or longer

KEY FACTS

- Predisposing factors include nasal polyps, septal deformity, dental infections and defects in mucociliary clearance

CLINICAL PRESENTATION
SYMPTOMS

- Rhinorrhea
- Nasal congestion
- Facial pain/pressure/fullness
- Hyposmia
- Mucopurulent drainage

SIGNS

- Mucopus in the nasopharynx
- Endoscopic findings of discharge, oedema or polyps

INVESTIGATIONS
- Nasal endoscopy
- CT scan to identify mucosal thickening

MANAGEMENT
- Antibiotics to clear infection
- Topical steroids
- FESS

COMPLICATIONS OF SINUSITIS
- **Orbital complications–Chandler's classification**
  - Preseptal cellulitis
  - Orbital cellulitis
  - Subperiosteal abscess
  - Orbital abscess
  - Cavernous sinus thrombosis
- **Pott's puffy tumour**
  - A life-threatening complication
  - Osteomyelitis of the frontal bone with subperiosteal abscess causing swelling and edema over the forehead and scalp
- **Intracranial complications**
  - Meningitis
  - Extradural abscess
  - Subdural abscess
  - Brain abscess
  - Cavernous sinus thrombosis
- **Mucocele**
  - Accumulation of sterile mucus with increased viscosity
  - Expansion of cyst can cause bony erosion and displacement of adjacent structures such as the orbit
  - Diagnosis on CT

HEAD AND NECK ANATOMY

ORAL CAVITY SUBSITES
- Lip
- Alveolar margin
- Floor of mouth
- Buccal mucosa
- Anterior 2/3 tongue
- Hard palate
- Retromolar trigone

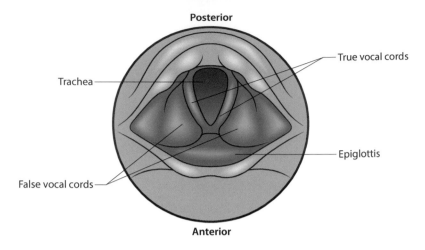

Figure 16.6   Anatomy of the Vocal cords.

LARYNX (VOICE BOX)
- **Supraglottic subsites**
  - Inferior surface of the epiglottis to the vestibular folds (false vocal cords)
- **Glottic subsites**
  - Contains vocal folds (true vocal cords) and 1 cm below them
- **Subglottis**
  - Inferior border of the glottis to the inferior border of the cricoid cartilage

PHARYNX
- **Nasopharyngeal borders**
  - Roof with sphenoid sinus superiorly
  - Lateral walls include the Eustachian tube, torus tuberis and fossa of Rosenmuller
  - Inferior border–free border of the soft palate
- **Oropharyngeal subsites**
  - Posterior 1/3 tongue and vallecula
  - Soft palate and uvula
  - Palatine and lingual tonsil
  - Posterior pharyngeal wall from the free border of the soft palate downwards to the horizontal plane of the vallecula
- **Hypopharyngeal subsites**
  - Posterior pharyngeal wall (from the level of epiglottis to cricoid cartilage)
  - Piriform sinus
  - Postcricoid region

RISK FACTORS
- Tobacco use (smoking and chewing)
- Excessive alcohol intake
- Human papilloma virus (HPV)

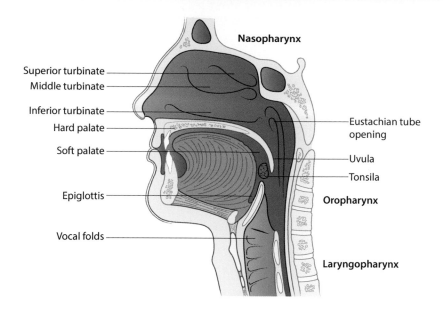

Figure 16.7 Anatomy of the pharynx.

- Radiation exposure
- Previous head and neck cancer
- Betel nut (paan) chewing

AETIOLOGICAL FACTORS

- HPV types considered high risk: 16, 18, 31, 33, 35, 39, 45, 51, 52, 56, 58, 59, 66
- 90% HPV 16 targeting reticulated tissue of the tonsils (lingual and palatine)

HUMAN PAPILLOMA VIRUS

KEY FACTS

- HPV type 16 (90%) is most commonly seen in squamous cell carcinoma (SCC) of the head and neck
- The virus targets the reticulated epithelium of the tonsils (lingual and palatine tonsils)
- Affects a younger patient population
- HPV-mediated SCC is associated with superior prognosis including a lower rate of recurrence and higher overall survival
- **Gardasil vaccine:** Is for type 6, 11, 16, 18
- HPV is a double stranded DNA
- Viral DNA is within the nucleus of the infected epithelium and infects stratified squamous epithelium, which have a high proliferation capacity

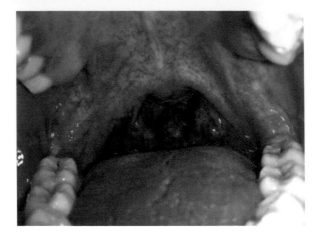

Figure 16.8   Left oropharyngeal SCC HPV+ve. Courtesy of Prof JP O'Neill

- HPV oncogene E6 binds to p53 (tumour suppressor gene) and E7 binds to Rb (retinoblastoma)
- High number of HPV-DNA replication occurs once the cell is close to the surface

INVESTIGATIONS

- Hematological investigation
- Radiological (CXR, CT neck and thorax, MRI and PET imaging)
- Laryngoscopy and oesophagoscopy for biopsy and to rule out a second primary
- Biopsy of lesion for tissue histology
- Fine needle aspiration cytology for suspicious nodal enlargement

NUTRITIONAL STATUS

- 40% are clinically malnourished on presentation
- Increased risk of aspiration pneumonia
- Consider nasogastric tube feeding in the immediate setting
- Percutaneous endoscopic or radiological inserted gastrostomy tube for long-term use

AIRWAY CONCERNS

- If concerned about an acute airway obstruction due to tumour, consider urgent endotracheal intubation, emergency cricothyroidotomy or tracheostomy

SPEECH REHABILITATION

- Electrolarynx
- Blom-Singer valve with tracheo-oesophageal puncture

STAGING

- TNM system

MANAGEMENT

- Multidisciplinary meeting discussion
- Single modality or combined therapy
- Surgical resection
- Radiotherapy (primary or adjuvant therapy)
- Concurrent chemotherapy
- Palliative care

LARYNGEAL CANCER

FUNCTION OF THE LARYNX

- Phonation
- Prevent aspiration during deglutition

HISTOLOGICAL SUBTYPES

- SCC (90%):
  - Approximately 98% of LSSC arise in the glottic or supraglottic region with glottic LSSC been more common.
  - Subglottic LSSC make up 2% of cases.
- Variants of SCC (spindle cell ca, verrucous ca, basaloid ca, adenosquamous ca)
- Neuroendocrine tumours (carcinoid tumour)
- Lymphoma
- Metastasis (regional or distant)

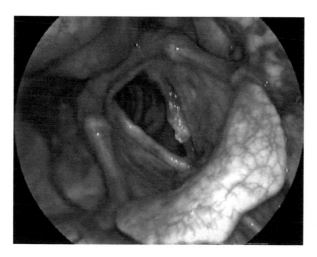

Figure 16.9   Endoscopic view of a left T1a tumor of the glottis. Courtesy of Prof JP O'Neill

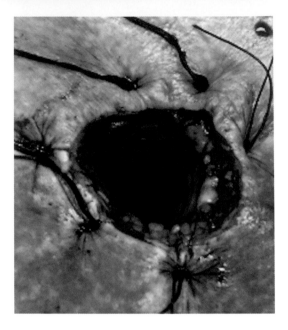

Figure 16.10   Perioperative picture of stoma suturing during total laryngectomy with insertion of a trachea-oesophageal prosthesis. Courtesy of Prof JP O'Neill

MANAGEMENT

- Stages I and II can be treated with **single modality therapy**
  - Surgery vs Radiotherapy
- Stages III and IV often require **combined therapy:**
  - Surgery and adjuvant radiotherapy
  - Surgery with adjuvant chemotherapy and radiotherapy
  - Chemotherapy and radiotherapy

SURGICAL OPTIONS

- Transoral laser microsurgery
- Hemilaryngectomy with voice preservation
- Supraglottic, or supracricoid laryngectomy
- Total laryngectomy

ORAL CANCER

HISTOLOGICAL SUBTYPES

- SCC (90%)
- Variants of SCC (spindle cell ca, verrucous ca, basaloid ca, adenosquamous ca)

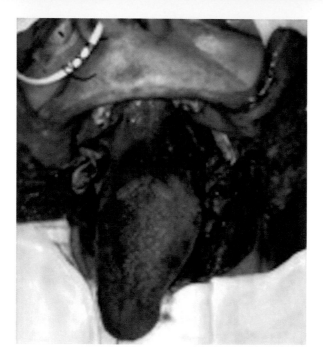

Figure 16.11 Salvage left oropharyngectomy with lip-split and mandibulotomy. Courtesy of Prof JP O'Neill

TREATMENT

- Surgery with or without radiotherapy is preferred for oral cavity cancer
- Adjuvant radiotherapy is considered for positive margins or perineural invasion
- Modified radical neck dissection is indicated in cases of positive nodal metastasis

OROPHARYNGEAL CANCER

KEY FACTS

- Majority are SCC
- Risk factors include alcohol, smoking and HPV infection

MANAGEMENT

- Early stage is treated with single modality
- Advanced stage can be treated with concurrent chemotherapy and radiotherapy
- Salvage surgery

NASOPHARYNGEAL CARCINOMA (NPC)

DEFINITION
- A genetic predisposition to environmental carcinogens leading to malignant transformation of nasopharyngeal epithelial cells

KEY FACTS
- Southeast Asia and Chinese population have high incidence of NPC
- NPC often arises from the fossa of Rosenmuller and spreads via direct extension

CLINICAL PRESENTATION
- Epistaxis
- Nasal obstruction
- Neck mass
- Cranial nerve dysfunction
- Unilateral middle ear effusion

STAGING
- Different from oral and oropharynx as primary treatment is chemo-radiotherapy

INVESTIGATION
- Biopsy of post nasal space examination under anesthesia
- Pan-endoscopy
- CT neck and thorax
- MRI skull base
- PET imaging

MANAGEMENT
- **Radiotherapy** is the mainstay of treatment
- Concurrent chemotherapy is used for disease with an advanced stage

SURGICAL PROCEDURES

TONSILLECTOMY

INDICATIONS
- **Recurrent tonsillitis:** Documented episodes of community managed tonsillitis or requiring hospital care
  - **7 episodes in 1 year**
  - **5–6 episodes per year over 2 years**
  - **3 episodes per year over 3 year**
  - **2 or more episodes of peritonsillar abscess**

- Suspected neoplasm
- Gross enlargement causing dysphagia or sleep apnoea
- Part of a staged surgical procedure

COMPLICATIONS

- Primary bleeding (within 24 hours) or secondary bleeding
- Pain including referred pain to the ear
- Damage of teeth
- General anesthetic complications
- Temporomandibular joint dislocation
- Infection
- Pulmonary complications (pneumonia, embolism)

MANAGEMENT OF TONSILLECTOMY BLEED

- Airway, breathing, circulation
- Persistent bleeding or if the patient is hemodynamically unstable, emergency operative
- Sporadic or intermittent bleeding in a hemodynamically stable patient can be managed with a trial conservation period
- Conservative management includes
  - Hospital admission for observation
  - FBC, group and screen
  - Nil per oral (NPO)
  - IV fluids
  - IV antibiotics
  - Analgesia
  - Hydrogen peroxide gargles

VENTILATION (TYMPANOSTOMY) TUBES

DEFINITION

- Small tube inserted into the tympanic membrane in order to keep the middle ear aerated for a prolonged period of time.

INDICATIONS

- Otitis media with effusion
- Recurrent acute otitis media
- Persistent Eustachian tube dysfunction
- Barotrauma
- Acute otitis media with bulging tympanic membrane or facial paralysis

TYPES

- Grommet tube
- T-shaped tube (stay for longer duration)

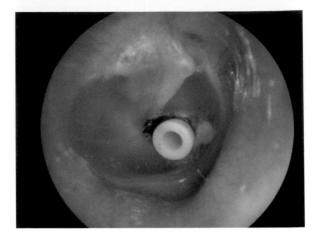

Figure 16.12 Grommet in situ, left tympanic membrane. Image courtesy of Mr Michael Saunders

COMPLICATIONS

- Otorrhea
- Residual tympanic membrane perforation
- Tympanosclerosis
- Injury to incudostapedial joint
- Bleeding (high dehiscent jugular bulb)
- Tube blockage
- Early extrusion of tube

MASTOIDECTOMY

DEFINITION

- Operative procedure to gain access to mastoid air cells, middle and inner ear structures

INDICATIONS

- Cholesteatoma
- Chronic suppurative otitis media
- Acute mastoiditis
- Temporal bone malignancy
- Cochlear implant surgery

TYPES

- Cortical mastoidectomy
- Radical mastoidectomy

COMPLICATIONS

- Facial nerve dysfunction
- Hearing loss (of varying severity including dead ear)
- Tinnitus
- Vertigo (due to lateral semicircular canal damage or fistula formation)
- Intracranial complications (meningitis, subdural or extradural abscess)
- Sigmoid sinus thrombosis

PAROTIDECTOMY

INDICATIONS FOR SUPERFICIAL PAROTIDECTOMY

- Benign parotid tumours or low-grade malignant tumours involving the superficial lobe
- Preservation of facial nerve

INDICATIONS FOR TOTAL PAROTIDECTOMY

- High-grade parotid gland malignancy
- Deep lobe involvement
- Facial nerve involvement

COMPLICATIONS

- Facial nerve paresis
- Bleeding and formation of a hematoma
- Greater auricular nerve dysfunction, leading to loss of sensation of the ear lobe
- Frey's syndrome:
  - Gustatory sweating due to regeneration of damaged auriculotemporal nerve.
  - This results in aberrant parasympathetic innervation of cutaneous sweat glands.

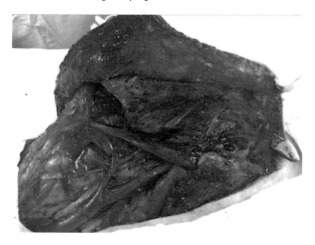

Figure 16.13   Left parotidectomy and left modified radical neck dissection (preservation of internal jugular vein). Courtesy of Prof JP O'Neill

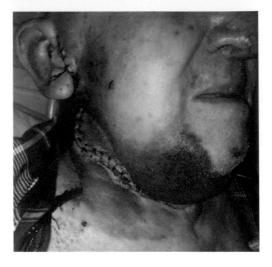

Figure 16.14 Right neck hematoma and ecchymosis post parotidectomy and neck dissection. Courtesy of Prof JP O'Neill

- Sialocele
- Cutaneous salivary gland fistula

NECK DISSECTION

DEFINITION
- Surgical excision of the cervical lymph nodes

KEY FACTS
- For management of head and neck malignancy
- The type of neck dissection undertaken depends on the anatomical location of the primary tumour and nodal status

TYPES
- **Radical neck dissection**
  - Excision of node level I–V
  - Sternocleidomastoid (SCM)
  - Internal jugular vein
  - Spinal accessory nerve
- **Modified radical neck dissection**
  - Excision of node level I–V
  - Type 3–spinal accessory nerve, internal jugular vein and SCM are spared
  - Type 2–spinal accessory nerve and internal jugular vein are spared
  - Type 1–spinal accessory nerve is spared

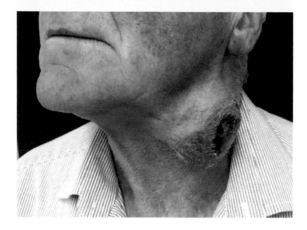

Figure 16.15 Left-sided lymphadenopathy with skin involvement, biopsy +ve for metastatic SCC. Courtesy of Prof JP O'Neill

- **Selective neck dissection**
  - Involves excision of nodes at risk of disease metastasis

COMPLICATIONS

- Wound infection and breakdown
- Flap necrosis
- Frozen shoulder syndrome due to sacrifice of spinal accessory nerve
- Vagus nerve injury
- Marginal mandibular nerve injury
- Hematoma
- Thoracic duct injury leading to chyle leak and fistula
- Cerebral and facial oedema due to internal jugular vein ligation
- Respiratory complications (pneumothorax, phrenic nerve injury, embolism, pneumonia)
- Major vessel damage (carotid artery)

MCQs FOR SELF-ASSESSMENT

SURGICAL SCORES AND CLASSIFICATION SYSTEMS

Chapter 1— Principles of Surgery:
- SIRS Criteria
- qSOFA Score

Chapter 3— Upper Gastrointestinal Surgery:
- Rockall Score
- DeMeester Score

Chapter 4— Hepatobiliary Surgery:
- Charcot's Triad
- Reynold's Pentad
- Ranson Criteria
- Modified Glasgow Criteria

Chapter 5— Colorectal Surgery:
- Alvarado Score
- Hinchey Classification
- Duke's Classification

Chapter 7— Peripheral Vascular Surgery:
- Rutherford-Fontaine Classification
- AAA Surveillance Figures
- ABPI Interpretation
- Well's Probability Score for DVT

Chapter 12— Major Trauma:
- Haemorrhagic Shock Classification: Signs and Symptoms
- GCS

Chapter 13— Plastic Surgery:
- The American ABCDE System for Presentation of Malignant Melanoma
- The Glasgow System
- Breslow Thickness

Chapter 14— Orthopaedic Surgery:
- Garden Classification (Intracapsular Neck of Femur Fractures)
- Denis–Weber Classification (Fibular Fracture)

Chapter 15— Neurosurgery:
- MRC Grading for Strength Examination
- Key Muscle Myotomes

Chapter 16— Otorhinolaryngology (ENT):
- Centor Score

PRINCIPLES OF SURGERY

SIRS CRITERIA
- Identifies patients who may be septic
- To meet the SIRS criteria, the patient must have:
  - A suspected infection AND two or more of the following:
    1. Acutely altered mental status
    2. Respiratory rate >20 breaths/minute
    3. Heart rate >90 beats/minute
    4. Temperature <36°C or >38.3°C
    5. WCC <4 × 10^6/L or >12 × 10^6/L

qSOFA SCORE
- Sequential organ failure assessment
- A qSOFA score of 2 or more indicates sepsis
- qSOFA score looks at the following organ systems:
  - Respiratory system: Looks at PaO_2/FiO_2
  - Haematologic: Looks at platelets
  - Hepatic: Looks at bilirubin
  - Cardiovascular: Hypotension
  - Neurologic: Glasgow Coma Score
  - Renal: Creatinine

UPPER GASTROINTESTINAL SURGERY

ROCKALL SCORE
- Assesses the risk of mortality after an upper GI bleed

	0	1	2	3
(A) Age	<60	60–79	80+	
(B) Shock	Nil	HR > 100	SBP < 100	
(C) Co-Morbidity	Nil major	Nil major	IHD/CCF Major morbidity	Renal failure Liver failure
(D) Diagnosis	Mallory-Weiss tear	All other diagnoses	GI malignancy	
(E) Evidence of Bleeding	None	None	Blood Spurting vessel Adherent clot	

DEMEESTER SCORE
- A pH study for dysphagia
- A composite measure of reflux episodes and length of occasions that pH is <4

HEPATOBILIARY SURGERY

CHARCOT'S TRIAD

- The presence of the following suggests ascending cholangitis:
  1. Constant severe right upper quadrant pain
  2. Obstructive jaundice
  3. Fever

REYNOLD'S PENTAD

- Charcot's triad with
  1. Hypotension
  2. Altered mental status

RANSON CRITERIA

- To assess the severity and associated mortality of acute pancreatitis
- Criteria on admission–1 point for each of the following:
  1. Age > 55
  2. WCC >16 × 10^9/L
  3. Glucose > 10 mmol/L
  4. LDH > 350 IU/L
  5. AST > 250 IU/L
- After 48 hours of admission–1 point for each of the following:
  1. Fall in haematocrit >10%
  2. Increase in urea >1.98 mmol/L
  3. Calcium < 2 mmol/L
  4. pO_2 < 8 kPa
  5. Base deficit > 4 mmol/L
  6. Fluid needs > 6 L in 48 hours
- Interpretation–predicted mortality rates (MR)
  - 0–2 points: 1% predicted MR
  - 3–4 points: 15% predicted MR
  - 5–6 points: 40% predicted MR
  - >7 points: 100% predicted MR

MODIFIED GLASGOW CRITERIA

- Three or more positive criteria within 48 hours of admission = severe attack and high dependency care referral is warranted
- Mnemonic–PANCREAS
  - PaO_2 < 8 kPa
  - Age > 55
  - Neutrophils/WCC > 15000 × 10^9/L
  - Corrected calcium < 2 mmol/L
  - Raised blood urea > 16 mmol/L
  - Enzymes elevated, AST > 200 U/L, LDH > 600 U/L
  - Albumin < 32 g/L
  - Sugar, blood glucose > 10 mmol/L

COLORECTAL SURGERY

ALVARADO SCORE

- Best employed as a tool to exclude appendicitis
- Score 0–3: Low risk
- Score 4–6: Observe, may need intervention
- Score 7–9: Male to proceed to appendectomy. Female to diagnostic laparotomy

Symptoms	Score	Signs	Score	Lab Values	Score
Abdominal pain	1	RIF tenderness	2	Leukocytosis > 10000	2
Anorexia	1	Rebound Tenderness	1	Neutrophils > 75%	1
Nausea and vomiting	1	Temperature > 37.5°C	1		

HINCHEY CLASSIFICATION

- For classification of acute diverticulitis
- It helps to determine the most suitable management

Hinchey Classification of Acute Diverticulitis	
1A	Paracolic phlegmon
1B	Pericolic/mesenteric abscess
II	Diverticulitis with walled-off abscess
III	Purulent peritonitis (perforated abscess cavity)
IV	Faeculent peritonitis

DUKE'S CLASSIFICATION

- For staging of colorectal cancer
- **Duke's A**–confined to bowel wall only
- **Duke's B**–through the bowel wall
- **Duke's C**–positive lymph nodes
- **Duke's D**–metastases

Duke's Classification	
Duke's A	Confined to bowel wall only
Duke's B	Through bowel wall
Duke's C	Positive lymph nodes
Duke's D	Metastases

PERIPHERAL VASCULAR SURGERY

RUTHERFORD-FONTAINE CLASSIFICATION

- Classification of chronic peripheral arterial disease

Rutherford-Fontaine Classification	
I	Asymptomatic
II	Intermittent Claudication: • IIA–Claudication distance >200 m • IIB–Claudication distance <200 m
III	Rest pain
IV	Tissue loss–ulcers, gangrene, necrosis

ABDOMINAL AORTIC ANEURYSM (AAA) SURVEILLANCE FIGURES

- Current UK screening/surveillance guidelines

3 cm–4.4 cm	Annual surveillance ultrasound scan
4.5 cm–5.4 cm	Three-monthly ultrasound scan surveillance
5.5 cm or greater	Surgical repair (open versus endovascular)

ABPI INTERPRETATION

- Ankle-brachial pressure index (ABPI) interpretation isratio of peak systolic doppler ankle pressure to arm pressure

ABPI Index	
1.1–0.9	Normal
0.9–0.5	Intermittent claudication
<0.5	Rest pain
<0.3	Tissue loss (ulcer, gangrene, necrosis)
>1.1	Calcified arteries (typically seen in people with diabetes, falsely elevated)

WELL'S PROBABILITY SCORE FOR DVT

- If 2 points or more then DVT is likely
- If 1 point or less then DVT is unlikely

Well's Probability Score for DVT	
Active malignancy	1 point
Paresis, paralysis or recent plaster immobilisation of lower limbs	1 point
Localised tenderness along the deep venous system	1 point
Entire leg swollen	1 point
Calf swelling >3 cm and larger than asymptomatic side	1 point
Pitting oedema	1 point
Collateral superficial veins	1 point
Previously documented DVT	1 point
Alternative diagnosis as likely as DVT	Minus 2 points

MAJOR TRAUMA

HAEMORRHAGIC SHOCK CLASSIFICATION: SIGNS AND SYMPTOMS

- Signs and symptoms of haemorrhage by class

Parameter	Class 1	Class 2 (Mild)	Class 3 (Moderate)	Class 4 (Severe)
Approximate blood loss	<15% Up to 750 ml	15–30% 750–1500 ml	31–40% 1500–2000 ml	>40% >2000 ml
Heart rate	<100	100–120	120–140	>140
Blood pressure	Normal	Normal	Decreased	Decreased
Pulse pressure	Normal/Increased	Decreased	Decreased	Decreased
Respiratory rate	14–20	20–30	30–40	>35
Urine output (ml/hr)	>30	20–30	5–15	Negligible
Glasgow Coma Scale	Normal	Normal	Reduced	Reduced
CNS mental state	Slightly anxious	Slightly anxious	Anxious, Confused	Confused, lethargic
Base deficit (mEq/L)	0 to −2	−2 to −6	−6 to −10	−10 or less
Need for blood products	Monitor	Possible	Yes	Massive transfusion protocol

THE GLASGOW COMA SCALE (GCS)

- Used for rapid neurological evaluation
- The GCS runs from 3 to 15, i.e. 3 is the lowest possible score
- A GCS of 8 or less indicates a need to intubate the patient

The Glasgow Coma Scale (GCS):

- Used for rapid neurological evaluation
- The GCS runs from 3-15, i.e. 3 is the lowest possible score
- A GCS of 8 or less indicates a need to intubate the patient

Assessment Area	Score
Eye-opening (E):	
• Spontaneous	4
• To sound	3
• To pressure	2
• None	1
• Non-testable	NT
Verbal response (V):	
• Orientated	5
• Confused	4
• Words	3
• Sounds	2
• None	1
• Non-testable	NT
Motor Response (M):	
• Obeys commands	6
• Localising	5
• Normal flexion	4
• Abnormal flexion	3
• Extension	2
• None	1
• Non-testable	NT

Note: GCS Score = (E[4] + V[5] + M[6]) = Best possible score 15; worst possible score 3. *If an area cannot be assessed, no numerical score is given for that region, and it is considered "non-testable." Source: www.glasgowcomascale.org

PLASTIC SURGERY

THE AMERICAN SYSTEM–ABCDE SYSTEM

- Check to see if moles have any of these features that are suspicious of malignant melanoma
- <u>Asymmetry:</u>
  - One side does not match the other

- Border:
  - Edges of the mole are irregular
- Colour:
  - More than one colour apparent
- Diameter:
  - Large mole >6 mm, increases over time
- Evolution:
  - Mole has changed in appearance/evolved

THE GLASGOW SYSTEM

- A 7-point checklist to help identify moles that are suspicious for malignant melanoma
- A mole with a score of 3 or more needs a specialist referral

Major (2 Points)	Minor (1 Point)
Change in size	Diameter of 7 mm or more
Irregular pigment	Inflammation
Irregular border	Oozing, bleeding, crusting
	Itching, altered sensation

BRESLOW THICKNESS

- A measure of the depth of the tumour–measures distance in mm from the epidermis to the maximum depth of the tumour
- The Breslow thickness is the single most important prognostic variable for malignant melanoma
- If the Breslow thickness is 0.8 mm or more, a sentinel lymph node biopsy is usually indicated

Depth	5-Year Survival (%)
In situ	95–100
<1 mm	95–100
1–2 mm	80–95
2–4 mm	60–75
>4 mm	50

ORTHOPAEDIC SURGERY

GARDEN CLASSIFICATION

- Classifies intracapsular neck of femur fractures to determine the best management
- Garden 1: Incomplete fracture, not displaced but impacted
- Garden 2: Complete, non-displaced fracture
- Garden 3: Complete fracture, partially displaced
  - Risk of avascular necrosis of the femoral head after fixation; therefore, management is hemiarthroplasty or total hip replacement

- Garden 4: Complete fracture, fully displaced
  - High risk of avascular necrosis; therefore, total or hemiarthroplasty is recommended

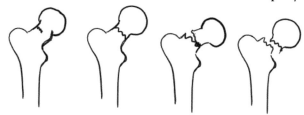

DENIS–WEBER CLASSIFICATION

- Normal ankle joint:
  - The syndesmosis consists of the ligament complex at the distal tibiofibular joint and the lower thickened portion of the interosseous membrane
- Weber A:
  - Fracture distal to the level of the syndesmosis
  - Usually treated in a below-knee walking cast
- Weber B:
  - Fracture is at the level of the syndesmosis
  - Some possibility of syndesmosis and disruption and instability
  - Needs surgical fixation if significant displacement
  - If not significantly displaced, then non-weight bearing below-knee cast for treatment
- Weber C:
  - Fracture proximal to the level of the syndesmosis
  - High likelihood of syndesmosis disruption and instability
  - Needs surgical fixation

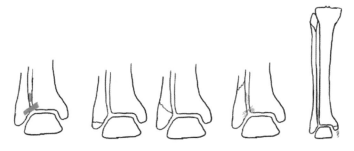

NEUROSURGERY

MRC GRADING FOR STRENGTH EXAMINATION

- The Medical Research Council's scale for measuring muscle power
- Carried out as part of the neurological examination
- Grades the power of individual muscle groups based on the movement of a single joint
- The scale runs from 0 to 5

Grade	Strength
0	No active contraction
1	Flicker of contraction
2	Contraction producing movement if gravity eliminated
3	Weak contraction and movement against gravity
4	Active movement against some resistance

KEY MUSCLE MYOTOMES

Upper Limb	
Myotomes	Muscles
C5	Elbow flexors
C6	Wrist extensors
C7	Elbow extensors
C8	Finger flexors
T1	Finger abductors (little finger)
Lower Limb	
Myotomes	**Muscles**
L2	Hip flexors
L3	Knee extensors
L4	Ankle dorsi-flexors
L5	Long toe extensors
S1	Ankle plantar flexors

OTORHINOLARYNGOLOGY (ENT)

CENTOR SCORE

- Indicates the likelihood of infection being bacterial tonsillitis versus viral tonsillitis
- Therefore, Centor score helps guide the need for antibiotic treatment
- A score of 0–2: Do not treat with antibiotics
- A score of 3–4: Treat with antibiotics

Signs and/or Symptoms	Score
Presence of tonsillar exudate	1
Tender cervical lymphadenopathy	1
History of fever	1
Absence of cough	1

FURTHER READING

CHAPTER 1

1. Oxford Medical Education—General Management: History Taking (2016).
2. Brown W, Loudon KW, Fisher J, Marsland LB. 2020. Pass the PSA [e-Book]. Elsevier Health Sciences.
3. British Columbia: Warfarin Therapy—Management during Invasive Procedures and Surgery (2015).
4. Teach me Surgery Online.

CHAPTER 2

5. Dabbas N, Adams K, Pearson K, Royle G. 2011. Frequency of abdominal wall hernias: is classical teaching out of date? JRSM Short Rep 2:5.
6. Davis BS, Dunn DP, Hostetler VC. 2017. Beyond hernias: a multimodality review of abdominal wall pathology. Br J Radiol 90:20160719.
7. Balla A, Batista Rodríguez G, Buonomo N, et al. 2017. Perineal hernia repair after abdominoperineal excision or extralevator abdominoperineal excision: a systematic review of the literature. Tech Coloproctol 21:329.
8. World Society of Emergency Surgery (WSES): Guidelines for emergency repair of complicated abdominal wall hernias, update (2017).

CHAPTER 3

9. Patti M. Gastroesophageal Reflux Disease Treatment & Management: Approach Considerations, Lifestyle Modifications, Pharmacologic Therapy [Internet]. Emedicine. medscape.com. 2021 [cited 12 January 2021]. Available from: https://emcdicine.medscape.com/article/176595-treatment
10. Esophageal Cancer: Practice Essentials, Background, Anatomy [Internet]. Emedicine. medscape.com. 2021 [cited 12 January 2021]. Available from: https://emedicine.medscape.com/article/277930-overview
11. Saliba G, Hayami M, Klevebro F, Nilsson M. 2020. Surgical treatment of Siewert type II gastroesophageal junction cancer: esophagectomy, total gastrectomy or other options? Annals of Esophagus 3:18.
12. Stomach Cancer Surgery Perth | Gastrectomy | Abdominal Surgery [Internet]. The Surgeons Collective Perth. 2021 [cited 12 January 2021]. Available from: https://www.thesurgeonscollective.com.au/treatments/stomach-cancer-surgery-total-partial-gastrectomy-perth
13. Minimally Invasive Laparoscopic Esophagectomy, Esophageal Cancer Treatment [Internet]. Expert Bariatric, Metabolic Surgeon for Weight Loss Surgery in Delhi | Dr Randeep Wadhawan. 2021 [cited 12 January 2021]. Available from: https://www.randeepwadhawan.com/oesophagectomy-cancer-of-the-oesophagus/

14. Dunn C, Patel T, Bildzukewicz N, Henning J, Lipham J. 2020. Which hiatal hernia's need to be fixed? Large, small or none? Annals of Laparoscopic and Endoscopic Surgery 5:29.

15. [Internet]. Marlin-prod.literatumonline.com. 2021 [cited 12 January 2021]. Available from: https://marlin-prod.literatumonline.com/cms/asset/a2ef514d-7db9-4561-a6e7-6a0ee1f8b780/gr3.jpg

16. Internal Clinical Guidelines, T. 2014. National Institute for Health and Care Excellence: Clinical Guidelines. Dyspepsia and Gastro-Oesophageal Reflux Disease: Investigation and Management of Dyspepsia, Symptoms Suggestive of Gastro-Oesophageal Reflux Disease, or Both. London: National Institute for Health and Care Excellence (UK).

17. Lordick F, Mariette C, Haustermans K, Obermannova R, Arnold D. 2016. Oesophageal cancer: ESMO Clinical Practice Guidelines for diagnosis, treatment and follow-up. Ann Oncol 27:v50–v57.

18. Pennathur A, Gibson MK, Jobe BA, Luketich JD. 2013. Oesophageal carcinoma. Lancet 381:400–412.

19. Rahman MW, Sumon SM, Amin MR, Kahhar MA. 2013. Rockall score for risk stratification in adult patients with non-variceal upper gastrointestinal hemorrhage. Mymensingh Med J 22:694–698.

20. Schlottmann F, Patti MG. 2017. Primary esophageal motility disorders: beyond achalasia. Int J Mol Sci 18(7):1399.

CHAPTER 4

21. Teach Me Surgery Online.

22. Oxford Handbook of Clinical Surgery (4th Edition) Greg McLatchie, Neil Borley, Joanna Chikwe. Oxford Medical Publications.

23. Essential Med Notes 2020: Comprehensive Medical Reference & Review for USMLE II and MCCQE (January 2020), Sara Mirali, Ayesh Seneviratne.

24. Surgery at a Glance. John Wiley & Sons, Jan 22, 2013 [Medical], p. 208, Pierce A. Grace, Neil R. Borley.

25. Roy-Chowdhury N, Chopra S, Grover S. 2018. Diagnostic Approach to the Adult with Jaundice or Asymptomatic Hyperbilirubinemia. [online] Uptodate.com. Available at: https://www.uptodate.com/contents/diagnostic-approach-to-the-adult-with-jaundice-or-asymptomatic-hyperbilirubinemia?search=jaundice&source=search_result&selectedTitle=1~150&usage_type=default&display_rank=1 [Accessed 30 Oct 2018].

26. Swaroop Vege S, Whitcomb D, Grover S. 2018. Clinical Manifestations and Diagnosis of Acute Pancreatitis. [online] Uptodate.com. Available at: https://www.uptodate.com/contents/clinical-manifestations-and-diagnosis-of-acute-pancreatitis?search=acute%20pancreatitis&source=search_result&selectedTitle=2~150&usage_type=default&display_rank=2 [Accessed 30 Oct. 2018].

27. Freedman S, Whitcomb D, Grover S. 2018. Clinical Manifestations and Diagnosis of Chronic Pancreatitis in Adults. [online] Uptodate.com.

Available at: https://www.uptodate.com/contents/clinical-manifestations-and-diagnosis-of-chronic-pancreatitis-in-adults?search=chronic%20pancreatitis&source=search_result&selectedTitle=1~150&usage_type=default&display_rank=1 [Accessed 30 Oct. 2018].

28. Uptodate.com. 2018. Clinical Manifestations, Diagnosis, and Staging of Exocrine Pancreatic Cancer. [online] Available at: https://www.uptodate.com/contents/clinical-manifestations-diagnosis-and-staging-of-exocrine-pancreatic-cancer?search=pancreatic%20cancer&source=search_result&selectedTitle=1~150&usage_type=default&display_rank=1 [Accessed 30 Oct. 2018].

CHAPTER 5

29. Liang MK, Anderson RE, Jaffe BM, Berger DH. 2015. The appendix. In: Schwartz's Principles of Surgery, Tenth Edition, Schwartz SI, Brunicardi CF (Eds), McGraw-Hill Companies, New York.

30. Salminen P, Paajanen H, Rautio T, Nordström P, Aarnio M, Rantanen T, Tuominen R, Hurme S, Virtanen J, Mecklin JP, Sand J, Jartti A, Rinta-Kiikka I, Grönroos JM. 2015. Antibiotic Therapy vs Appendectomy for Treatment of Uncomplicated Acute Appendicitis: The APPAC Randomized Clinical Trial. JAMA 313(23):2340.

31. UpToDate—Management of Acute Appendicitis.

32. UpToDate—Overview of the Management of Primary Colon Cancer.

33. PathologyOutlines.com. Anus and perianal area, Cornish T, Gonzalez R, Ladoulis C, Riddle N, Rishi A, Weisenberg E. Revised: 31 August 2018, © 2002–2018.

CHAPTER 6

34. Endoscopy for the Diagnosis of Inflammatory Bowel Disease, Jeffrey Daniel Jacobs and Scott Lee–Submitted: March 7 2018. Reviewed: June 20 2018. Published: November 5 2018–DOI: 10.5772/intechopen.79657.

35. El Salvador Atlas of Gastrointestinal Endoscopy. GastrointestinalAtlas.com

36. UpToDate overview of imaging techniques in the diagnosis and management of inflammatory bowel diseases. Katarzyna B. Biernacka, Dobromiła Barańska, Piotr Grzelak, Elżbieta Czkwnianc, Katarzyna Szabelska-Zakrzewska. 2019. Prz Gastroenterol 14(1):19–25. doi: 10.5114/pg.2019.83423

37. Peppercorn M, Kane S. 2018. Clinical Manifestations, Diagnosis and Prognosis of Crohn Disease in Adults. [online] Uptodate.com. Available at: https://www.uptodate.com/contents/clinical-manifestations-diagnosis-and-prognosis-of-crohn-disease-in-adults?search=crohns%20disease%20adult&source=search_result&selectedTitle=2~150&usage_type=default&display_rank=2 [Accessed 30 Oct. 2018].

38. Fleshner, P. 2018. Surgical Management of Ulcerative Colitis. [online] Uptodate.com. Available at: https://www.uptodate.com/contents/surgical-management-of-ulcerative-colitis?search=ulcerative%20colitis%20treatment&source=search_result&selectedTitle=4~150&usage_type=default&display_rank=4 [Accessed 30 Oct. 2018].

CHAPTER 7

39. Alguire P, Scovell S. 2018. Overview and management of lower extremity chronic venous disease. [online] UpToDate. Available at: https://www.uptodate.com/contents/overview-and-management-of-lower-extremity-chronic-venousdisease?search=chronic%20venous%20insufficiency&source=search_result&selectedTitle=1~150&usage_type=default&display_rank=1 [Accessed 28 Oct. 2018].

40. Neschis DG, Golden MA. 2017. Clinical features and diagnosis of lower extremity peripheral artery disease. [online] UpToDate. Available at: https://www.uptodate.com/contents/clinical-features-and-diagnosis-of-lower-extremity-peripheral-artery-disease?search=peripheral%20arterial%20disease&source=search_result&selectedTitle=1~150&usage_type=default&display_rank=1 [Accessed 28 Oct. 2018].

41. Chaer R. 2018. Endovascular repair of abdominal aortic aneurysm. [online] UpToDate. Available at: https://www.uptodate.com/contents/endovascular-repair-of-abdominal-aortic-aneurysm?search=abdominal%20aortic%20aneurysm&source=search_result&selectedTitle=7~150&usage_type=default&display_rank=7 [Accessed 28 Oct. 2018].

42. Eidt J. 2018. Open surgical repair of abdominal aortic aneurysm. [online] UpToDate. Available at: https://www.uptodate.com/contents/open-surgical-repair-of-abdominal-aortic-aneurysm?search=abdominal%20aortic%20aneurysm&source=search_result&selectedTitle=6~150&usage_type=default&display_rank=6 [Accessed 28 Oct. 2018].

43. Berger J, Davies M. 2018. Overview of lower extremity peripheral artery disease. [online] UpToDate. Available at: https://www.uptodate.com/contents/overview-of-lower-extremity-peripheral-artery-disease?search=vascular%20surgery&source=search_result&selectedTitle=1~150&usage_type=default&display_rank=1 [Accessed 28 Oct. 2018].

CHAPTER 8

44. Breast-Conserving Therapy. UpToDate. https://tinyurl.com/y6f9rtex

45. Surgical Treatment of Breast Cancer. https://emedicine.medscape.com/article/1276001-overview

46. Breast Cancer Risk Factors. https://emedicine.medscape.com/article/1945957-overview#a6

47. European Guidelines on Breast Cancer Screening and Diagnosis.

48. Genes Dis. 2018 May 12;5(2):77–106. doi: 10.1016/j.gendis.2018.05.001. eCollection 2018 Jun. Breast Cancer Development and Progression: Risk Factors, Cancer Stem Cells, Signaling Pathways, Genomics, and Molecular Pathogenesis. Feng Y, Spezia M, Huang S, Yuan C, Zeng Z, Zhang L, Ji X, Liu W, Huang B, Luo W, Liu B, Lei Y, Du S, Vuppalapati A, Luu HH, Haydon RC, He TC, Ren G.

49. Am Soc Clin Oncol Educ Book. 2018 May 23;(38):457–467. doi: 10.1200/EDBK_201313. New and Important Changes in the TNM Staging System for Breast Cancer. Hortobagyi GN, Edge SB, Giuliano A.

50. Breast Cancer Treatment (PDQ®): Health Professional Version. Authors PDQ Adult Treatment Editorial Board. Source PDQ Cancer Information Summaries [Internet]. Bethesda (MD): National Cancer Institute (US), 2002–2018 May 31.

51. Surg Pathol Clin. 2018 Mar;11(1):17–42. doi: 10.1016/j.path.2017.09.003. Epub 2017 Dec 1. A Diagnostic Approach to Fibroepithelial Breast Lesions. Tan BY, Tan PH.

52. J Adolesc Health. 2018 Sep 29. pii: S1054-139X(18)30281–30287. doi: 10.1016/j.jado-health.2018.06.028. [Epub ahead of print] The Effect of Surgical Treatment for Gynecomastia on Quality of Life in Adolescents. Nuzzi LC, Firriolo JM, Pike CM, Cerrato FE, DiVasta AD, Labow BI.

CHAPTER 9

53. Standring S, Borley NR, et al., eds. 2008. Gray's anatomy: the anatomical basis of clinical practice (40th ed.). London: Churchill Livingstone.

54. Stathopoulos P, Gangidi S, Kotrotsos G, Cunliffe D. 2015. Graves' disease: a review of surgical indications, management, and complications in a cohort of 59 patients. International Journal of Oral and Maxillofacial Surgery.

55. Adigbli G, King J. 2015. Airway management of a life-threatening post-thyroidectomy haematoma. BMJ Case Rep 2015.

56. Dossett, Lesly; Rudzinski, Erin; Blevins, Lewis; Chambers, Eugene. 2007. Malignant Pheochromocytoma of the Organ of Zuckerkandl Requiring Aortic and Vena Caval Reconstruction. Endocrine Practice.

57. Ross D, Burch H, Cooper D, Greenlee M, Laurberg P, Maia A, Rivkees S, Samuels M, Sosa J, Stan M, Walter M. 2016. 2016 American Thyroid Association Guidelines for Diagnosis and Management of Hyperthyroidism and Other Causes of Thyrotoxicosis. Thyroid 26(10):1343–1421.

58. Tuttle, R. 2018. Differentiated thyroid cancer: Overview of management. [online] Uptodate.com. Available at: https://www.uptodate.com/contents/differentiated-thyroid-cancer-overview-of-management?topicRef=7860&source=see_link [Accessed 15 Oct. 2018].

59. Fuleihan G, Silverberg S. 2017. Primary hyperparathyroidism: Clinical manifestations. [online] Uptodate.com. Available at: https://www.uptodate.com/contents/primary-hyperparathyroidism-clinical-manifestations?search=hyperparathyroidism&source=search_result&selectedTitle=3~150&usage_type=default&display_rank=3 [Accessed 15 Oct. 2018].

60. Young W. 2018. Clinical presentation and diagnosis of pheochromocytoma. [online] Uptodate.com. Available at: https://www.uptodate.com/contents/clinical-presenta-tion-and-diagnosis-of-pheochromocytoma?search=pheochromocytoma&source=search_result&selectedTitle=1~150&usage_type=default&display_rank=1 [Accessed 15 Oct. 2018].

61. Nieman L. 2018. Primary therapy of Cushing's disease: Transsphenoidal surgery and pituitary irradiation. [online] Uptodate.com. Available at: https://www.uptodate.com/contents/primary-therapy-of-cushings-disease-transsphenoidal-surgery-and-pitu-itary-irradiation?search=Cushing%27s%20disease%20pituitary&source=search_res ult&selectedTitle=1~150&usage_type=default&display_rank=1 [Accessed 15 Oct. 2018].

62. Pearce, Elizabeth N. Diagnosis and management of thyrotoxicosis. BMJ 2006; 332, (7554): 1369–1373. doi:10.1136/bmj.332.7554.1369

63. Pal, Pooja et al. "Bone Metastases in Follicular Carcinoma of Thyroid." Indian journal of otolaryngology and head and neck surgery: official publication of the Association of Otolaryngologists of India 2018; 70(1):10–14. doi:10.1007/s12070-017-1170-x

CHAPTER 10

64. Weider JA. Pocket Guide to Urology, 5th edition. ISBN 978-0-9672845-6-9

65. NICE guideline [CG97] Lower Urinary Tract Symptoms in Men: Management 2015. www.nice.org.uk/guidance/cg97

66. Foster HE, Dahm P, Kohler TS, et al. 2019. Surgical Management of Lower Urinary Tract Symptoms Attributed to Benign Prostatic Hyperplasia: AUA Guideline Amendment. J Urol 202:592.

67. Türk C, Neisius A, Petrik A, et al. 2018. Guidelines on Urolithiasis. European Association of Urology. ISBN 978-94-92671-04-2

68. NICE guideline [NG118] Renal and Ureteric Stones: Assessment and Management 2019. www.nice.org.uk/guidance/ng118

69. Ljungberg B, Albiges L, Bensalah K, Bex A, et al. 2020. Guidelines on Renal Cell Carcinoma. European Association of Urology. www.uroweb.org

70. Chang SS, Boorjian SA, Chou R, 2016; et al. 2016. Diagnosis and Treatment of Non-Muscle Invasive Bladder Cancer: AUA/SUO Guideline. J Urol 196:1021.

71. Khadra MH, Pickard RS, Charlton M, et al. 2000. A Prospective Analysis of 1,930 Patients with Hematuria to Evaluate Current Diagnostic Practice. J Urol 163:524.

72. NICE Guideline. Bladder Cancer: Diagnosis and Management 2015. www.nice.org.uk/guidance/ng2

73. Mottet N, Cornford P, et al. Guidelines on Prostate Cancer 2014. European Association of Urology. www.uroweb.org

74. Ballentine Carter, H., Peter C. Albertsen, Michael J. Barry, et al. Early Detection of Prostate Cancer 2018. American Urological Association.

75. Andrew Stephenson, Scott E. Eggener, Eric B. Bass. Diagnosis and Treatment of Early-Stage Testicular Cancer: AUA Guideline (2019).

76. Kidney Disease: Improving Global Outcomes (KDIGO) Transplant Work Group. KDIGO Clinical Practice Guideline for the Care of Kidney Transplant Recipients. Am J Transplant 2009; 9 Suppl 3:S1–S155. doi:10.1111/j.1600-6143.2009.02834.x

77. Bamoulid J, Staeck O, Halleck F, Khadzhynov D, Brakemeier S, Dürr M, Budde K. 2015. The Need for Minimization Strategies: Current Problems of Immunosuppression. Transpl Int 2015; 28(8):891–900. doi: 10.1111/tri.12553. Epub 2015 Mar 18. PMID: 25752992.

CHAPTER 11

78. Demmy T, Dexter E. 2020. Overview of minimally invasive thoracic surgery–UpToDate. Available at: https://www.uptodate.com/contents/overview-of-minimally-invasive-thoracic-surgery?search=cardiothoracic surgery&source=search_result&selectedTitle=3~15 0&usage_type=default&display_rank=3

79. Gaasch W. 2020. Indications for valve replacement in aortic stenosis in adults–UpToDate. Available at: https://www.uptodate.com/contents/indications-for-valve-replacement-in-aortic-stenosis-in-adults?search=aortic stenosis&source=search_result&selectedTitle=2~150&usage_type=default&display_rank=2

80. Huggins JT, Carr SR, Woodward GA. 2020. Thoracostomy tubes and catheters: Indications and tube selection in adults and children–UpToDate. Available at: https://www.uptodate.com/contents/thoracostomy-tubes-and-catheters-indications-and-tube-selection-in-adults-and-children?search=chest tube insertion&source=search_result&selectedTitle=1~150&usage_type=default&display_rank=1

81. Light RW, Lee GY. 2020. Pneumothorax in adults: Epidemiology and etiology–UpToDate. Available at: https://www.uptodate.com/contents/pneumothorax-in-adults-epidemiology-and-etiology?search=pneumothorax&source=search_result&selectedTitle=1~150&usage_type=default&display_rank=1

82. Meyer T. 2020. Auscultation of cardiac murmurs in adults–UpToDate. Available at: https://www.uptodate.com/contents/auscultation-of-cardiac-murmurs-in-adults?search=heart murmurs&source=search_result&selectedTitle=2~150&usage_type=default&display_rank=2

83. NEJM. 2014. Chest tube insertion NEJM–YouTube, New England Journal of Medicine. Available at: https://www.youtube.com/watch?reload=9&v=69A6mdtfSek&has_verified=1

84. Light RW. 2018. Primary spontaneous pneumothorax in adults. 4/5/2018 ed. UpToDate. Available at: https://www-uptodate-com/contents/primary-spontaneous-pneumothorax-in-adults?search=pneumothorax&source=search_result&selectedTitle=1~150&usage_type=default&display_rank=1#references

85. Kumar P, Clark M, Camm AJ, Bunce NH. 2012. Cardiovascular Disease, Clinical Medicine, Eighth Edition, pp. 723–751.

86. Aranki S, 2018. Coronary artery bypass graft surgery: Graft choices—UpToDate. Available at: https://www.uptodate.com/contents/coronary-artery-bypass-graft-surgery-graft-choices?search=%20Coronary%20artery%20bypass%20graft%20surgery:%20Graft%20choices%20&source=search_result&selectedTitle=1~150&usage_type=default&display_rank=1

87. Nishimura RA, Otto CM, Bonow RO, et al. 2017. 2017 AHA/ACC Focused Update of the 2014 AHA/ACC Guideline for the management of patients with valvular heart disease: A report of the AHA/ACC Task Force on Clinical Practice. 15/3/17 ed. AHAjournals.Org. Available at: https://www.ahajournals.org/lookup/doi/10.1161/CIR.0000000000000503

CHAPTER 12

88. Injuries and violence: the facts. Geneva: World Health Organization, 2010.

89. Advanced Trauma Life Support (ATLS), Tenth Edition. USA: American College of Surgeons, 2018.

90. American College of Surgeons Committee on Trauma (2012). Initial Assessment and Management, Advanced Trauma Life Support, Ninth Edition, pp. 2–28.

91. American College of Surgeons Committee on Trauma (2012). Thoracic Trauma, Advanced Trauma Life Support, Ninth Edition, pp. 94–110.

92. American College of Surgeons Committee on Trauma (2012). Abdominal and Pelvic Trauma, Advanced Trauma Life Support, Ninth Edition, pp. 122–147.

93. Raja A, Zane RD. 2018. Initial Management of Trauma in Adults. UpToDate. Available at: https://www.uptodate.com/contents/initial-management-of-trauma-in-adults?search=Initial%20Management%20of%20Trauma%20in%20Adults&source=search_result&selectedTitle=1~150&usage_type=default&display_rank=1

CHAPTER 13

94. Karimkhani C, Green AC, Nijsten T, Weinstock MA, Dellavalle RP, Naghavi M, Fitzmaurice C. 2017. The global burden of melanoma: results from the Global Burden of Disease Study 2015. Br J Dermatol 177(1):134–140. doi: 10.1111/bjd.15510. Epub 2017 Jun 12. PMID: 28369739; PMCID: PMC5575560.

95. In 2015, global cases were 5 in 100,00 persons per year.

96. British Association of Dermatologists. Available at: http://www.bad.org.uk/healthcare-professionals

97. Buzaid AC, Gershenwald JE. Tumor node metastasis (TNM) staging system and other prognostic factors in cutaneous melanoma. Available at: https://www.uptodate.com/contents/tumor-node-metastasis-tnm-staging-system-and-other-prognostic-factors-in-cutaneous-melanoma

98. Hettiaratchy S, Papini R. 2004. Initial management of a major burn: II—assessment and resuscitation. 329(7457):101–103.

99. Hettiaratchy S, Papini R. 2004. Initial management of a major burn: I—overview. 328(7455):1555–1557.

100. Notebook G. NICE urgent referral guidance for suspected malignant melanoma. Available at: https://www.gpnotebook.co.uk/simplepage.cfm?ID=-221249461

101. Rutkove SB. Overview of upper extremity peripheral nerve syndromes. Available at: https://www.uptodate.com/contents/overview-of-upper-extremity-peripheral-nerve-syndromes

102. Thornton JF, Gosman AA. 2004. Skin grafts and skin substitutes and principles of flaps. Selected Readings in Plastic Surgery 10(1):78.

CHAPTER 14

103. British Orthopaedic Association. 2017. British Orthopaedic Association | BOA Standards for Trauma (BOASTs), Audit Standards for Trauma.

104. British Orthopaedic Association and British Geriatrics Society. 2007. The care of patients with fragility fracture. Available at: https://www.bgs.org.uk/sites/default/files/content/attachment/2018-05-02/Blue Book on fragility fracture care.pdf

105. National Institute for Health and Care Excellence. 2014. "Osteoarthritis: care and management", Osteoarthritis: Care and Management. Available at: https://www.nice.org.uk/guidance/cg177/resources/osteoarthritis-care-and-management-pdf-35109757272517

106. National Institute for Health and Care Excellence. 2016. "Fractures (non-complex): assessment and management", NICE.Org.UK.

107. Rockwood and Green's. 2015. Fractures in Adults, Volume 2; Charles M. Court-Brown, James D. Heckman, Margaret M. McQueen, William M. Ricci, Paul Tornetta (III), Michael D. McKee, Wolters Kluwer Health, 2015.

CHAPTER 15

108. HSE guidance: Bleeding in the brain. https://www.hse.ie/eng/health/az/b/bleeding-in-the-brain/complications-of-subarachnoid-haemorrhage.html

109. BMJ Best Practice, Subarachnoid Haemorrhage. Bestpractice.bmj.com/topics/en-gb/3000106

110. Kumar P, Clark, Jarman P. 2012. "Neurological Disease", Clinical Medicine (ed. 8), pp. 1067–1150.

111. Lissauer T, Clayden G, Newton RW, Stevens M. 2012. "Illustrated Textbook of Paediatrics", Chapter on Malignant Disease: Brain Tumours (ed. 4), p. 372.

112. Singer RJ, Ogilvy CS, Rordorf G. 2018. Treatment of aneurysmal subarachnoid haemorrhage. [UpToDate] Available at: https://www.uptodate.com/contents/treatment-of-cerebral-aneurysms?search=Clinical%20management%20and%20diagnosis%20of%20aneurysmal%20subarachnoid%20haemorrhage%20%26%20Treatment%20of%20aneurysmal%20subarachnoid%20haemorrhage&source=search_result&selectedTitle=1~150&usage_type=default&display_rank=1

CHAPTER 16

113. Sataloff RT, Sclafani AP. 2015. Sataloff's Comprehensive Textbook of Otolaryngology: Head & Neck Surgery: Facial Plastic and Reconstructive Surgery (Vol. 3). JP Medical Ltd.

114. Bull PD, Clarke R. 2002. Lecture Notes on Diseases of the Ear, Nose and Throat. Blackwell Science.

115. Scholes MA, Ramakrishnan VR. 2015. Ent Secrets. Elsevier Health Sciences.

116. Woo P. 2009. Stroboscopy. Plural Publishing.

117. Hussain SM. ed. 2018. ENT, Head & Neck Emergencies: A Logan Turner Companion. CRC Press.

INDEX

Note: Locators in *italics* represent figures and **bold** indicate tables in the text.

A

Abdominal aortic aneurysms (AAAs), 151
    aneurysm, types of, 155
    clinical features, 153
    complications of AAA repair, 154–155
    definition, 151
    differential diagnosis, 153
    endoleak, 155, **155**
    investigations, 153
    management, 153–154
    risk factors, 152
    surveillance, 152, **153**, 379
Abdominal trauma, 258
    categories, 258–259
    initial examination, 259–260
    investigations, **260**
    resuscitative laparotomy, indications for, 261
    urgent laparotomy, indications for, 261
ABPI, *see* Ankle-brachial pressure index
Achalasia, 57
    complications, 59
    definition, 57
    epidemiology, 58
    investigations, 58
    management, 59
    pathogenesis and aetiology, 58
Acoustic neuroma
    clinical presentation, 355
    definition, 355
    investigations, 355
    management, 356
Acute abdomen, differential diagnosis of, 7, *8*,
        9–10, *10*
    diffuse abdominal pain, 12
    epigastric pain, 7–11
    left iliac fossa (LIF) pain, 14
    LUQ pain, 11
    right iliac fossa (RIF) pain, 12–14
    right/left flank pain, 12
    right upper quadrant (RUQ) pain, 11
    suprapubic pain, 14
    umbilical pain, 12

Acute otitis media (AOM)
    clinical presentation, 351
    complications, 351
    definition, 350
    pathogens, 351
Acute urinary retention (AUR), 211
    aetiology, 211
    clinical presentation, 211
    epidemiology, 211
    investigations, 212
    treatment, 212
        self-intermittent catheterisation
            (SIC), 213
        suprapubic catheterisation, 213
        urethral catheterisation, 212–213
Adenocarcinoma, 60, 64, *64*, 108, 136
Advanced Trauma Life Support (ATLS®) System
        (Tenth Edition), 250
    general information, 250–252
    primary survey, adjuncts to, 254
    secondary survey, 254
    trauma triad of death, **253**
AIN, *see* Anal intraepithelial neoplasia
Airway concerns, 364
Allergic rhinitis
    clinical presentation, 357
    definition, 357
    investigations, 357
    management, 357
    typical allergens, 357
Allergies, 4
Alvarado scoring system, 103, **103**, 378
Amaurosis fugax, 162
American system – ABCDE system, 381
Anaemia, 137
Anal cancer
    anal intraepithelial neoplasia (AIN), 123
    anatomy of anal canal defining the types of
        tumours, 123
    clinical features, 123
    investigations, 124
    lymphatic drainage, 123
    management, 124
    risk factors, 123
    treatment, 124
    types of tumours of, 123

Anal fissure
    aetiology, 117
    clinical features, 117
    definition, 117
    examination
        acute anal fissure, 117
        chronic fissure, 118
    management, 118
    types, 117
Anal fistula
    aetiology, 119
    clinical assessment, 119
    clinical features, 119
    definition, 119
    Goodsall's rule, *120*
    investigations, 119
    management, 121
    primary tracks, *120*
    surgical management options, 121
    types, *120*
Anal intraepithelial neoplasia (AIN), 123
Anaplastic thyroid cancer
    aetiology, 196
    definition, 196
    investigations, 196
    treatment, 196–197
Anastrozole, 177
Ankle-brachial pressure index (ABPI), 148, 379
Ankle fractures, 304, *305*, *306*
    classifications, 304
    clinical presentation, 304
    complications, 306
    Maisonneuve fracture, 306, *307*
Anorectal abscess
    classification, 118
    clinical features, 118
    definition, 118
    investigations, 119
    management, 119
Anterior cord syndrome, 332
Anterior shoulder dislocation, 298
Antibiotics, 103
AOM, *see* Acute otitis media
Aortic regurgitation (AR), 240
    aetiology, 240
    clinical presentation, 240–241
    indications for surgery, 241
    investigations, 241
    prognosis, 241
Aortic stenosis (AS), 238
    aetiology, 238
    clinical presentation, 238
    indications for surgery, 238
    investigations, 238
    prognosis, 239
    surgical approach, 238
Appendicitis, 12–13
Appendicitis, acute, 101
    Alvarado score, 103
    carcinoid tumour of appendix, 104
    clinical features, 101–102
    complications, 104
    differential diagnosis, 102
    investigations, 102
    management, 103
    pathophysiology, 101
    special tests, 102
AR, *see* Aortic regurgitation
Arterial atherosclerosis, balloon angioplasty of, *149*
Arterial ulcer, *164*
AS, *see* Aortic stenosis
Asymptomatic gallstones, 78
Atherosclerosis, 147
AUR, *see* Acute urinary retention
Axillary node clearance, 177

B

Back pain, 312
Barrett's oesophagus, 46, *47*
    aetiology, 47
    definition, 46
    management, 47
Basal cell carcinoma versus squamous cell
        carcinoma, 268–269
Bascom's operation, 122
Battle sign, *323*
BCT, *see* Breast-conserving therapy
Benign breast disease
    breast cysts, 179
    breast infections, 179
    fat necrosis, 180
    fibroadenoma, 179
    fibrocystic disease, 179
    gynaecomastia, 180
Benign prostatic hyperplasia
    clinical presentation, 213–214
    complications of surgery, 215
    definition, 213
    investigations, 214
    treatment, 214–215
Beta-blocker, 193
Bile, 76
Biliary colic, 11
    clinical features, 78–79
    investigations, 79
    management, 79
    pathogenesis, 78

Bladder cancer, 221
  aetiology, 221
  clinical presentation, 221
  epidemiology, 221
  investigations, 222
  prognosis, 223
  treatment, 222–223
Blood products, administration of, 27
Blunt cardiac injury, **259**
Body mass index (BMI), 18–19
Bowel habit, altered, 6
Bowel obstruction, 12, 111
  aetiology, 112–113, *112*
  causes, 113
  classification, 111
  clinical presentation, **112**
  complicated, 111–112
  definition, 111
  investigations, 113
  management, 114
  specific management, 114
Brain, anatomy of, *336*
Brain tumours, 334
  clinical presentation, 335
  investigations, 337
  management, 338–339
  pathogenesis, 337
  pathophysiology, 337–338
Breast cancer, 171
  aetiology, 171
  clinical features, 172
  ductal carcinoma in-situ, 172
  invasive ductal carcinoma, 172
  invasive lobular carcinoma, 172
  investigations, 173
  medical management, 177–178
  pathological features, 171
  screening, 178
  surgical management, 175–177
  triple assessment, 173–174, *173*
BreastCheck, 178
Breast-conserving therapy (BCT), 175
Breast disease, benign, *see* Benign breast
    disease
Breslow thickness, 382
Brown-Sequard syndrome, 332
Burns, 270
  aetiology, 270
  assessing depth, 270–271
  complications, 273
  emergency burn care, 270
  management, 272–273
  resuscitation, 271
  severity of burn injury, 270

C

CABG, *see* Coronary artery bypass grafting
Carbimazole, 193
Carcinoid tumour of appendix, 104
Cardiac (myocardial infarction (MI)/
    pericarditis), 8
Cardiothoracic surgery, 233
  aortic regurgitation (AR), 240–241
  aortic stenosis (AS), 238–239
  chest tube insertion, 243–244
  coronary artery bypass grafting (CABG),
    235–236
  mitral regurgitation (MR), 239
  mitral stenosis (MS), 240
  pneumothorax, 241
  pre-operative investigations for, 235
  primary spontaneous pneumothorax,
    241–243
  secondary spontaneous
    pneumothorax, 243
  valvular heart disease, 237
Carotid artery disease, 162
  carotid endarterectomy, 163
  clinical features, 162
  definitions, 162
  investigations, 162
  management, 162–163
Carotid duplex scan, 162
Cauda equina syndrome, 332
  clinical presentation, 312
  definition, 312
  diagnosis, 312
  treatment, 312
CBF, *see* Cerebral blood flow
CD, *see* Crohn's disease
Centor score, 384
Central control, 184–185
Cerebral blood flow (CBF), 320–321
Cerebral herniation, 321, *322*
Cerebrovascular accident (CVA), 162
Chagas disease, 59
Chandler's classification, 361
Charcot's triad, 377
Chemical burns, 270
Chemotherapy, 177
Chest tube insertion, 243
  definition, 243
  technique, 244
  tube placement, confirmation of, 244
Cholangitis, ascending
  aetiology, 85
  clinical presentation, 86
  definition, 85

investigations, 86
pathophysiology, 85
prognosis, 87
treatment, 86–87
Cholecystitis, acute
    clinical presentation, 80
    definition, 79
    investigations, 80
    management, 80–81
    pathophysiology, 80
Cholecystitis, chronic
    complications, 83
    investigations, 83
    management, 83
    presentation, 83
Cholecystitis/cholangitis, 11
Cholecysto-duodenal fistula, 84
Cholesteatoma
    aetiology, 353
    classification, 353
    clinical presentation, 353
    definition, 353
    investigations, 354
    management, 354–355
Chronic airway and alveolar diseases, 243
Cilostazol, 149
Claudication, 6
Clavicle fracture
    complications, 298
    treatment, 298
Closed active drains, 18
Closed fracture, 289
Closed passive drains, 18
Cold thermal, 270
Colles' fracture, 293
Colloids, 24
Colon, 109, 137
Colorectal cancer, 108
    clinical presentation, 109
    emergency presentations, 109
    investigations, 109
    management
        chemotherapy, 110–111
        follow-up, 111
        palliative treatment, 111
        potentially curative treatment, 110
        tumour location, surgical options based on, 110
    morphology, 108–109
    pathological staging, 110
    pathophysiology, 108
    risk factors, 108
    staging, 109
    TNM staging, **110**

Colorectal surgery, 99
    acute appendicitis, 101–104
    anal cancer, 123–124
    anal fissure, 117–118
    anal fistula, 119–121
    anorectal abscess, 118–119
    bowel obstruction, 111–114
    colorectal cancer, 108–111
    defunctioning stoma, 128
    diverticular disease, 104–107
    end colostomy, 127–128, 127
    end ileostomy, 126
    haemorrhoids, 115–116, 115
    high-output stoma, 131–132
    loop colostomy, 128
    loop ileostomy, 124–125
    necrosis, 130
    parastomal hernia, 130–131, 131
    perianal disorders, 114
    pilonidal sinus and abscess, 121–122
    skin complications, 132
    stoma complications, 128
    stoma retraction, 129–130
    stomas, 124
    stoma stenosis, 129
Compartment syndrome
    causes, 284
    complications, 285
    description, 283
    diagnosis, 284
    management, 285
    presentation, 284
Concussion, 320
Conn's syndrome
    clinical features, **202**
    complications, **202**
    definition, 202
    investigations, 202
    treatment, 203
Coronary artery bypass grafting (CABG)
    complications, 236
    indications for surgery, 235
    procedure, 235
    prognosis, 236
    selection of conduits, 236
Cortisol excess and Cushing's disease
    causes, 201
    investigations, 201
    post-operative management, 201–202
    treatment, 201
Cranial trauma, 319
    assessment of head injury, 322–323
    cerebral blood flow (CBF), 320–321
    cerebral herniation, 321, 322

concussion, 320
head injuries, aetiology of, 320
head injury, application in, 321
investigations, 324
management, 324
Munro-Kellie doctrine, 321, *321*
scalp layers, 319, *319*
skull fractures, 320
Crohn's disease (CD)
clinical features
mucosal inflammation, 138
perianal problems, 138
transmural inflammation, 138
upper GI tract, 139
epidemiology, 136
extraintestinal manifestations, 140
fistulising features, 139
inflammatory features, 138
pathophysiology, 136
stenosing features, 139
surgical management, 143
pre-operative preparation, 144
treatment options, **142**
Crystalloid fluids, 24
types, **25**
Cullen's sign, 88
Cushing's disease
causes, 201
clinical features, **200**
investigations, 201
post-operative management, 201–202
treatment, 201
CVA, *see* Cerebrovascular accident

D

DAI, *see* Diffuse axonal injury
Deep inguinal ring, 36
Deep vein thrombosis (DVT), 159
aetiology, 159
clinical features, 160
definition, 159
investigations, 160
management, 161
prophylaxis, 160
risk factors, 160
thrombolysis, 161–162
Wells probability score, **161**
Defunctioning stoma, 128
Demeester score, 376
Denis–Weber classification, 304, 382
Diabetic foot, 165
aetiology, 166
clinical features, 166

features, 165
investigations, 166
management, 166
neuropathic ulcers, 167
risk factors, 166
Diaphragmatic rupture, **258**
Diffuse abdominal pain, differential diagnosis of
acute mesenteric ischaemia, 12
bowel obstruction, 12
chronic mesenteric ischaemia, 12
gastroenteritis, 12
Diffuse axonal injury (DAI), 320
Diffuse oesophageal spasm
investigations, 59
management, 59
presentation, 59
Dinner fork deformity, *293*
Direct hernias, 35
Distal radial fracture, 292
complications, 295
eponyms, 292
risk factors, 292
treatment, 294
Diverticular disease, 104
aetiology, 105
classification, 107
clinical presentation, 105
complications
acute diverticulitis, investigations for,
106–107
classification, 107
diverticular fistula, 106
management, 107
pericolic/paracolic abscess, 105
peritonitis, 105
stricture formation, 106
definition, 104
epidemiology, 104
Diverticular fistula, 106
Diverticulitis, 14, 106–107
Drains, 17
complications, 17
types, 18
Drug history, 4
Duke's classification, 110, 378
Duodenal ulceration, 50
Dupuytren's contracture, *279*
Dupuytren's disease, *278*
aetiology, 278
complications (surgery), 280
definition, 278
Dupuytren's diathesis (DD), 279
epidemiology, 278
management, *280*

presentation, 278
surgical indications, 279
DVT, *see* Deep vein thrombosis
Dyspepsia, 5
Dysphagia, 5, 55, **56**, **57**
causes, 55–56
definition, 55
Dysuria, 7

E

Ear, foreign body in, 344
Ectopic pregnancy, 13
Electrical burns, 270
End colostomy, 127, *127*
associated colorectal surgeries, 127–128
clinical features, 127
End ileostomy
associated colorectal surgery, 126
clinical features, 126
Endocrine disorders, 181
anaplastic thyroid cancer, 196–197
anatomical review, 183–185
Conn's syndrome, 202–203
cortisol excess and Cushing's disease,
200–201
follicular thyroid cancer, 195, **195**
Graves' disease, 192–194
medullary thyroid cancer, 195
neck swelling, differential diagnosis of,
186–187, **186**
papillary thyroid cancer, 194–195
phaeochromocytoma, 199–200, **199**
primary hyperparathyroidism, 197–198
secondary and tertiary hyperparathyroidism,
199
thyroid cancer, **194**, **196**
thyroid disease, types of, 185–186, **185–186**
thyroid disorders, investigation of, 187–189
thyroidectomy, **189**
thyrotoxicosis, 189–191, **190**, **191**
Endoleak, 155, **155**
Endovascular aneurysm repair (EVAR), 154
ENT; *see also* Otorhinolaryngology
ear, foreign body in, 344
nose, foreign body in, 344
upper oesophagus, foreign body in, 344
Enterohepatic circulation, 72
Epididymo-orchitis, acute, 228
aetiology, 228
clinical presentation, 228
definition, 228
investigations, 229
management, 229

Epigastric pain, differential diagnosis
of, 7–10
cardiac (myocardial infarction (MI)/
pericarditis), 8
gastro-oesophageal reflux disease
(GORD), 8
pancreatitis, 7
peptic ulcer disease/gastritis, 7
ruptured AAA, 11
Epistaxis, 356
blood vessels involved, 356
clinical presentation, 356
investigations, 357
local causes, 356
management, 357
systemic causes, 356
ESWL, *see* Extracorporeal shock wave lithotripsy
EVAR, *see* Endovascular aneurysm repair
Exophthalmos, *192*
Extracorporeal shock wave lithotripsy
(ESWL), 218
Extradural haemorrhage, 324
clinical presentation, 324
management, 324
mechanism of injury, 324
Extraintestinal manifestations, 139, *139*
extraintestinal manifestations of CD and
UC, 140
investigations, 140
management, 141

F

Family history, 4
Fat necrosis, 180
Femoral hernia, **39**
clinical features, 39
differential diagnosis, 39
epidemiology, 38
management, 39
surgical anatomy, 39
Fibroadenoma, 179
Fibrocystic disease, 179
Fine needle aspiration cytology (FNAC), 174
Flaps, 277
Fluids, in surgical patients
assessing fluid balance, 23
blood products, administration of, 27
challenge, 26
common indications, 23
compartments, 24
requirements, 24
special circumstances, 26
special surgical circumstances, 26

types
  advantages, 24
  colloids, 24
  crystalloids, 24
FNAC, *see* Fine needle aspiration cytology
Follicular thyroid cancer
  epidemiology, **195**
  metastatic activity, 195
  pathological features, 195
Foreign body
  in ear, 344
  in nose, 344
  in upper oesophagus, 344
Fracture fixation, principles of, 291, *291*
Fracture healing, stages in, 291
Fracture reduction, 289, 290
Fractures, types of, *289*
Fracture treatment, principles in, 290
Full-thickness skin graft, **276**

G

Gallbladder
  gangrene, 82
  perforated, 82–83
Gallbladder empyema
  definition, 81
  investigations, 81
  management, 82
  presentation, 81
Gallstone disease, 76
  aetiology, 76
  common presentations, **77–78**
  pathophysiology of gallstones, 76–77
Gallstone ileus
  aetiology, 84
  clinical presentation, 84
  diagnosis, 84
  treatment, 84
Gangrene of gallbladder
  diagnosis, 82
  management, 82
  presentation, 82
Gardasil vaccine, 363
Garden classification, 382
Gastric cancer, 63
  adenocarcinoma, risk factors for, 64
  classification and aetiology, 63
  investigations, 64
  management, 64–65
  partial/total gastrectomy complications, 65, *65*
  pathophysiology, 63–64
  prognosis, 66

Gastric ulceration, 51
Gastrinoma, 50
Gastroenteritis, 12
Gastro-oesophageal reflux disease (GORD), 5, 8
  clinical features, 45
  complications, 46
  definition, 45
  epidemiology, 45
  investigations, 45–46
  management, 46
  pathophysiology, 45
  risk factors, 45
Gastrostomy, 19, *19*
GCS, *see* Glasgow Coma Scale
Germ cell tumours, classification of, **225**
Glasgow Coma Scale (GCS), 252, *253*, 381
Glasgow criteria, modified, 377
Glasgow system, 266, 382
Goitre, *187*
Goodsall's rule, *120*
GORD, *see* Gastro-oesophageal reflux disease
Graves' disease
  definition, 192
  investigations, 193
  management of
    medical, 193
    radioactive iodine, 193
    surgery, 193–194
Grey Turner's sign, 88
Gynaecomastia, 180

H

Haematemesis, 5
Haematuria, 7
Haemorrhage: signs and symptoms of, **252**
Haemorrhagic Shock Classification, 381
Haemorrhoidectomy, 116
Haemorrhoids, 115, *115*
  aetiology, 115
  complications, 115
  definition, 115
  four degrees of, 115
  investigations, 116
  management, 116
Hand trauma
  amputations, 281
  fractures, 281
  tendon injuries, 280
Head and neck anatomy
  aetiological factors, 363
  larynx (voice box), 362
  oral cavity subsites, 361

pharynx, 362
risk factors, 362–363
Head and neck masses, 347
    parapharyngeal abscess, 348
    peritonsillar abscess (quinsy), 347
    retropharyngeal abscess, 348
Head injury
    aetiology, 320
    application in, 321
    assessment, 322–323
Heller's cardiomyotomy, 59
Hepatic jaundice, 76
Hepatitis, 11
Hepatobiliary surgery, 69
    acute cholecystitis, 79–81
    asymptomatic gallstones, 78
    biliary colic, 78–79
    cholangitis, ascending, 85–87
    cholecystitis, chronic, 83
    gallbladder empyema, 81–82
    gallstone disease, 76–77, **77–78**
    gallstone ileus, 84
    gangrene of gallbladder, 82
    jaundice, 71–76, **72**
    mucocoele, 83–84
    obstructive jaundice, 84–85
    pancreatic cancer, 95–97, **96**
    pancreatitis, acute, 87–92
    pancreatitis, chronic, 92–95, **93**
    perforated gallbladder, 82–83
Hepatobiliary symptoms, 6
Hepatocellular jaundice, 71
Hernia, 31
    classification, **33**
    definition, 33
    femoral hernia, 38–39, **39**
    general pathology
        irreducible/incarcerated, 34
        reducible, 34
        strangulated, 34
    hiatus hernia, 47
        definition, 47
        investigations, 48
        management, 49
        types, **48**
    incidence (relative), 33
    incisional hernia, 40–41
    inguinal hernia, 34–38, **36**, **37**
    obturator hernia, 42, *42*
    paraoesophageal hernia, *49*
    spigelian hernia, 41–42, *41*
    umbilical hernia, 40, *40*
    uncommon types of
        pantaloon hernia, 34

Richter's hernia, 33, *34*
    sliding hernia, 33
Hesselbach's triangle, 36
Hiatus hernia, 47, *48*
    definition, 47
    investigations, 48
    management, 49
    types, **48**
High-output stoma, 131
    aetiology, 131
    complications, 131–132
    definition, 131
    management, 132
Hinchey classification, 107, **107**, 378
Hip fracture, 301
    classification, *301*
    complications, 302
Homan's sign, 160
Hueston's tabletop test, 279
Human papilloma virus, 363
    airway concerns, 364
    investigations, 364
    management, 365
    nutritional status, 364
    speech rehabilitation, 364
    staging, 364
Humeral fracture
    complications, 296
    mechanisms of injury, 295–296
    Neer classification, 296
    treatment, 296
Hyperparathyroidism
    primary, 197
        aetiology, 197
        clinical features, **198**
        diagnosis, 197–198
        presentation, 198
        treatment, 198
    secondary, 199
        clinical features, **199**
    tertiary, 199
        clinical features, **199**
Hyperthyroidism, clinical presentation of, **185**
Hypertrophic scar, *275*
Hypervolaemic signs, 23
Hypoalbuminemia, 137
Hypokalaemia, 137
Hypothyroidism, clinical presentation of, **185**
Hypovolaemic signs, 23

I

IBD, *see* Inflammatory bowel disease
Important nearby structures, 183–184

Incisional hernia, 40
  aetiology, 40–41
  clinical presentation, 41
  management, 41
Indirect hernias, 35
Infectious flexor tenosynovitis
  complications, 285
  complications, 285
  Kanavel's cardinal signs, 285
  management, 285
Inflammatory bowel disease (IBD), 14, 133
  Crohn's disease (CD), 136, 138–140, 143, 144
  definition, 135
  epidemiology, 135
  extraintestinal manifestations, 139–141, *139*
  pathophysiology, 136
  types, **135**
  ulcerative colitis (UC), 135–137, 140, 142, 143
Infra-renal abdominal aortic aneurysm, *152*
Inguinal hernia, 13, *36*, **37**
  clinical presentation, 37
  complications of repairing, 38
  differential diagnosis, 37
  epidemiology, 34
  investigations, 37
  management, 37–38
  surgical anatomy
    deep inguinal ring, 36
    inguinal ligament, 36
    superficial inguinal ring, 36
  types, 35, *35*
Inguinal ligament, 36
Intergluteal pilonidal disease, 121
Ivor Lewis procedure, 62, *62*

J

Jaundice, 6
  aetiology, 71
  definition, 71
  differential diagnosis, 73
  investigations, 73–74
  liver function tests in, **73**
  management, 75–76
  pathophysiology, 71–72
  prognosis, 76
  symptoms and signs of, **72**
  types, **72**
Jejunostomy, 19

K

Kanavel's cardinal signs, 285
Karydakis procedure, 122

Keloid scar, *275*
Kiesselbach's plexus, 356

L

Laparoscopic cholecystectomy, 82
Laparoscopic herniorrhaphy, 38
Lapatinib, 177
Laryngeal cancer
  function of larynx, 365
  histological subtypes, 365
  management, 366
  surgical options, 366
Larynx (voice box), 362
Laxatives, **23**
Lead-pipe colon, 136
Left iliac fossa (LIF) pain, 14
Leg ulcers, 163
  causes, 163–165
  definition, 163
Leriche syndrome, 147
LIF pain, *see* Left iliac fossa pain
Limb ischaemia, Rutherford-Fontaine
      classification for, **148**
Lipodermatosclerosis, 158
Little's area, 356
Liver function tests in jaundice, **73**
Loop colostomy, 128
Loop ileostomy, 124, *125*
  associated colorectal surgery, 125
  clinical features, 124
  clinical relevance, 125
Lower GI symptoms
  altered bowel habit, 6
  rectal bleeding, 6
  tenesmus, 6
Lower limb injuries, 301
  ankle fractures, 304–306, *305*, *306*
  back pain, 312
  cauda equina syndrome, 312
  compartment syndrome in orthopeadics,
      308–309
  hip fracture, 301–302, *301*
  open fractures, 307–308
  osteoarthritis (OA), 313–315
  pelvic fractures, 309–310, *311*
  sciatica, 313
  septic arthritis, 311
  slipped upper femoral epiphysis (SUFE),
      303–304
  tibial fracture, 307
Lower limb ischaemia, acute, 150
  aetiology, 150
  complications, 150

definition, 150
management, 150
reperfusion, complications of, 150
types of amputation, 150
LUQ pain, differential diagnosis of, 11
Lymphatic drainage, 114

M

Maisonneuve fracture, 306, *307*
Major trauma
common aetiology, 249
definition, 249
global burden of fatal injury, 249
global injury mortality by cause, 249
Malignant lung and chest diseases, 243
Malignant melanoma, 265
clinical presentation, 265–266,
265, **266**
definition, 265
differential diagnosis, 266
incidence, 265
management, 267–268
pathological subtypes, 266
risk factors, 265
staging, 266–267
Mammogram, 174
Mastoidectomy
complications, 371
definition, 370
indications, 370
types, 370
McKeown procedure, 62
Median nerve, 281–282
Medications in surgery, **22**
pre-operative drug alterations, 21, **21**
warfarin
guidelines for administration of, **21**
patients on, 21
reversing, 22
Medullary thyroid cancer, 195
Mesenteric ischaemia
acute, 12
chronic, 12
Mirizzi's syndrome, 84, 85
Mitral regurgitation (MR), 239
aetiology, 239
clinical presentation, 239
indications for surgery, 239
investigations, 239
prognosis, 239
surgical approach, 239
Mitral stenosis (MS), 240
clinical presentation, 240

investigations, 240
prognosis, 240
surgical approach, 240
MR, *see* Mitral regurgitation
MS, *see* Mitral stenosis
Mucocoele
aetiology, 83
management, 84
presentation, 84
Munro-Kellie doctrine, 321, *321*
Muscle myotomes, 330, **330**, 384

N

Nasal polyps
clinical presentation, 358
investigations, 359
management, 359
Nasojejunal tubes, 19
Nasopharyngeal carcinoma (NPC)
clinical presentation, 368
definition, 368
investigation, 368
management, 368
staging, 368
Neck, anatomy of, *187*
Neck dissection
complications, 373
definition, 372
types, 372–373
Neck swelling, differential diagnosis of,
186–187, **186**
Necrosis
aetiology, 130
clinical features, 130
management, 130
Needle core biopsy, 174
Nephrostomy, 209–210, *209*
Neurosurgery, 317
brain tumours, 334–339
cranial trauma, 319–324
extradural haemorrhage, 324
spinal cord injury, 332
spinal injury, 329–332
subarachnoid haemorrhage (SAH), 328–329,
328, **328**
subdural haemorrhage,
326–327, *327*
Nose, foreign body in, 344
NPC, *see* Nasopharyngeal carcinoma
Nutrition in surgical patients, 18
body mass index (BMI), 18–19
nutritional support, types of, 19
poor nutrition, 18

O

OA, *see* Osteoarthritis
Obstructive jaundice
  clinical presentation, 85
  diagnosis, 85
  management, 85
  pathophysiology, 84
Obstructive jaundice, 75–76
Obturator hernia, 42, *42*
Obturator sign, 102
Odynophagia, 55
  causes, 56
  definition, 55
Oesophageal cancer, 60
  adenocarcinoma, 60, *64*
  clinical features, 61
  investigations, 61
  management, 62–63
  risk factors, **61**
  squamous cell carcinoma (SCC), 60
Oesophageal dysmotility, 60
Oesophageal motility disorders, 57
  primary, 57
  secondary, 57
Oesophago-gastro-duodenoscopy (OGD), *66*
  explain to patient what the procedure
    involves, 66
  intravenous sedation used, 67
  preparation, 67
  risks associated with, 67
OGD, *see* Oesophago-gastro-duodenoscopy
OME, *see* Otitis media with effusion
Oncotype DX test, 178
Open fractures, 289
  definition, 307
  management, 308
Open passive drains, 18
Open wire-guided excisional biopsy, 174
Oral cancer
  histological subtypes, 366
  treatment, 367
Oropharyngeal cancer, 367
Orthopaedics, principles of, 289
  definitions, 289
  fracture fixation, principles of, 291
  fracture healing, stages in, 291
  fracture reduction, 290
  fracture treatment, principles in, 290
  general fracture management, 290
Orthopaedic surgery, 287
  lower limb injuries, 301
    ankle fractures, 304–306, *305*, *306*
    back pain, 312

    cauda equina syndrome, 312
    compartment syndrome in orthopeadics,
      308–309
    hip fracture, 301–302, *301*
    open fractures, 307–308
    osteoarthritis (OA), 313–315
    pelvic fractures, 309–310, *311*
    sciatica, 313
    septic arthritis, 311
    slipped upper femoral epiphysis (SUFE),
      303–304
    tibial fracture, 307
  upper limb injuries
    anterior shoulder dislocation, 298
    clavicle fracture, 298
    distal radial fracture, 292–295
    humeral fracture, 295–296
    posterior shoulder dislocation, 299
    scaphoid fracture, 300
Orthopeadics, compartment syndrome in, 308
  clinical features, 309
  treatment, 309
Osteoarthritis (OA), 313
  characteristics of osteoarthritis on
    radiographs, 314
  clinical presentation, 314
  investigations, 314
  management, 314
  total hip arthroplasty (THA), 314
  total knee arthroplasty (TKA), 315
Otitis externa
  clinical presentation, 350
  definition, 349
  management, 350
  pathogens, 350
  risk factors, 350
Otitis media with effusion (OME)
  clinical presentation, 352
  complications, 352
  definition, 351
  investigations, 352
  management, 352
  risk factors, 352
Otology, 348
Otoplasty, 349
Otorhinolaryngology (ENT), 341
  acoustic neuroma, 355–356
  acute otitis media (AOM), 350–351
  acute rhinosinusitis, 359–360
  allergic rhinitis, 357
  cholesteatoma, 353–355
  chronic rhinosinusitis, 360–361
  chronic suppurative otitis media, 352–353
  epistaxis, 356–357

head and neck anatomy, 361–363
head and neck masses, 347–348
human papilloma virus, 363–365
laryngeal cancer, 365–366
mastoidectomy, 370–371
nasal polyps, 358–359
nasopharyngeal carcinoma (NPC), 368
neck dissection, 372–373
oral cancer, 366–367
oropharyngeal cancer, 367
otitis externa, 349–350
otitis media with effusion (OME), 351–352
otology, 348
parotidectomy, 371–372
pinna (auricular) hematoma, 348–349
prominent ears, 349
rhinology, 356
sinusitis, 359
surgical procedures, 368
tonsillectomy, 368–369
tonsillitis, acute, 345–347
ventilation (tympanostomy) tubes, 369–370

P

PAD, *see* Peripheral arterial disease
Pain, 3–4
Pancreatic cancer, 95
    aetiology, 95
    differential diagnosis, 96
    investigations, 96
    management, 96–97
    pathophysiology, 95
    prognosis, 97
    symptoms and signs, **96**
Pancreatitis, 7
Pancreatitis, acute
    aetiology, 87–88
    clinical presentation, 88
    complications, 90–91
    definition, 87
    differential diagnosis, 88
    investigations, 89
    management, 91–92
    pathophysiology, 88
    prognosis, 92
    risk scoring, 89
Pancreatitis, chronic
    aetiology, 92–93
    definition, 92
    differential diagnosis, 93
    investigations, 93–94
    management, 94–95
    pathophysiology, 93

prognosis, 95
    symptoms and signs, **93**
Pantaloon hernia, 34, 35
Papillary thyroid cancer
    metastatic activity, 194
    pathological features, 194
    prognostic factors, 194–195
Paraoesophageal hernia, *49*
Parapharyngeal abscess, 348
Parastomal hernia, *131*
    aetiology, 130–131
    definition, 130
Parathyroid glands, 183
Parks' classification, 120
Parotidectomy
    complications, 371–372
    superficial parotidectomy, indications for, 371
    total parotidectomy, indications for, 371
Past medical history, 4
PCNL, *see* Percutaneous nephrolithotomy
Peau d'orange, *173*
Pelvic fractures, 309, *311*
    complications, 310
    initial management, 310
    types, 310
Pelvic inflammatory disease (PID), 13
Pentoxifylline, 149
Peptic ulcer disease, 7, 50
    aetiology, 50
    clinical features, 50–51
    complications, 51–52
    definition, 50
    investigations, 51
    management, 51
    managing complications of
        gastric outlet obstruction, 62
        haemorrhage, 62
        perforation, 62
Percutaneous nephrolithotomy (PCNL), 218
Perforated gallbladder
    clinical presentation, 82
    investigations, 83
    management, 83
Perianal disorders, 114
Pericolic/paracolic abscess, 105
Peripheral arterial disease (PAD), 147
    aetiology, 147
    definition, 147
    differential diagnoses, 148
    investigations, 148
    management, 149
    risk factors, **147**
    signs and symptoms, 147–148
    symptoms

claudication, 6
rest pain, 6–7
Peripherally inserted central venous catheter (PICC) line, 20
Peripheral vascular disease, 145
abdominal aortic aneurysms (AAAs), 151–155
acute lower limb ischaemia, 150
carotid artery disease, 162–163
deep vein thrombosis (DVT), 159–162
diabetic foot, 165–167
leg ulcers, 163–165
peripheral arterial disease (PAD), 147–149
ruptured AAA, 156–157
varicose veins, 157–159, 157
Peritonitis, 105
Peritonsillar abscess (quinsy), 347
PFA, see Plain film of abdomen
Phaeochromocytoma, 199
aetiology, 199
definition, 199
investigations, 200
presentation, 200
treatment, 200
Pharynx, 362
Pharynx, anatomy of, 363
PICC line, see Peripherally inserted central venous catheter line
PID, see Pelvic inflammatory disease
Pilonidal sinus and abscess, 121
aetiology, 121
clinical features, 122
definition, 121
examination, 122
investigations, 122
management, 122
pathogenesis, 121
Pinna (auricular) hematoma, 348
clinical presentation, 349
management, 349
Pinnaplasty, 349
Plain film of abdomen (PFA), 84
Plastic surgery, 263
basal cell carcinoma versus squamous cell carcinoma, 268–269
burns, 270–273
compartment syndrome, 283–285
Dupuytren's disease, 278–280, 278
hand trauma, 280–281
infectious flexor tenosynovitis, 285
malignant melanoma, 265–268, 265
trigger finger, 286
upper limb compression neuropathy, 281–283
wound healing, 273–277
Pneumonia, 11

Pneumothorax
classification, 241
definition, 241
Posterior interosseous syndrome, 283
Posterior shoulder dislocation, 299
management, 299
Post-hepatic (obstructive) jaundice, 71
Pott's puffy tumour, 361
Pre-hepatic (haemolytic) jaundice, 71
Pre-operative drug alterations, 21, 21
Pretibial myxoedema, 192
Primary spontaneous pneumothorax, 241
clinical features, 242
complications, 242
investigations, 242
management, 243
surgery, 243
Principles of surgery, 1
acute abdomen, differential diagnosis of, 7–14, 8, 9–10, 10
common surgical symptoms, 3–5
drains, 17–18
fluids in surgical patients, 23–27
hepatobiliary symptoms, 6
lower GI symptoms, 6
medications in surgery, 21–22, 22
nutrition in surgical patients, 18–19
peripheral arterial disease symptoms, 6–7
sepsis, 27–29
surgical incisions/scars, 16, 17
upper GI symptoms, 5
urology symptoms, 7
Prominent ears
clinical presentation, 349
definition, 349
management, 349
Propylthiouracil (PTU), 193
Prostate cancer
aetiology, 223
clinical presentation, 223
epidemiology, 223
histology grading, 224
investigations, 223–224
treatment, 224–225
Prostatic hyperplasia. benign, see Benign prostatic hyperplasia
Pseudopolyposis, 136
Psoas sign, 102
PTU, see Propylthiouracil
Pulmonary contusion, 257

Q

QSOFA score, 27, 27

R

Raccoon eye, *323*
Radial nerve, 283
Radial tunnel syndrome, 283
Ranson criteria, 377
RCC, *see* Renal cell carcinoma
Rectal bleeding, 6
Recurrent laryngeal nerve, 184
Renal cell carcinoma (RCC), 219
    aetiology, 219
    clinical presentation, 219
    epidemiology, 219
    investigations, 220
    paraneoplastic syndromes, 219–220
    signs, 219
    symptoms, 219
    treatment, 221
Renal transplant, 229
    aetiology, 229
    complications, 231
    contraindications to renal transplant, 229
    drugs used in, **230**
    during heterotopic transplant, 230
    maintenance immunosuppressive therapy, 230
    pre-transplant workup, 230
Rest pain, 6–7
Resuscitative laparotomy, indications for, 261
Retroperitoneal space, 88
Retropharyngeal abscess, 348
Reynold's pentad, 377
Rheumatic heart disease, 240
Rhinology, 356
Rhinosinusitis, acute
    clinical presentation, 360
    definition, 359
    investigations, 360
    management, 360
Rhinosinusitis, chronic
    clinical presentation, 360
    definition, 360
    investigations, 361
    management, 361
    sinusitis, complications of, 361
Richter's hernia, 33, *34*
RIF pain, *see* Right iliac fossa pain
Right iliac fossa (RIF) pain
    appendicitis, 12–13
    ectopic pregnancy, 13
    inflammatory bowel disease, 14
    inguinal hernia, 13
    pelvic inflammatory disease (PID), 13
    ruptured ovarian cyst, 13
    ureteric stone, 13

Right/left flank pain, differential
    diagnosis of, 12
Right upper quadrant (RUQ) pain
    biliary colic, 11
    cholecystitis/cholangitis, 11
    hepatitis, 11
    pneumonia, 11
Rockall score, 55, **55**, 376
Rome criteria, 78
Rovsing's sign, 102
Ruptured AAA, 11, 156
    clinical features, 156
    management, 156–157
Ruptured ovarian cyst, 13
RUQ pain, *see* Right upper quadrant pain
Rutherford-Fontaine classification, **148**, 379

S

SAH, *see* Subarachnoid haemorrhage
Scalp layers, 319, *319*
Scaphoid fracture, 300
SCC, *see* Squamous cell carcinoma
Schwann cells, 355
Sciatica
    clinical presentation, 313
    defintion, 313
    investigations, 313
    management, 313
Scleroderma, 60
Secondary spontaneous pneumothorax
    aetiology, 243
    thoracic surgery, notes on, 243
Self-intermittent catheterisation (SIC), 213
Sensory dermatomes, 330, *331*
Sentinel node biopsy, 177
Sepsis
    adjunctive investigations, 28
    diagnosis, 27
    septic shock, 28–29
    severe sepsis management, 28, **28**
Septic arthritis, 311
    investigations, 311
    treatment, 311
Sequential Organ Failure Assessment (SOFA)
    score, 27, 376
SIC, *see* Self-intermittent catheterisation
Sick day rules, 21
Sinusitis, 359
Sinusitis, complications of, 361
SIRS criteria, 176
Skin complications, 132
    aetiology, 132
    management, 132

Skin grafts, 276
  types, **276**
Skip lesions, 136
Skull fractures, 320
Sliding hernia, 33
Slipped upper femoral epiphysis (SUFE), 303
  clinical presentation, 303
  management, 304
  X-ray features, 303
Smith's fracture, *294*
Social history, 4–5
SOFA score, *see* Sequential Organ Failure
        Assessment score
Speech rehabilitation, 364
Sphincter, external, 114
Sphincter, internal, 114
Spigelian hernia, 41–42, *41*
Spinal cord injury, 332
  initial management, 332
  spinal cord syndromes, 332
Spinal injury, 329
  clinical examination, 330–332
  general anatomy pointers, 329
  general principles, 329
  vertebral column, assessment of injuries
        to, 329
Split-thickness skin graft, **276**
Squamous cell carcinoma (SCC), 60, 363
Stenosing flexor tenosynovitis), 286
Stoma complications, 128
Stoma retraction
  aetiology, 129
  clinical features, 129
  definition, 129
  management, 130
Stomas, definition of, 124
Stoma stenosis
  aetiology, 129
  clinical presentation, 129
  definition, 129
  management, 129
Strength examination, MRC grading
        for, 382
Stricture formation, 106
Subarachnoid haemorrhage (SAH), 328, *328*
  clinical features, **328**
  definition, 328
  investigations, 328–329
  management of aneurysmal SAH, 329
Subdural haemorrhage, 326, *327*
  clinical presentation, 326
  mechanism of injury, 326
  risk factors, 326
  treatment, 327

SUFE, *see* Slipped upper femoral epiphysis
Superficial inguinal ring, 36
Suppurative otitis media, chronic
  definition, 352
  management, 353
Suprapubic catheter, 208
Suprapubic catheterisation, 213
Suprapubic pain, differential diagnosis
        of, 14
Surgical incisions/scars, *16*, *17*
Surgical procedures, 368
Symptomatic carotid artery disease, clinical
        features of, 162
Symptoms, surgical, 3
  allergies, 4
  drug history, 4
  family history, 4
  pain, 3–4
  past medical history, 4
  presenting complaint, 3
  social history, 4–5
  systems review, 5
Systemic connective tissue diseases, 243

T

Tamoxifen, 177
TAPP repair, *see* Transabdominal preperitoneal
        patch repair
Tenesmus, 6
Tension pneumothorax, 254, *255*
TEP repair, *see* Totally extraperitoneal repair
Testicular pain, acute, 227
Testicular torsion, 227
  clinical presentation, 227
  epidemiology, 227
  management, 227
Testicular tumours
  aetiology, 225
  clinical presentation, 226
  epidemiology, 225
  investigations, 226
  prognosis, 226
  treatment, 226
TFTs, *see* Thyroid function tests
THA, *see* Total hip arthroplasty
Thermal burns, 270
Thoracic aortic injury, **258**
Thoracic trauma, 254
  management
    ATLS protocol, 254–255
    secondary survey, 257
    underwater seal drain, 256–257
Thyroid acropachy, *192*

Thyroid cancer
anaplastic, *see* anaplastic thyroid cancer
epidemiology, **194**
follicular, *see* follicular thyroid cancer
medullary, *see* medullary thyroid cancer
papillary, *see* papillary thyroid cancer
signs and symptoms, **196**
types, **194**
Thyroid disease, types of, 185–186, **185–186**
Thyroid disorders, investigation of
biopsy, 189
bloods, 187–188
imaging, 188–189
single nodule, surveillance of, 189
Thyroidectomy, **189**
Thyroid eye disease, **192**
Thyroid function tests (TFTs), **185**, **188**
Thyroid gland, 183
Thyroid hormones, central control of, *184*
Thyrotoxicosis
causes, **190**
clinical presentation, **190**
definition, 189
definitive management, 191
general management, 191, **191**
investigation, 190
TIA, *see* Transient ischaemic attack
Tibial fracture, 307
TKA, *see* Total knee arthroplasty
Tonsillectomy
complications, 369
indications, 368–369
management, 369
Tonsillitis, acute
clinical presentation, 346
complications, 347
definition, 345–346
investigations, 346
management, 347
pathogens, 346
Torsion of appendix testis/hydatid of morgagni, 228
aetiology, 228
clinical presentation, 228
management, 228
Total hip arthroplasty (THA), 314
Total knee arthroplasty (TKA), 315
Totally extraperitoneal (TEP) repair, 38
Total parenteral nutrition (TPN), 19–20
TPN, *see* Total parenteral nutrition
Tracheobronchial rupture, **258**
Transabdominal preperitoneal patch (TAPP) repair, 38
Transient ischaemic attack (TIA), 162

Transurethral resection of bladder tumour (TURBT), 222
Trastuzumab, 177
Trauma, 247
abdominal trauma, 258–261, **260**
Advanced Trauma Life Support (ATLS®) System (Tenth Edition), 250–254
major trauma, 249
thoracic trauma, 254–257
Trendelenburg test, 158–159
Trigger finger, 286
complications from surgery, 286
management, 286
T Tube, 18
TURBT, *see* Transurethral resection of bladder tumour

U

UC, *see* Ulcerative colitis
Ulcerative colitis (UC)
clinial features, 137
epidemiology, 135
extraintestinal manifestations, 140
pathophysiology, 136
surgical management, 142–143
treatment options, **142**
Ulnar nerve, 282–283
Umbilical hernia, *40*
aetiology, 40
management, 40
types, 40
Umbilical pain, differential diagnosis of, 12
Upper gastrointestinal bleeding, 53
clinical presentation, 53
definition, 53
differential diagnosis, **53**
investigations, 54
management of unstable upper GI bleed, 54–55
physical exam, 53
Rockall score, 55, **55**
Upper gastrointestinal surgery, 43
achalasia, 57–59
Barrett's oesophagus, 46–47, *47*
Chagas disease, 59
diffuse oesophageal spasm, 59
dysphagia, 55–56, **56**, *57*
gastric cancer, 63–66
gastro-oesophageal reflux disease (GORD), 45–46
hiatus hernia, 47–49, *48*, **48**
odynophagia, 55–56
oesophageal cancer, 60–63, *61*

oesophageal motility disorders, 57
oesophago-gastro-duodenoscopy (OGD),
      66–67, 66
peptic ulcer disease, 50–62
scleroderma and oesophageal dysmotility, 60
upper gastrointestinal bleeding, 53–55, **53**
Upper gastrointestinal symptoms
   dyspepsia, 5
   dysphagia, 5
   gastro-oesophageal reflux disease (GORD)/
      heartburn, 5
   haematemesis, 5
Upper limb compression neuropathy
   median nerve, 281–282
   radial nerve, 283
   ulnar nerve, 282–283
Upper limb injuries
   anterior shoulder dislocation, 298
   clavicle fracture, 298
   distal radial fracture, 292–295
   humeral fracture, 295–296
   posterior shoulder dislocation, 299
   scaphoid fracture, 300
Upper oesophagus, foreign body in, 344
Ureteric stone, 13
Ureteroscopy, 218
Urethral catheterisation, 212–213
Urgent laparotomy, indications for, 261
Urinary tract stones, 215
   acute episode, management, 217–218
   aetiology, 215–216
   clinical presentation, 216, **216**
   differential diagnosis, **216**
   investigations, 217
   types, **216**
   urolithiasis, complications of, 217
Urological devices, 207
   nephrostomy, 209–210, *209*
   suprapubic catheter, 208
   urinary catheters, 207–208, *207*, *208*
   urostomy/ileal conduit, 210
Urology, 205
   acute epididymo-orchitis, 228–229
   acute testicular pain, 227
   acute urinary retention (AUR), 211–213
   benign prostatic hyperplasia, 213–215
   bladder cancer, 221–223
   common urological devices, 207–210

prostate cancer, 223–225
renal cell carcinoma, 219–221
renal transplant, 229–231
testicular torsion, 227
testicular tumours, 225–226
torsion of the appendix testis/hydatid of
   morgagni, 228
urinary tract stones, 215–218
Urology symptoms
   dysuria, 7
   haematuria, 7
Urostomy/ileal conduit, 210

V

Valvular heart disease, 237
   choice of valve type, 237
Varicose veins, 157, *157*
   aetiology, 157–158
   clinical features, 158
   complications, 158
   complications of surgery, 159
   definition, 157
   diagnosis and investigations, 158
   management, 159
   Trendelenburg test, 158–159
Ventilation (tympanostomy) tubes
   complications, 370
   definition, 369
   indications, 369
   types, 369
Vertebral column, assessment of injuries to, 329
Vocal cords, anatomy of, *362*

W

Warfarin
   guidelines for administration, **21**
   patients on, 21
   reversing, 22
Wartenberg syndrome, 283
Well's probability score for DVT, 380
Wound healing
   classification, 273
   disordered, 275–276
   phases, *274*
   wound management, 276–277